D0821176

OUTLINE OF
ORTHOPAEDICS

OUTLINE OF ORTHOPAEDICS

BY

JOHN CRAWFORD ADAMS

M.D.(London), M.S.(London), F.R.C.S.(England)

Consultant Orthopaedic Surgeon, St Mary's
Hospital, London ; Civil Consultant in Orthopaedic
Surgery, Royal Air Force ; Deputy Editor, Journal
of Bone and Joint Surgery.

SEVENTH EDITION
SECOND REPRINT

CHURCHILL LIVINGSTONE
EDINBURGH AND LONDON
1971

CHURCHILL LIVINGSTONE

Medical Division of Longman Group Limited

Distributed in the United States of America by Longman Inc., New York and
by associated companies, branches and representatives throughout the world.

© E. & S. LIVINGSTONE LIMITED, 1956, 1958, 1960, 1961, 1964, 1967
© LONGMAN GROUP LIMITED, 1971

*All rights reserved. No part of this publication may
be reproduced, stored in a retrieval system, or transmitted
in any form or by any means, electronic, mechanical,
photocopying, recording or otherwise, without the prior
permission of the publishers (Churchill Livingstone,
23 Ravelston Terrace, Edinburgh).*

First Edition	1956
Second Edition	1958
Third Edition	1960
Fourth Edition	1961
Reprinted	1963
Fifth Edition	1964
Reprinted	1966
Sixth Edition	1967
Reprinted	1968
First E.L.B.S. Edition published . . .	1969
Reprinted	1969
Seventh Edition	1971
Reprinted	1973
Reprinted	1974

ISBN 0 443 00786 1

Made and Printed in Great Britain

Preface to the Seventh Edition

FOR this new edition the text has again been drastically revised. Some sections—for instance those on rheumatoid arthritis, gout, spina bifida, and the treatment of degenerative arthritis of the hip and knee—have been largely rewritten. Many of the illustrations have been improved and a number of new ones have been added. The bibliography has also been extended and brought up to date.

I am grateful to the staff of Messrs Churchill Livingstone for their ready help and advice.

J. C. ADAMS.

LONDON,
May 1971.

Preface to the First Edition

THIS book is intended primarily to help students who are studying for the qualifying examinations. I hope that it may also be of use to practitioners whose work brings them into occasional contact with orthopaedic problems, and to physiotherapists and orthopaedic nurses.

My endeavour has been to present an easily read account of our present knowledge and thought on orthopaedic surgery in the shortest possible compass consistent with accuracy, and without resorting to the style of a synopsis. Rarities that are unimportant to the undergraduate student have been omitted, and descriptions of operative technique have been cut down to the barest essentials. Fractures have been excluded because the publishers and I believe that they could be considered more appropriately in a companion volume.

v

Despite limitations of space I thought it right to include some notes on the methods of examining joints and limbs, because I believe that a clear exposition of clinical methods is the most important contribution that the orthopaedic surgeon can make to the student's surgical training.   If the examination candidate can examine a limb competently and elicit the physical signs correctly, his battle is more than half won : and the knowledge will stand him in good stead throughout his clinical career.

J. C. ADAMS.

LONDON,
November 1955.

NOTE ON TERMINOLOGY

The anatomical nomenclature used in this book conforms to that recommended by the International Anatomical Nomenclature Committee and approved at the Eighth International Congress of Anatomists at Wiesbaden in 1965.   This nomenclature, which differs only in minor respects from the earlier Birmingham revision of the Basle nomenclature, has been adopted at most schools of anatomy, and it is to be hoped that it will become the standard terminology acceptable alike to anatomists and surgeons.

The recommended method of recording and expressing joint movement conforms to that laid down by the American Academy of Orthopaedic Surgeons in the booklet published by the Academy in 1965 and approved by most of the Orthopaedic Associations of the English-speaking world.   The guiding principle of the method is that for any joint the extended ' anatomical position ' is regarded as zero degrees, and movement at the joint is measured from this starting position.   For example, in the knee the straight position is described as zero degrees and the fully flexed position is expressed as (say) 145 degrees of flexion.

Contents

CHAPTER   PAGE

       INTRODUCTION 1

   I. CLINICAL METHODS 5

  II. GENERAL SURVEY OF ORTHOPAEDIC DISORDERS 34

 III. NECK AND CERVICAL SPINE . . . 148

 IV. TRUNK AND SPINE 173

  V. SHOULDER REGION 222

 VI. UPPER ARM AND ELBOW 245

VII. FOREARM, WRIST, AND HAND . . . 264

VIII. HIP REGION 308

 IX. THIGH AND KNEE 354

  X. LEG, ANKLE, AND FOOT 393

     REFERENCES AND BIBLIOGRAPHY . . . 445

     INDEX 465

Introduction

THE term orthopaedic is derived from the Greek words
ορθος (straight) and παις (child). It was originally
applied to the art of correcting deformities by Nicolas
Andry, a French physician, who in 1741 published a book
entitled *Orthopaedia : Or the Art of Correcting and Preventing
Deformities in Children : By such Means, as may easily be put in
Practice by Parents themselves, and all such as are Employed in
Educating Children.*

In Andry's time orthopaedic surgery in the form known to-day
did not exist. Surgery was still primitive. Indeed, except for
sporadic attempts by ingenious individuals, it is probable that
little real progress had been made since the days of Hippocrates.

That is not to say that surgeons were unintelligent or that
they lacked a capacity for careful study and research. Early
writings prove that many of them were shrewd observers, and
from the time of John Hunter (1728-93) onwards this was
increasingly true. Take, for example, the words of Sir Astley
Cooper (1768-1848) in his *Treatise on Dislocations and Fractures
of the Joints* : " Nothing is known in our profession by guess ;
and I do not believe, that from the first dawn of medical science
to the present moment, a single correct idea has ever emanated
from conjecture. It is right, therefore, that those who are studying
their profession should be aware that there is no short road to
knowledge ; that observations on the diseased living, examinations
of the dead, and experiments upon living animals are the only
sources of true knowledge ; and that inductions from these are
the sole basis of legitimate theory."

The enthusiasm and the capacity for study were there. The
real obstacle to progress was the lack of the essential facilities that
we now take so much for granted—anaesthesia, asepsis, powerful
microscopes, and x-rays. Any surgical operation that could not
be completed within a few minutes was out of the question when
the patient's consciousness could be clouded only by intoxication
or exsanguination. And when every major operation was inevitably

1

followed by suppuration which often proved fatal it is small wonder that operations were seldom advised except in an attempt to save life.

Thus orthopaedic surgery, until relatively recent times, was limited to the correction of deformities by rather crude pieces of

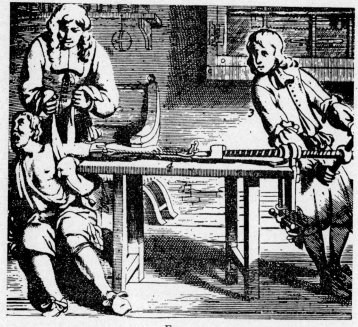

FIG. 1
An early method of reducing a dislocated shoulder.
(From Scultetus: *Armamentarium Chirurgicum*, 1693.)

apparatus, to the reduction of fractures and dislocations by powerful traction (Fig. 1), and to amputation of limbs (Fig. 2).

LANDMARKS OF SURGERY IN THE NINETEENTH CENTURY

Fundamental advances in surgery were in fact dependent upon the development of other branches of science and of industry which provided, for instance, the high-powered microscope and the x-ray tube. It is therefore not surprising that, after centuries of stagnation, the facilities that were lacking were all made available within the span of a single life-time, at the period of the Industrial Revolution.

The first epoch-making advance was the introduction of anaesthesia. The credit for this should be given jointly to Crawford Long, of Athens, Georgia, who was the first to use

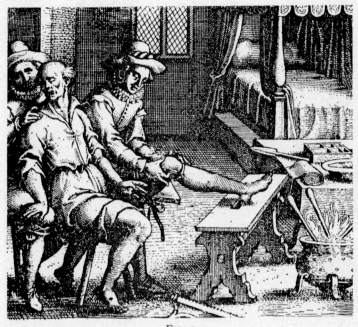

FIG. 2

A seventeenth-century amputation scene.
(From Fabricius: *Opera*, 1646.)

ether in 1842 but delayed publication of his observations for seven years ; and to W. T. G. Morton, of Boston, Massachusetts, whose use of ether anaesthesia was reported in 1846.

A few years later Louis Pasteur (1822-95), working in Paris and equipped at last with an adequate microscope, was carrying out his fundamental research on bacteria as a cause of disease. Then in 1867 Joseph Lister (1827-1912), on the basis of Pasteur's work, introduced his antiseptic surgical technique which allowed the surgeon, for the first time in history, to look for primary healing of his operation wounds. Finally, in 1895, came Roentgen's report from Würzburg in Germany of his discovery of x-rays, which within a short time were put to practical use in surgical diagnosis.

THE EMERGENCE OF ORTHOPAEDICS AS A DISTINCT SPECIALITY

Thus at the dawn of the twentieth century the stage was set for the phenomenally rapid evolution of surgery that has been witnessed by many still alive to-day. With the consequent widening of the scope of surgical practice orthopaedic surgery, at first encompassed by the general surgeon, began to branch off as a distinct science and art ; but it was not until after the first world war that it came to be widely recognised as a separate speciality.

In Great Britain many of the fundamental principles of orthopaedics had been propounded, just before the twentieth century began, by Hugh Owen Thomas[1] (1834-91) of Liverpool. But Thomas was not primarily concerned with operative surgery, and it was left to his nephew, Sir Robert Jones (1857-1933) to set orthopaedic surgery upon the sound foundation that it now enjoys. During and after the first world war Robert Jones trained many of the surgeons, British and American, who were among the first to devote their professional lives entirely to the practice of orthopaedics.

To-day the tempo of advance has inevitably slowed, after the first great surge of discovery. Yet there remain a great many problems still to be solved, and in this challenge lies the peculiar fascination that orthopaedic surgery holds for its devotees.

THE PRESENT SCOPE OF ORTHOPAEDIC SURGERY

The orthopaedic surgeon is concerned with diseases and injuries of the trunk and limbs. His field is not confined to the bones and joints ; it includes in addition the muscles, tendons, ligaments, bursae, nerves, and blood vessels. He is not concerned with injuries of the skull, which fall within the province of the neurosurgeon ; or with injuries of the jaws, which are the responsibility of the faciomaxillary or dental surgeon.

[1] Thomas's name is remembered in the widely used Thomas's knee splint and in Thomas's test for fixed flexion at the hip.

References, page 445.

CHAPTER ONE

Clinical Methods

IN this chapter an attempt will be made to indicate the correct line of approach to an orthopaedic problem, with particular reference to diagnosis and treatment.

As in all branches of medicine and surgery, proficiency in diagnosis can be acquired only from long experience. There is no short cut to a familiarity with physical signs or to skill in radiographic interpretation. Nevertheless the inexperienced surgeon who tackles the problem methodically step by step will often give a better account of himself than his more experienced colleague who makes a ' snap ' diagnosis after no more than a cursory investigation.

In the choice of treatment the development of a sound judgment is also largely a matter of experience. Yet more than that is needed. Other essential qualities are common sense and a sympathetic appreciation of human problems. There are surgeons who never acquire a sound judgment however long their apprenticeship. Others seem to have a natural aptitude that quickly matures under proper guidance and training.

DIAGNOSIS OF ORTHOPAEDIC DISORDERS

Diagnosis depends first upon an accurate determination of all the abnormal features from 1) the history ; 2) clinical examination ; 3) radiographic examination ; and 4) special investigations. Secondly, it depends upon a correct interpretation of the findings.

HISTORY

In the diagnosis of many orthopaedic conditions the history is of first importance. In cases of torn meniscus in the knee, for instance, the diagnosis sometimes depends upon the history alone. Except in the most obvious conditions, a detailed history is always required.

First the exact nature of the patient's complaint is determined. Then the development of the symptoms is traced step by step from their earliest beginning up to the time of the consultation. The patient's own views on the cause of the symptoms are always worth recording : often they prove to be correct. Enquiry is made into activities that have been found to improve the symptoms or to make them worse, and into the effect of any previous treatment. Facts that often have an important bearing on the condition are the age and present occupation of the patient, his previous occupations, his hobbies and recreational activities, and previous injuries.

When a detailed history of the local symptoms has been obtained, do not omit to enquire whether there have been symptoms in other parts of the body, and whether the general health is affected. Ask also about previous illnesses.

Finally, in cases that seem trivial, a tactful enquiry why the patient decided to seek advice, and to what extent he is worried by his disability, will often give a valuable clue to the underlying problem. It should be remembered that very often a patient seeks advice not because he is handicapped by his disability (which is often insignificant) but because he fears the development of some serious disease such as cancer, tuberculosis, or progressive crippling deformity.

CLINICAL EXAMINATION

The part complained of is examined according to a rigid routine which is never varied. If this is done familiarity with the routine will ensure that no step in the examination is forgotten. Accuracy of observation is essential : it can be acquired only by much practice and by diligent attention to detail.

The examination of the part complained of does not complete the clinical examination. It sometimes happens that symptoms felt in one part have their origin in another. For example, pain in the leg is often caused by a lesion in the spine, and pain in the knee may have its origin in the hip. The possibility of a distant lesion must therefore be considered and an examination made of any region under suspicion.

Finally, localised symptoms may be the first or only manifestation of a generalised or widespread disorder. A brief examination is therefore made of the rest of the body with this possibility in mind.

Thus the clinical examination may be considered under **three** headings : 1) examination of the part complained of ; 2) investigation of possible sources of referred symptoms ; and 3) general examination of the body as a whole.

EXAMINATION OF THE PART COMPLAINED OF

The following description of the steps in the clinical examination is intended only as a guide. The technique of examination will naturally be varied according to individual preference. Nevertheless, it is useful to stick to a particular routine, for a familiarity with it will ensure that no step in the examination is forgotten.

Exposure for Examination

It is essential that the part to be examined should be adequately exposed and in a good light. Many mistakes are made simply because the surgeon does not insist upon the removal of enough clothes to allow proper examination. When a limb is being examined the sound limb should always be exposed for comparison.

Inspection

Inspection should be carried out systematically, with attention to the following four points : 1) **The bones :** Observe the general alignment and position of the parts to detect any deformity, shortening, or unusual posture. 2) **The soft tissues :** Observe the soft-tissue contours, comparing the two sides. Note any visible evidence of general or local swelling, or of muscle wasting. 3) **Colour and texture of the skin :** Look for redness, cyanosis, pigmentation, shininess, or other changes. 4) **Scars or sinuses :** If a scar is present, determine from its appearance whether it was caused by operation (linear scar with suture marks), injury (irregular scar), or suppuration (broad, adherent, puckered scar).

Palpation

Again there are four points to consider. 1) **Skin temperature :** By careful comparison of the two sides judge whether there is an area of increased warmth or of unusual coldness. An increase of local temperature denotes increased vascularity. The usual cause is an inflammatory reaction ; but it should be remembered that a rapidly growing tumour may also bring about marked local hyperaemia. 2) **The bones :** The general shape and outline of the bones are investigated. Feel in particular for thickening, abnormal prominence, or disturbed relationship of the normal landmarks. 3) **The soft tissues :** Direct particular attention to the muscles (are they in spasm, or wasted ?), to the joint tissues (is the synovial membrane thickened, or the joint distended with fluid ?), and to the detection of any local swelling (? cyst ; ? tumour) or general swelling of the part. 4) **Local tenderness :** The exact site of any local tenderness should be mapped out and an attempt made to relate it to a particular structure.

Determining the cause of a diffuse joint swelling. The question often arises : what is the cause of a diffuse swelling of a joint ? The answer can be supplied after careful palpation. For practical purposes a *diffuse* swelling of the joint as a whole can have only three causes : 1) thickening of the bone end ; 2) fluid within the joint ; and 3) thickening of the synovial membrane. In some cases two or all three causes may be combined, but they can always be differentiated by palpation. *Bony thickening* is detected by deep palpation through the soft tissues, the bone outlines being compared on the two sides. A *fluid effusion* generally gives a clear sense of fluctuation between the two hands. *Synovial thickening* gives a characteristic boggy sensation—rather as if a layer of soft sponge-rubber had been placed between the skin and the bone. It is nearly always accompanied by a well marked increase of local warmth, for the synovium is a very vascular membrane.

Measurements

Measurement of limb length is often necessary, especially in the lower limbs, where discrepancy between the two sides is important. Measurement of the circumference of a limb segment on the two sides provides an index of muscle wasting, soft-tissue swelling or bony thickening. Details will be given in the chapters on individual regions.

Estimation of Fixed Deformity

Fixed deformity exists when a joint cannot be placed in the neutral (anatomical) position. Its causes are described on page 38. The degree of fixed deformity at a joint is determined by bringing the joint as near as it will come to the neutral position and then measuring the angle by which it falls short.

Movements

In the examination of joint movements information must be obtained on the following points : 1) What is the range of active movement ? 2) Is passive movement greater than active ? 3) Is movement painful ? 4) Is movement accompanied by crepitation ?

In measuring the range of movement it is important to know what is the normal. With some joints the normal varies considerably from patient to patient ; so it is wise always to use the unaffected limb for comparison. Limitation of movement in all directions suggests some form of arthritis, whereas selective limitation of movement in some directions with free movement in others is more suggestive of a mechanical derangement.

Except in two sets of circumstances passive movement will usually be found equal to the active. The passive range will exceed the active only in the following conditions : 1) when the muscles responsible for the movement are paralysed ; and 2) when the muscles or their tendons are torn, severed or unduly slack.

Power

The power of the muscles responsible for each movement of a joint is determined by instructing the patient to move the joint against the resistance of the examiner. With careful comparison of the two sides it is possible to detect gross impairment of power. By general convention, the strength of a muscle is recorded according to the Medical Research Council grading as follows : o = no contraction ; 1 = a flicker of contraction ; 2 = slight power, sufficient to move the joint only with gravity eliminated ; 3 = power sufficient to move the joint against gravity ; 4 = power to move the joint against gravity plus added resistance ; 5 = normal power.

In the occasional instances when more precise information is required muscle strength can be measured against weights, spring balances, or deflection bars.

Stability

The stability of a joint depends partly upon the integrity of its articulating surfaces and partly upon intact ligaments. When a joint is unstable there is abnormal mobility—for instance, lateral mobility in a hinge joint. It is important, when testing for abnormal mobility, to ensure that the muscles controlling the joint are relaxed ; for a muscle in strong contraction can often conceal ligamentous instability.

Peripheral Circulation

Symptoms in a limb may be associated with impairment of the arterial circulation. Time should therefore be spent in assessing the state of the circulation by examination of the colour and temperature of the skin, the texture of the skin and nails, and the arterial pulses. This examination is particularly important in the case of the lower limb. Further details are given on page 394.

Tests of Function

It is next necessary to test the function of the part under examination. How much does the disorder affect the part in its fulfilment of everyday activities ? Methods of determining this vary according to the part affected. To take the lower limb as an example, the best test of function is to observe the patient standing, walking, running, and jumping. Special tests are required to investigate certain functions—for example, the Trendelenburg test for abductor efficiency at the hip (p. 318).

INVESTIGATION OF POSSIBLE SOURCES OF REFERRED SYMPTOMS

When the source of the symptoms is still in doubt after careful examination of the part complained of, attention must be directed to possible extrinsic disorders with referred symptoms. This will entail examination of such other regions of the body as might be responsible. For instance, in a case of pain in the shoulder it might be necessary to examine the neck for evidence of a lesion interfering with the brachial plexus, and the thorax and abdomen for evidence of diaphragmatic irritation, because either of these conditions may be a cause of shoulder pain. Again, in a case of pain in the thigh the examination will often have to include a study of the spine, abdomen, pelvis, and genito-urinary system as well as a local examination of the hip and thigh.

GENERAL EXAMINATION

The mistake is sometimes made of confining the attention to the patient's immediate symptoms and failing to assess the patient as a whole. It should be made a rule in every case, however trivial it may seem, to form an opinion not only of the patient's general physical condition but also of his psychological outlook. In simple and straight-forward cases this general survey may legitimately be brief and rapid, but it should never be omitted.

RADIOGRAPHIC EXAMINATION

The correct interpretation of radiographs becomes easier if the films are examined methodically according to an inflexible routine. In this way abnormalities are far less likely to be missed than they are if one simply gazes hopefully but haphazardly into the viewing box. The following routine is suggested. 1) Set the films in the anatomical position on a viewing box ; simply to hold the films up against the light is to invite mistakes. 2) Note what part of the body is shown and by which projections the films have been made. 3) Stand back from the viewing box to assess the *general density* of the bones (Fig. 3) : judge from experience whether the density seems normal, or whether it is reduced (rare-faction [1]) or increased (sclerosis). 4) Look more closely for any *local changes of density*. 5) Examine the *cortex* of each bone : run the eye round the outline of the bone, looking for breaks in the continuity of the cortex, and for irregularities or areas of erosion ; then examine the substance of the cortex for thickening, thinning, alteration of texture, or new bone formation. 6) Examine the *medulla* of each bone : look for alterations of texture and for areas of destruction or sclerosis. 7) Examine the *joints* : look for

---

[1] The term rarefaction is used here to include osteoporosis and osteomalacia. Pathologically, *osteoporosis* implies increased porosity of bone from attenuation of its trabeculae : the matrix is deficient as well as the bone salts. In *osteomalacia*, which is distinct pathologically, the matrix remains but its mineralisation is deficient, the trabeculae being composed largely of osteoid tissue. Radiologically, there is nothing to distinguish osteoporosis from osteomalacia : in both states the bone looks ' thin.' For this radiological appearance the all-embracing term *rarefaction* is the most appropriate.

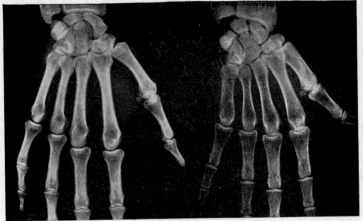

FIG. 3

To show the importance of assessing bone density in the study of radiographs. The two hands were exposed simultaneously on the same film. The one on the left is the hand of a normal person. That on the right is the hand of a patient with osteomalacia complicating idiopathic steatorrhoea. Note the marked general rarefaction of the bones.

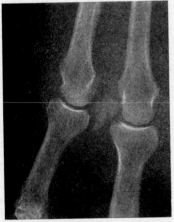

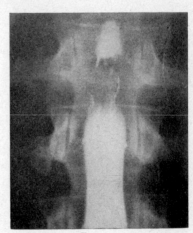

FIG. 4   FIG. 5

Figure 4—It is important to study the soft-tissue areas as well as the bones. The shadow between the metacarpal heads in this radiograph is a calcified deposit. It might at first be mistaken for a displaced fragment of bone, but it is distinguished from bone by the fact that it is homogeneous and lacks the trabecular pattern that is characteristic of bone. Figure 5—Myelography is an important aid in the study of certain spinal lesions, especially tumours. This example shows a filling defect due to an intrathecal tumour.

narrowing of the so-called joint space (more correctly, the cartilage space), for erosion, irregularity or roughening of the joint surfaces, for peripheral new bone formation (osteophytes), and for loose bodies. 8) Examine the *soft tissues* so far as they are shown : look for areas of ossification or calcification (Fig. 4), for relatively dense shadows that might denote an abscess or other fluid collection or a solid mass of tissue, and for areas of relative transradiancy that might denote the presence of gas or fat.

The mistake is often made, when an abnormality has been discovered, of disregarding the rest of the film. It should never be forgotten that two or more separate abnormalities may be present on one film : the routine method of inspection should always be completed regardless of any lesion already discovered. Plenty of time should be spent on the examination of radiographs, and the trap of jumping to hasty conclusions before the films have been properly examined should be avoided at all costs.

Special Radiographic Techniques

In the routine radiography of most parts of the body plain antero-posterior and lateral films are all that are required. In cases of difficulty special techniques will give more complete information than the plain films alone.

Tomography. By moving film and x-ray tube in opposite directions during the exposure the structures in the plane corresponding to the axis of movement remain in sharp definition, whereas the structures superficial and deep to that plane are blurred by the movement. By this technique the parts can be shown, as it were, in serial ' slices ' cut at varying depths from the surface. Tomography is particularly useful in regions such as the spine where, in plain films, the part to be studied is often obscured by overlapping shadows.

Stereoscopic films. These give a three-dimensional picture which is helpful in the study of such regions as the skull, shoulder, spine, and pelvis.

Contrast radiography. In this technique a radio-opaque fluid is injected into cavities or tissue spaces before the radiographs are taken, thereby defining clearly the limits and outline of the space. Methods in common use are : *myelography*, to outline the spinal theca (Fig. 5) ; *arthrography*, to outline the cavity of a joint ; *arteriography*, to show the arterial tree (Fig. 6) ;

venography, to show the network of veins; and *sinography*, to define the course and ramifications of a sinus. In some techniques air can be used as the contrast medium instead of a radio-opaque fluid.

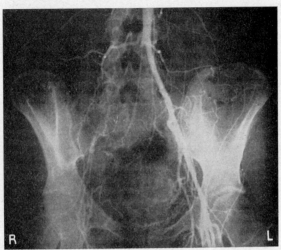

FIG. 6

Arteriography provides clear evidence about the state of the arterial tree. This example shows occlusion of the right common iliac artery at its origin from the aorta.

Cineradiography. By linking a cine camera or video-tape recorder to the x-ray image intensifier a moving picture of a joint can be obtained and stored for future reference. This technique is often helpful in showing the pattern of joint movement, especially in the spinal column. Thus it may show more reliably than any other method whether a particular spinal joint is mobile or immobile—for instance after attempted surgical fusion.

SPECIAL INVESTIGATIONS

More often than not the diagnosis can be established without the aid of special investigations. In any case the possibilities should be narrowed down to as few as possible before such investigations are ordered. If doubt then exists, appropriate tests are ordered to support or weaken each possible diagnosis. The tests most commonly employed in orthopaedic diagnosis may be summarised as follows.

Haematological : Erythrocyte sedimentation rate ; haemoglobin estimation and red blood corpuscle counts ; leucocyte counts (total and differential) ; clotting time of blood ; sternal marrow puncture.

Biochemical : Examination of the urine ; examination of the cerebrospinal fluid ; serum calcium estimation ; serum inorganic phosphate estimation ; alkaline phosphatase estimation ; acid phosphatase estimation ; blood uric acid estimation ; serum protein estimation ; serum protein electrophoresis.

Serological and bacteriological : Wassermann or Kahn reaction ; Mantoux test; gonococcal fixation test; agglutination tests for typhoid and paratyphoid organisms and for brucella abortus; Rose-Waaler sheep-cell agglutination test; latex fixation test; bacteriological examination of fluid or solid specimens.

Histological: Examination of specimens obtained by aspiration biopsy or by open operation.

Electrical (' electrodiagnosis ') : Nerve conduction tests ; strength-duration curves ; electromyography.

Nerve conduction tests are used to determine whether or not a nerve is able to transmit an electrical impulse. The principle is to apply a stimulating electrode over a point on the nerve trunk distal to the lesion, and to observe whether or not the muscles supplied by the nerve will contract in response to the stimulus. The nerves of the sound limb are examined first, to determine the threshold of current required to cause a muscle contraction. If in the affected limb a current at least twice as great as the threshold fails to produce a muscle contraction, nerve conduction is absent. A nerve conduction test provides a simple method of determining whether or not a clinical paralysis is due to a complete lesion of the nerve. If nerve conduction is present the lesion cannot be complete. Nerve conduction tests may also be used to determine the site of an incomplete lesion in the nerve trunk. There will be good nerve conductivity so long as the stimulating electrode lies distal to the lesion, and severely reduced or (in most cases) absent conductivity the moment the electrode becomes proximal to the lesion.

Strength-duration curves record the excitability of nerve and muscle. Surface electrodes are applied over the muscle to be tested, and a graph is constructed by plotting the minimal voltage that is required to cause the muscle to contract, against the duration of the stimulus in milliseconds (Fig. 7). These curves are valuable in indicating the state of innervation of a muscle, and especially in showing the progress of denervation or of re-innervation after injury or disease. A normal muscle will respond to stimuli varying in duration from 300 milliseconds to less than 1 millisecond—often down to 0·3 or even 0·1 of a millisecond—without any increase in the voltage. When the duration of the stimulus is decreased even further a progressive increase in the voltage is required in order to produce a contraction. A curve plotted from such a muscle (A in Fig. 7) is termed a nerve curve, because the muscle contraction is caused by stimulation of the motor nerve entering the muscle. A muscle that is totally denervated will respond to low-voltage stimuli only when the duration of the stimulus is

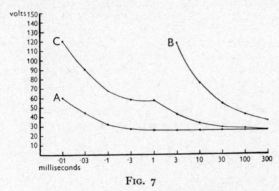

FIG. 7

Typical strength-duration curves for normal muscle, denervated muscle, and partly denervated muscle. Curve A represents the electrical reactions of the normal right tibialis anterior muscle of a young man. Note that the muscle responds to stimuli as short as 0·3 milliseconds without an increase of voltage. Curve B represents the same patient's left tibialis anterior, paralysed in consequence of a lesion of the common peroneal nerve. The curve is typical of total denervation: the muscle responds only to long-duration stimuli, and as the duration is decreased the voltage necessary to produce a contraction rises steeply. Curve C represents the deltoid muscle of a patient who had sustained a dislocation of the shoulder with injury to the axillary nerve. The curve shows partial denervation: the upward kink is a characteristic feature.

relatively long—that is, in the order of 100 milliseconds or more. With stimuli shorter than 100 milliseconds the voltage must be progressively increased to produce a contraction, and a response cannot be elicited at all with stimuli shorter than 1 millisecond. The curve from such a denervated muscle (B in Fig. 7) is termed a muscle curve, because the contraction depends upon direct stimulation of the muscle fibres and is not a response to stimulation of the motor nerve. The curve of a partly innervated muscle (for instance, one that is recovering after a nerve injury, or one that is paretic from poliomyelitis) lies between the normal or nerve curve and the curve of denervation, and it is characterised by an upward kink, denoting superimposition of the two basic types of curve (C in Fig. 7). If progressive recovery is occurring the curve will be seen on serial examinations to be becoming flatter, with a shift towards the left. Conversely, if the process of denervation is progressive, the curve will become steeper and will be shifted to the right. Failure of a muscle to respond at all to a high-voltage long-duration stimulus indicates that the muscle has become fibrotic (absolute degeneration).

In *electromyography* the electrical changes occurring in a muscle are picked up by a needle electrode, suitably amplified, and studied in the form of sounds through a loud-speaker, or of tracings recorded optically. Normal muscle is electrically ' silent ' at rest, but shows electrical discharges on contraction. Partly denervated or totally denervated muscle shows spontaneous contractions of individual fibres (fibrillation potentials). Different wave forms and sounds are characteristic of various disorders of the nervous system and of muscle. By electromyography it is possible to determine with certainty whether a lesion is in the anterior horn cell, in the peripheral nerve or in the muscle.

INTERPRETATION OF THE FINDINGS

When the study of the patient is complete the abnormal findings elicited from the history, clinical examination, radiographic examination, and appropriate special investigations should be assembled together to form a composite clinical picture. This can then be matched against the recognised disorders of the region under consideration. It is comforting to remember that the number of disorders that commonly affect a particular region is limited. Often the number is not large. Theoretically, therefore, if all the possibilities are listed and thereafter confirmed or eliminated one by one the correct diagnosis must always be revealed.

In practice, of course, diagnosis is not so simple as that. But it is nevertheless true that if the problem is tackled logically, step by step, in the manner described, a correct conclusion can be formed in the great majority of cases. The only essentials are a capacity for painstaking enquiry, with strict attention to detail, accurate observation, and a working knowledge of the salient features of the common disorders.

Psychogenic or Stress Disorders

This heading is included to issue a word of warning. When the cause of a patient's symptoms remains obscure despite a thorough investigation there is a prevalent tendency—it has almost become fashionable—to discount the genuineness of the symptoms and to ascribe them to ' hysterical,' ' functional,' or ' psychogenic ' factors, or simply to stress. This must be deplored as a dangerous policy that has led on countless occasions to the overlooking of a serious organic disease.

Just because we fail to discover the cause of a particular symptom it by no means follows that the symptom is imaginary or psychogenic ; it usually means only that we are not sufficiently skilled in diagnosis. Admittedly, true hysterical disorders are encountered from time to time in orthopaedic practice, but they are few and far between. Much more often a long-continued organic pain leads to a distracted state of mind that is wrongly interpreted as a hysterical manifestation. It is far safer to err on the side of disregarding possible psychogenic factors than to overlook an organic lesion on the supposition that the symptoms are imaginary.

TREATMENT OF ORTHOPAEDIC DISORDERS

Orthopaedic treatment falls into three categories : 1) No treatment—simply reassurance or advice ; 2) non-operative treatment ; 3) operative treatment. In every case these three possibilities of treatment should be considered one by one in the order given. At least half of the patients attending orthopaedic out-patient clinics (excluding cases of fracture) do not require treatment : all that they need is reassurance and advice. In many cases the sole reason for the patient's attendance is that he fears that he may have cancer, tuberculosis or other serious disease. If he can be reassured that there is no evidence of serious disease he goes away satisfied, and his symptoms immediately become less disturbing.

If active treatment seems to be required it is a good general principle that whenever practicable a trial should be given first to non-operative measures. Most orthopaedic operations fall into the category of ' luxury ' rather than life-saving procedures. Consequently the patient should seldom be persuaded to submit himself to operation : rather should he have to bully the surgeon into performing it. When one is undecided whether to advise conservative treatment or operation it is wise always to err on the side of non-intervention.

METHODS OF NON-OPERATIVE TREATMENT
Rest
Since the days of H. O. Thomas (p. 4), who emphasised its value in diseases of the spine and limbs, rest has been one of the mainstays of orthopaedic treatment. Complete rest demands recumbency in bed or immobilisation of the diseased part in plaster. But by ' rest ' the orthopaedic surgeon does not necessarily mean complete inactivity or immobility. Often he means no more than ' relative rest,' implying simply a reduction of wonted activity and avoidance of strain.

Support
Rest and support often go together ; but there are occasions when support is needed but not rest—for example, to stabilise a joint rendered insecure by muscle paralysis, or to prevent the development of deformity. When support is to be temporary it can be provided by a plaster-of-Paris case or splint. When it is to be prolonged or permanent an individually made surgical appliance is required. Examples in common use are steel-reinforced lumbar corsets, spinal braces, walking calipers, below-knee steels with ankle straps, and drop-foot springs.

Physiotherapy
Physiotherapy in its various forms occupies an important place in the non-operative—and in the post-operative—treatment of orthopaedic disabilities. Being easily prescribed, and entailing no trouble to the surgeon, it is no doubt often misused : much treatment is given that can have no beneficial effect except perhaps psychologically. Occasionally, too, an unskilled physiotherapist by over-enthusiastic stretching or forcing has retarded rather than hastened the patient's recovery. But it is unrealistic on these accounts to condemn all physiotherapy as valueless or dangerous, as some surgeons do. Enlightened teaching has helped to produce an awareness among present-day physiotherapists of the hazards as well as the merits of their art, and a correct emphasis is being

placed upon the value in many conditions of active rather than of passive treatment—in other words, of helping the patient to help himself. This approach is particularly rewarding in the rehabilitation of patients after injury or after operation, and in such diseases as poliomyelitis and cerebral palsy.

When it is used, physiotherapy should be pursued thoroughly. Half-hearted treatment at infrequent intervals is a waste of time. Ideally it should be practised daily. The following are the most important forms in which physiotherapy is given.

Active exercises. Exercises may be given for three purposes : 1) to mobilise joints, 2) to strengthen muscles, and 3) to improve coordination or balance. In *mobilising exercises* the patient's active efforts to move the joint may be assisted by gentle pressure by the physiotherapist's hand (assisted active exercises). In *muscle-strengthening exercises* the patient is encouraged to contract the weakened muscles against the resistance of weights or springs, the resistance being increased as the muscles gain power. *Exercises to improve coordination* are of particular importance in cerebral palsy.

Passive joint movements. The chief use of passive movements is to preserve full mobility when the patient is unable to move the joint actively—that is, when the muscles are paralysed or severed. They are important in poliomyelitis and after nerve injuries—especially to preserve mobility in the hand. Certain movements that are not under the control of the patient may also be used passively for treatment purposes—notably distraction, which is commonly employed, for instance, in the treatment of prolapsed cervical disc and of certain other painful conditions of the spinal column (see also under Manipulation on p. 22).

Electrical stimulation of muscles. If a muscle has its nerve supply intact electrical stimulation is of relatively little importance in increasing muscle strength : active exercises are generally much more effective. Nevertheless, electrotherapy does have a place when used in conjunction with exercises—for example, in improving the function of the intrinsic muscles of the foot, in restoring activity to a quadriceps muscle that has been inhibited after operation upon the knee, or in re-education after a tendon transfer operation. Since the nerve supply is intact the muscle may be stimulated through its motor nerve by ' faradism ' (that is, by shocks of short duration induced by the make-and-break of an induction coil or by an electronic stimulator).

If the muscle is denervated (for instance, after a peripheral nerve injury) it may be stimulated electrically, while recovery of nerve function is awaited, in order to retard the process of fibrosis that occurs after about two years in any denervated muscle. Such a muscle can be stimulated only by ' galvanism ' (that is, by shocks of relatively long duration which stimulate the muscle fibres directly, not through its motor nerve). There is no object in prescribing this treatment if recovery of nerve function within two years cannot be hoped for.

Local heat. Possibly by increasing the blood flow, or possibly in some other way, heat produces a soothing effect on many aching pains of ' rheumatic ' or ' fibrositic ' type, but the effect is often only short-lived. Surface heat is applied by an *infra-red* or *radiant-heat* lamp. Deep heat is applied by *short-wave diathermy*, which produces the greatest heat at a point between the two electrodes. *Wax (paraffin) baths* provide a simple method of heating the hands.

Ultra-sound therapy. Ultra-sonic waves (at about a million cycles per second) projected as a beam from a transducer penetrate to a considerable depth. When the waves strike the tissues the energy is converted into heat. There is also said to be a micro-massage effect. This treatment is used for relief of pain in osteo-arthritis, in certain types of back pain and in some other painful conditions.

Massage. Massage has only a limited field of usefulness. In general, it is far less effective than active exercises in improving the circulatory return in cases of gravitational oedema. Nevertheless it is occasionally useful as a supplementary measure in such cases ; and it may also be of value in loosening subcutaneous scars.

Local Injections

The indications for local injections fall into two groups: 1) osteoarthritis or rheumatoid arthritis, in which the substance (usually hydrocortisone with or without a local anaesthetic solution) is injected directly into the affected joint with rigid aseptic precautions; and 2) extra-articular lesions of the type often ascribed (for want of more precise knowledge) to chronic strain, as exemplified by tennis elbow, tendonitis about the shoulder, and certain types of back pain. The response depends upon the nature of the basic lesion: permanent relief is often gained in extra-articular lesions such as tennis elbow, but in arthritis the benefit is often no more than temporary.

Drugs

Drugs have rather a small place in orthopaedic practice. Those used may be placed in seven categories: 1) antibiotics; 2) sulphonamides; 3) analgesics; 4) sedatives; 5) anti-inflammatory drugs; 6) hormone-like drugs; 7) specific drugs. *Antibiotics* are of immense importance in infective lesions, especially in acute osteomyelitis and acute pyogenic arthritis; but to be successful treatment must be begun very early. Antibiotics are also of definite value in certain chronic infections, notably in tuberculosis. *Sulphonamides*, though they have to some extent been superseded by antibiotics, are of value in preventing or treating infection by organisms that are sensitive to them. *Analgesics* should be used as little as possible. Many orthopaedic disorders are prolonged for many weeks or months, and it is undesirable to prescribe any but the mildest analgesics continuously over long periods, except for incurable malignant disease. *Sedatives* may be given if needed to promote sleep, but as with analgesics the rule should be to prescribe no more than is really necessary. *Anti-inflammatory drugs* are those that damp down the excessive inflammatory response that may occur especially in rheumatoid arthritis and related disorders. The most powerful are the steroids cortisone, prednisone and their analogues. These should be used with extreme caution and indeed should be avoided altogether whenever possible, because through their serious side effects they may sometimes do more harm than good. Examples of less powerful anti-inflammatory agents, which should be preferred to steroids except in rare circumstances, are aspirin, phenylbutazone, indomethacin and ibrufen. Many of these drugs also come into the category of analgesics. *Hormone-like drugs* include the corticosteroids noted above, and sex hormones or analogues used for control of certain metastatic tumours. Notable among the latter is stilboestrol, for the metastatic deposits of carcinoma of the prostate. *Specific drugs* work well in certain special diseases.

Examples are vitamin C for scurvy, vitamin D for rickets, colchicum for gouty arthritis, and salicylates for the arthritis of rheumatic fever.

Manipulation

Treatment by manipulation is practised widely by orthopaedic surgeons and by others in allied professions. Strictly, the term might legitimately be used to include the passive movements that form part of the daily activities of a physiotherapy department and which have already been referred to above ; but it is used here in a more restricted sense, to describe passive movements of joints, bones or soft tissues carried out by the surgeon—with or without an anaesthetic, and often forcefully—as a deliberate step in treatment.

The subject will be considered under three general headings : 1) manipulation for correction of deformity ; 2) manipulation to improve the range of movement at a stiff joint ; and 3) manipulation for relief of chronic pain in or about a joint.

Manipulation for correction of deformity. In this category manipulation has its most obvious application in the reduction of fractures and dislocations. It is also used to overcome deformity from contracted or short soft tissues—as, for example, in congenital club foot. Yet another example is the forcible subcutaneous rupture and dispersal of a ganglion over the dorsum of the wrist.

Technique. An anaesthetic may or may not be required, according to the nature of the condition that is being treated. In many instances— as in manipulation for a fracture or dislocation—the aim is to secure full reduction at the one sitting ; but in resistant deformities such as club foot repeated manipulation may be required at intervals of a week or so, a little further improvement being gained each time.

Subsequent management. After manipulation for a deformity that is liable to recur—as in most cases of displaced fracture and in chronic deformities of joints—the limb is usually immobilised on a splint or in plaster to maintain the correction. In cases of resistant deformity gradual yielding of the soft tissue allows re-application of the splint in a more favourable position each time it is changed.

Manipulation for joint stiffness. The type of case mainly concerned here is that in which a joint shows serious limitation of movement after an acute injury—usually a fracture of a limb bone. ' Frozen ' shoulder (periarthritis) in its non-active stage may also be included in this category. In such cases the stiffness is caused by adhesions either within the joint itself or, more often, in the soft tissues about or near the joint. Forcible manipulation by the surgeon is not required very often for stiffness of this type, because it will usually respond gradually to treatment by active exercises under the care of a physiotherapist, combined with increasing use of the limb.

Technique. Muscular relaxation should be secured by anaesthesia, supplemented if necessary by a relaxant drug. Great force should not be used : it is better to gain slight improvement by moderate force and then to repeat the manipulation after an interval. Excessive force may fracture a bone ; or it may cause fresh bleeding within the joint, thereby aggravating the stiffness.
Subsequent management. Manipulation for joint stiffness should always be followed by intensive active exercises designed to retain the increased range of movement.

Manipulation for relief of chronic pain. In this third category of case treatment by manipulation is somewhat empirical, because in many instances it is impossible to determine precisely the nature of the underlying pathology, and consequently the way in which manipulation acts is a matter of conjecture. Manipulation is used in such cases simply because previous experience has proved that it is often successful.

The painful conditions that respond best to manipulation are chronic strains, especially of the tarsal joints, the joints of the spinal column, and the sacro-iliac joints. A chronic strain may be the consequence of an acute injury that has not been followed by complete resolution, or it may be caused by long-continued mechanical overstrain. It is generally surmised that adhesions are present that prevent the extremes of joint movement (even though a restriction of movement may not be obvious clinically), that these adhesions are painful when stretched, and that the effect of manipulation is to rupture them. An alternative explanation that is advanced in certain cases is that there is a minor displacement of the joint surfaces or of an intra-articular structure (even though this can seldom be demonstrated radiologically), and that the effect of manipulation is to restore normal apposition.

Technique. Manipulation for relief of pain from chronic strain consists in putting the affected joint or joints forcibly through a full range of movement, usually while the patient is fully relaxed under an anaesthetic but sometimes without an anaesthetic. Longitudinal distraction of the joint is often a useful preliminary to the forcing of the extreme range.

Subsequent management. The manipulation should usually be followed by physiotherapy to maintain the function of the joint. It may be repeated after an interval if initial improvement does not progress to complete cure.

Dangers and safeguards in treatment by manipulation.

Manipulation may do harm if it is undertaken for the stiffness of inflammatory arthritis in an active stage, or if a tumour or other destructive disease exists close to the joint. This emphasises the importance of careful clinical and radiological examination— supplemented if necessary by other investigations such as deter- mination of the erythrocyte sedimentation rate—before treatment is begun. It is to be noted that manipulation is of no value for stiffness of the metacarpo-phalangeal joints and interphalangeal joints of the hand.

During the manipulation itself care must be taken to avoid disasters such as the fracture of a bone or massive displacement of an intervertebral disc. It is well known that a fracture— especially of the patella or humerus—may be caused easily by injudicious manipulation. This risk is greatly increased if the bone is already weak from the osteoporosis of disuse or from some other rarefying disease.

Radiotherapy

Radiotherapy—by x-rays or by the gamma rays of radio-active substances—may be used for certain benign conditions or for malignant disease. Because of its possible ill effects it should be advised only with caution for benign lesions, but it may sometimes be the mainstay of treatment in ankylosing spondylitis and in cases of giant-cell tumour of bone that are unsuitable for local excision. In malignant disease radiotherapy is usually palliative rather than curative. In conditions such as malignant bone tumours for which a tumour dose in the order of 7,000 roentgens may be required only the penetrating rays produced by a super-voltage x-ray plant or by a radio-active cobalt unit should be used. With such apparatus a high dose can be delivered to the tumour with the least possible damage to the skin.

OPERATIVE TREATMENT

The chief essential of any operation is that it should not make the patient worse than he was before he submitted to it. This is so obvious that the statement may sound almost absurd. Yet it is unfortunately true that a disturbing number of operations carried out for orthopaedic conditions do in fact cause more harm than good for one reason or another. Hence the selection of cases for operation, the choice of the most appropriate operation in given circumstances, the technical performance of the operation, and the post-operative management are matters of the highest importance, and they call for a high degree of judgment and skill. Herein lies much of the fascination of orthopaedic surgery.

A detailed account of operative techniques is unnecessary here. All that is required is a brief mention of the more important operations.

Osteotomy

Osteotomy is the operation of cutting a bone. It has almost supplanted *osteoclasis* (forcible bending or incomplete breaking of a bone), which formerly was often used to correct deformities of the long bones in children with rickets and which may still be suitable occasionally for that purpose.

Indications. The general indications for osteotomy are as follows : 1) to correct excessive angulation, bowing or rotation of a long bone ; 2) to permit angulation of a bone in order to compensate for mal-alignment at a joint ; 3) to permit elongation or shortening of a bone in the lower limb in order to correct a discrepancy of length between the two sides. In addition, there are certain special indications for osteotomy at the upper end of the femur: 4) to improve stability at the hip by altering the line of weight transmission (abduction osteotomy, p. 328) ; 5) to relieve the pain of an osteoarthritic hip (displacement osteotomy, p. 339) ; and 6) as an aid to arthrodesis of the hip,

2

by eliminating temporarily the leverage of the femur and thus helping to secure complete immobility at the joint while fusion is occurring.

Technique. If the bone is relatively soft (as in children) it may be divided simply with an osteotome or, in the case of a thin bone, by bone-cutting forceps. The strong cortex of the major long bones in an adult is not easily divided in that way because it tends to splinter ; so most surgeons weaken the bone by making multiple drill holes before applying the osteotome, or, where access is adequate, use a saw. When the bone has been divided and the necessary correction made it is often convenient to fix the fragments with a plate, nail-plate, or medullary nail : this may allow external splintage to be dispensed with. If internal fixation is not used the fragments must be held in position by a suitable splint or plaster until union has occurred.

Arthrodesis

The operation of arthrodesis, or joint fusion, has a wide application. The disability from a single stiff joint is usually slight, and patients readily adapt themselves to it. Even when two or three joints are fused function may be surprisingly good, depending upon the particular joints affected.

Indications. Arthrodesis is indicated mainly in the following conditions. 1) Advanced osteoarthritis with disabling pain, especially when confined to a single joint. 2) Quiescent tuberculous arthritis with destruction of the joint surfaces, to eliminate risk of recrudescence and to prevent deformity. 3) Instability from muscle paralysis, as after poliomyelitis. 4) For permanent correction of deformity, as in hammer toe.

Methods of arthrodesis. Arthrodesis may be intra-articular or extra-articular, or the two may be combined. In *intra-articular* arthrodesis the joint is opened and the bone ends are displayed. The articular cartilage (or what remains of it) is removed so that raw bone is exposed. The joint is placed in the desired position and immobilised (usually by metallic internal fixation as well as by a plaster-of-Paris splint) until clinical tests and radiographs show sound bony fusion.

In *extra-articular* arthrodesis the joint itself is left undisturbed, but it is ' by-passed ' by securing bone-to-bone fusion above or below the joint, usually through the medium of a bone graft. The method is applicable mainly to the spine, shoulder, and hip. It has a theoretical advantage in cases of infective joint disease, because any risk of reactivating or disseminating the infection by opening the joint is avoided.

Examples of the methods of arthrodesing the shoulder and hip are illustrated in Figures 8 and 9.

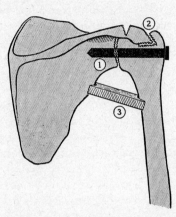 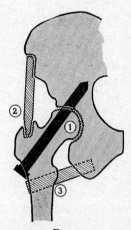

FIG. 8

Three methods of arthrodesis of the shoulder.   1.   Intra-articular arthrodesis with fixation by a nail.   2.   Extra-articular arthrodesis : acromion turned down into a slot in the greater tuberosity. 3. Extra-articular arthrodesis : strut graft between humerus and scapula.

FIG. 9

Three methods of arthrodesis of the hip.   1.   Intra-articular arthrodesis with fixation by a nail.   2. Extra-articular arthrodesis by ilio-femoral graft.   3. Extra-articular arthrodesis by ischio-femoral graft.

Position for arthrodesis.   The best position for arthrodesis should not be regarded as rigidly established for each joint : variations may be appropriate and desirable in individual cases— for instance, to conform to the requirements of the patient's work. The following is only a general guide. *Shoulder :* About 30 to 40 degrees of abduction and 40 degrees of medial rotation. *Elbow :* If only one elbow is affected, 90 degrees of flexion (or according to the requirements of the patient's work).   If both elbows are affected one should be in flexion above the right angle and the other about 20 degrees below the right angle.

If forearm rotation is lost the most useful position of the forearm is in 10 degrees of pronation. *Wrist :* Extended 20 degrees. *Interphalangeal joints :* Semiflexed. *Hip :* About 15 degrees of flexion ; no abduction or adduction. *Knee :* About 20 degrees of flexion. *Ankle :* In men, right angle ; in women, 20 to 30 degrees of plantarflexion, according to accustomed height of heel.

Arthroplasty

Arthroplasty is the operation for construction of a new movable joint. It is not applicable to every joint: in practice, its use is almost confined to the elbow, the hip, the knee, certain joints in the hand, and the metatarso-phalangeal joints in the foot.

Indications. The indications for arthroplasty are not well defined, for there is considerable diversity of opinion among different surgeons. Broadly, it has a use in the following conditions : 1) advanced osteoarthritis or rheumatoid arthritis with disabling pain, especially in the elbow, hip, hand and metatarso-phalangeal joints; 2) for the correction of certain types of deformity (especially hallux valgus); 3) quiescent tuberculous arthritis of the elbow, with destruction of the joint surfaces; 4) certain ununited fractures of the neck of the femur. It will be realised that in several of these conditions arthroplasty is an alternative to arthrodesis.

Methods of arthroplasty. Three methods are in general use. Each has its merits, disadvantages and special applications.

Excision arthroplasty. In this method one or both of the articular ends of the bones are simply excised, so that a gap is created between them (Fig. 10). The gap fills with fibrous tissue, or a pad of muscle or other soft tissue may be sewn in between the bones. By virtue of its flexibility the interposed tissue allows a reasonable range of movement, but the joint often lacks stability. The method is applicable to all the joints for which arthroplasty is practicable except the knee. It is used most commonly at the metatarso-phalangeal joint of the great toe, in the treatment of hallux valgus and hallux rigidus.

Cup arthroplasty. This method is applicable to ball-and-socket joints. In practice its use is virtually limited to the hip. The joint surfaces are refashioned to a true hemispherical form, and a highly polished cup of inert metal is interposed between them as a new lining (Fig. 11). Movement occurs at both surfaces of the cup, no attempt being made to fix it immovably to either joint surface. In the course of time the constant friction of the bones against the polished surface of the cup stimulates the development of a surface layer of smooth fibrocartilage. A serious disadvantage of cup arthroplasty is that the blood supply

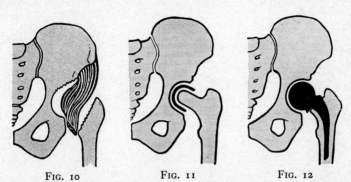

FIG. 10   FIG. 11   FIG. 12

Three methods of arthroplasty, as exemplified at the hip. Figure 10—Excision arthroplasty. Note the interposed soft tissue. Figure 11—Cup arthroplasty. Figure 12—Replacement arthroplasty: either the femoral head alone is replaced, as in the diagram, or both the femoral head and the acetabulum may be replaced.

of the bone within the cup is in jeopardy ; if the blood supply is inadequate the femoral head undergoes avascular necrosis and may collapse.

Replacement arthroplasty. This method is still in a stage of development. In principle one (or sometimes both) of the articulating bone ends is excised and replaced by an inert prosthesis of similar shape (Fig. 12). Ideally the prosthesis should remain rigidly fixed to the stump of bone to which it is fitted : loosening may cause failure. An acrylic filling compound or ' cement ' is often used to aid fixation. First developed for use in the hip (for ununited fractures of the femoral neck), the method has been adapted, with modifications, to other joints such as the knee and the metacarpo-phalangeal joints. In prosthetic replacement for arthritis there is a trend towards replacement of both the articulating surfaces (total replacement arthroplasty), but it is not yet known whether such prosthetic joints will last indefinitely.

Bone Grafting Operations

Bone grafts are usually obtained from another part of the patient's body (autogenous grafts or autografts). If it is impracticable or undesirable to take bone from the patient's own body, grafts from another human subject may be used (homogenous grafts, homografts or allografts). They are generally stored frozen under aseptic conditions in a 'bone bank' until required, but cadaveric bone sterilised by boiling or by irradiation is sometimes used. Grafts obtained from animals (heterogenous grafts or heterografts) may be satisfactory if they are specially treated to eliminate their antigenic properties. Recently, limited use has been made of animal bone (chiefly bovine) prepared commercially in sterile packs, but most surgeons believe that it is far inferior to the patient's own bone and cannot be relied upon to become incorporated with the host bone.

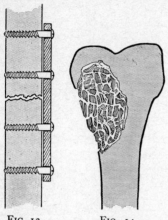

Fig. 13   Fig. 14

Examples of bone grafting techniques. Figure 13—Cortical slab graft held by four screws, as used to bridge an ununited fracture. Figure 14—Cancellous grafts used to fill a cavity in a bone.

Bone transferred as an autograft from one site to another does not survive wholly in a living state. For the most part the bone cells die, although a few that are near the surface may possibly survive. The purpose of the graft—as of allografts and heterografts—is mainly to serve as a scaffolding or temporary bridge upon which new bone is laid down. Thus the whole of a graft is eventually replaced by new living bone. This process of replacement is dependent upon adequate revascularisation of the graft ; so a graft that lies in a highly vascular bed is more likely to succeed than one that is surrounded by relatively ischaemic tissue.

Indications. Bone grafts are used mainly in three types of case : 1) in cases of ununited fracture, to promote union ; 2) in arthrodesis of joints, either to supplement an intra-articular arthrodesis or to promote extra-articular fusion ; 3) to fill a defect or cavity in a bone.

Technique. Bone for grafting may be obtained as a solid slab, or it may be used in the form of multiple slivers or of small chips.

Slab grafts. A slab graft is usually obtained from strong cortical bone : the subcutaneous part of the tibia is a common site. The graft is fixed to the recipient bone either by screws or by inlaying. Such a graft serves as an internal splint as well as a framework for the growth of new bone (Fig. 13).

Sliver grafts. Sliver or strip grafts are generally obtained from spongy cancellous bone—especially from the crest of the ilium. They are used mainly for ununited fractures. They are laid about the fracture, deep to the periosteum, and are held in place by suture of the soft tissues over them.

Chip grafts. These also are preferably obtained from cancellous bone. The chips are packed firmly into, or around, the recipient bone and are held in place simply by suture of the soft tissues over them (Fig. 14).

Tendon Transfer Operations

In the operation of tendon transfer, or tendon transplant, the insertion of a healthy functioning muscle is moved to a new site, so that the muscle henceforth has a different action. In this way the function of a paralysed or severed muscle can be taken over by one that is intact. In properly selected cases there need be no noticeable loss of power in the former sphere of action of the transferred muscle, because there is often considerable duplication or overlap in the function of individual muscles. Thus a tendon of flexor digitorum superficialis may be transferred to a new site without appreciably impairing the power of finger flexion, which can be adequately controlled by the flexor profundus. Similarly the extensor indicis can be spared for a new function without seriously interfering with the power of extension of the finger.

Indications. Tendon transfers have their main application in three groups of conditions : 1) in cases of muscle paralysis, to restore or improve active control of a joint by re-routing a healthy muscle to act in place of a paralysed one; 2) in cases of deformity from muscle imbalance, to maintain correction by switching healthy muscles to restore proper balance; and 3) in cases of ruptured or cut tendon, when direct suture of the ends is impracticable.

Technique.   The tendon to be transferred is divided at an appropriate point, re-routed in the direction of its new action, and secured to its new insertion.   If it is to be inserted into bone it is passed through a drill hole and held by suturing back on itself.   If it is to be united to a tendon stump the junction may be secured by end-to-end suture or, preferably, by interlacing the tendons one through the other and transfixing them with mattress sutures.

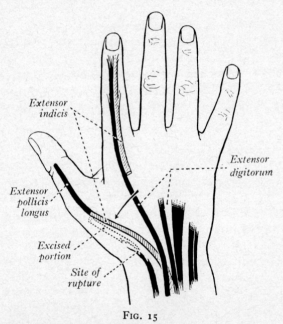

FIG. 15

Transfer of extensor indicis to replace a ruptured extensor pollicis longus. This transfer is to be preferred to direct suture when the ends of the ruptured tendon are frayed.

Examples. 1) In a case of radial paralysis, with loss of active extension of the wrist, fingers and thumb, function may be restored by the following tendon transfers : pronator teres is transferred to extensor carpi radialis brevis ; flexor carpi ulnaris is transferred to extensor digitorum and extensor pollicis longus, and palmaris longus is transferred to abductor pollicis longus. 2) In a case of congenital talipes equino-varus (p. 409) transfer of the tendon of the tibialis anterior or tibialis posterior to the outer side of the foot will help to prevent recurrence of the deformity. 3) In a case of rupture of the extensor pollicis longus, with extensive fraying of the tendon, direct repair may be impracticable. Function may be restored by transfer of the extensor indicis to the extensor pollicis longus (Fig. 15).

Tendon Grafting Operations

In tendon grafting a length of free tendon is used to bridge a gap between the severed ends of the recipient tendon.

Indications. The chief use of free tendon grafts is in the reconstruction of flexor tendons severed in the fibrous digital sheaths of the hand (p. 303).

Technique. The free tendon graft is usually obtained from the palmaris longus or from one of the toe extensors at the dorsum of the foot. Proximally, it is joined to the recipient tendon by sutures of stainless steel wire. Distally, it may be secured to the distal stump of the recipient tendon or it may be attached directly to bone through a drill hole.

Equalisation of Leg Length

If a patient's legs are of markedly unequal length, as in certain cases of congenital anomaly, previous poliomyelitis, or damage to a growth epiphysis, the discrepancy may be reduced or eliminated by operation. The methods available are: 1) leg lengthening; 2) leg shortening; and 3) arrest of epiphysial growth. *Leg lengthening* is suitable mainly for children. It is achieved by dividing the appropriate bone (usually the tibia, sometimes the femur) and then gradually elongating the limb in a special screw-distraction apparatus at the rate of about two millimetres a day. A maximum of about five centimetres may be gained. The procedure is time-consuming and trying for the patient, and should be reserved for carefully selected cases. *Leg shortening*, by removing an appropriate length from the shaft of the longer femur or tibia, is less hazardous but not to be undertaken lightly because it disturbs a limb that was previously normal. In a patient who is fairly tall, and especially in adults, it is often preferable to leg lengthening. *Arrest of epiphysial growth* (on the longer side) is applicable only to children with considerable growth still to come. It entails either destruction, or sealing by bone grafts or by metal staples, of the lower femoral epiphysis or of the upper tibial epiphysis, or both. The correction to be expected depends upon the amount of growth still to come from the corresponding epiphysis of the opposite (shorter) leg, which depends in turn upon the age at which the operation is undertaken.

References and bibliography, page 445.

2*

CHAPTER TWO

General Survey of Orthopaedic Disorders

THIS chapter is devoted to a broad preliminary review of the field of orthopaedics. The main groups of disorders will be described without a detailed consideration of their local manifestations. Against this general background the features of the common disorders as they affect each particular region will be discussed in the subsequent chapters.

Classification

Most orthopaedic disorders fall within the following groups:

INJURIES

DEFORMITIES
>   Congenital deformities
>   Acquired deformities

AFFECTIONS OF JOINTS
>   Arthritis
>   Dislocation and subluxation
>   Internal derangements

AFFECTIONS OF BONE
>   Infections of bone
>   Tumours of bone
>   Other local affections of bone
>   General affections of the skeleton

AFFECTIONS OF SOFT TISSUE
>   Inflammatory lesions of soft tissue
>   Tumours of soft tissue

NEUROLOGICAL DISORDERS
>   Poliomyelitis
>   Cerebral palsy
>   Spina bifida
>   Peripheral nerve lesions

INJURIES

Recent injuries of the limbs and spine form a subject for special study, and they are dealt with in textbooks on fractures. Injuries will be considered here only in so far as they contribute to persistent or recurrent disability.

CONGENITAL DEFORMITIES

Congenital deformities or malformations, by definition, are attributable to faulty development and are present at birth, though they may not be recognised until later. They vary from severe malformations that are incompatible with life and may be found in still-born infants, to minor abnormalities of structure that have no practical significance. Incidence varies in different countries and among different races : in Britain probably 2 or 3 per cent of infants are born with some significant developmental abnormality, but only about half of these affect the skeleto-motor system. Some of the better known anomalies are summarised in Table I.

Causes

An abnormality of development may be caused by 1) genetic abnormality, 2) environmental abnormality, or 3) combined genetic and environmental abnormalities. Studies of families and twins have helped geneticists to determine the influence of genetic and environmental factors, alone or combined, in the causation of many of the recognised malformations.

Genetic causes include mutation of a whole chromosome, as in mongolism (Down's syndrome), and mutation of a small part of a chromosome or of a single gene, as in achondroplasia. The defect is not necessarily always inherited from an affected parent, for it may arise from a fresh mutation in the germ cell.

Environmental causes are not well understood. Experiments in animals have shown that many different types of environmental influence—dietetic, hormonal, chemical, physical or infective—may cause abnormalities of development, and the system of the body that is mainly affected depends upon the timing of the environmental ' insult.' But except for a few specific agents acting early in pregnancy there is no conclusive evidence that similar influences are important causes of malformations in man. The specific agents whose influence is well attested include radiation, the virus of rubella, and certain drugs (notably aminopterin and thalidomide).

TABLE I

SOME OF THE BETTER KNOWN CONGENITAL DEFORMITIES OR ANOMALIES
OF ORTHOPAEDIC INTEREST, WITH THEIR SALIENT CLINICAL FEATURES.

(When a fuller description appears elsewhere in this book the relevant page number is given.
Conditions not thus designated are either so rare or of such little importance to the student that
further description is unnecessary.)

NAME OF DEFORMITY OR ANOMALY	CLINICAL OR PATHOLOGICAL FEATURES
Generalised	
Osteogenesis imperfecta (fragilitas ossium) (p. 104)	Fragile soft bones, easily broken or deformed. Blue sclerotics. Joint laxity. Otosclerosis.
Diaphysial aclasis (multiple exostoses) (p. 104)	Cartilage-capped bony outgrowths from metaphyses. Deficient remodelling. Stunted growth.
Dyschondroplasia (multiple chondromatosis ; Ollier's disease) (p. 106)	Masses of cartilage in long-bone metaphyses. Impaired growth. Deformity. Often unilateral.
Achondroplasia (chondro-dystrophy) (p. 107)	Short-limb dwarfing from defect of long-bone growth. Trident hand. Large head.
Osteopetrosis (Albers - Schönberg disease; 'marble bones')	Hard dense bones, but with increased liability to fracture. Anaemia from obliteration of medulla.
Gargoylism (Hurler's syndrome)	Dwarfing. Kyphosis from deformed vertebrae. Corneal opacity. Large liver and spleen. Mental deficiency.
Cranio-cleido dysostosis	Impaired ossification of skull. Deficient clavicles. Often deficient symphysis pubis.
Arthrogryposis multiplex congenita (amyoplasia congenita)	Stiff deformed limb joints from defective development of muscles. Hips often dislocated. Club feet.
Myositis ossificans progressiva (p. 108)	Ectopic ossification, often beginning in trunk but extending to limbs. Short big toe.
Vitamin-resistant rickets (p. 117)	Rachitic bone changes corrected only by massive doses of vitamin D. Hypophosphataemia not responsive to vitamin D.
Fanconi's syndrome (renal tubular rickets) (p. 118)	Rachitic rarefied bones with consequent deformity. Hypophosphataemia. Glycosuria ; amino-aciduria.
Neurofibromatosis (Recklinghausen's disease) (p. 108)	*Café-au-lait* areas or spots. Cutaneous fibromata. Neurofibromata on cranial or peripheral nerves. Often scoliosis.
Haemophilia (p. 60)	Prolonged blood clotting time. Bleeding into joints or soft tissue.
Gaucher's disease (p. 124)	Deposition of kerasin in reticulum cells, causing cyst-like appearance in bones, and large liver and spleen.
Congenital arterio-venous fistula	Hypertrophy and lengthening of limb. Bruit.

TABLE I—*continued*

NAME OF DEFORMITY OR ANOMALY	CLINICAL OR PATHOLOGICAL FEATURES
Trunk and Spine	
Congenital short neck (Klippel-Feil syndrome) (p. 153)	Short stiff neck with low hair-line. Fused or deformed cervical vertebrae.
Congenital high scapula (Sprengel's shoulder) (p. 153)	Scapula tethered high up, usually only on one side. Scapular movement impaired.
Cervical rib (p. 165)	Often symptomless. Vascular symptoms (partial ischaemia) or nerve symptoms (paraesthesiae, lower trunk paresis).
Hemivertebra (congenital scoliosis) (p. 180)	Defective development of vertebra (and often of adjacent structures) on one side. Scoliosis.
Spina bifida (spinal dysraphism) (p. 180)	Spina bifida occulta, meningocele or myelocele. Often leg deformities from paralysis or muscle imbalance. Often incontinence.
Limbs	
Congenital amputation	Part or whole of one or more limbs absent.
Phocomelia	Aplasia of proximal part of limb, the distal part being present ('seal-limb').
Constriction rings	Limb or digit constricted as if by a tight string. May be associated with syndactyly.
Absence of radius (radial club hand)	Hand deviated laterally from lack of normal support by radius. Thumb often absent.
Absence of thumb	Thumb alone may be absent, but other deformities may co-exist.
Absence of proximal arm muscles	Trapezius, deltoid, sternomastoid or pectoralis major absent.
Radio-ulnar synostosis	Forearm bones fused at proximal ends, preventing rotation.
Madelung's deformity (p. 276)	Head of ulna dislocated dorsally from lower end of radius. Radius bowed.
Syndactyly	Webbing of two or more digits.
Polydactyly	More than five digits.
Ectrodactyly	Lobster-claw appearance of hand, with pincer grip.
Congenital dislocation of hip (p. 321)	Neonatal : diagnostic click obtainable. Later infancy : shortening ; limited abduction. Radiographs diagnostic.
Congenital coxa vara (p. 350)	Defective ossification of femoral neck, with reduced neck-shaft angle.
Congenital short femur	Proximal end of femur deficient or rudimentary. Thigh short.
Absence of fibula	Leg under-developed on outer side. Foot small and everted; lateral two or three digital rays may be absent.
Congenital club foot (p. 409)	Foot inverted and plantarflexed (equinovarus), or everted and dorsiflexed (calcaneovalgus).
Congenital curled toe (p. 438)	Lateral angulation of one or more toes. Toe may lie over or under adjacent toe.

Combined genetic and environmental factors seem to be the usual cause of the more common congenital malformations in man, on the evidence of twin and family studies. It is thought probable that developing embryos react differently to environmental influences : some have a natural resistance whereas others are susceptible. A malformation is therefore likely to arise when an environmental ' insult ' is inflicted upon cells that have a genetically determined lack of resistance to it.

Practical Significance

Many of the recognised congenital abnormalities of the skeleto-motor system have little practical importance, either because they are very rare or because there is little that can be done for them : these will not all be considered further in this book. There are others, however, that present major problems to the orthopaedic surgeon and may demand energetic treatment. These include congenital dislocation of the hip (p. 321), congenital club foot (p. 409), spina bifida (p. 141), congenital scoliosis (p. 184), osteogenesis imperfecta (p. 104) and cervical rib (p. 165).

Inborn Predisposition to Disease in Adults

It is well recognised that, quite apart from the overt congenital anomalies discussed above, there exists in some patients a genetically determined predisposition to abnormalities developing in later life. Examples of orthopaedic conditions to which a susceptibility may exist include certain types of osteoarthritis (especially of the hips), ankylosing spondylitis, gouty arthritis, rheumatic fever, idiopathic scoliosis, osteochondritis dissecans, and Dupuytren's contracture.

ACQUIRED DEFORMITIES

Acquired deformities may be classified in two groups : those in which deformity arises at a joint, and those in which it arises in a bone.

DEFORMITY ARISING AT A JOINT

Deformity may be said to exist at a joint when the joint cannot be placed voluntarily in the neutral anatomical position.

Causes

The causes of deformity arising at a joint may be summarised as follows (Fig. 16).

Dislocation or subluxation. This is usually caused by injury, but it may occur as a congenital deformity, or it may follow disease of the joint (pathological dislocation).

Muscle imbalance. Unbalanced action of muscles upon a joint may hold it continuously in a particular arc of its range. In time, secondary contractures occur in the dominant muscles or in the soft tissues, preventing the joint from returning to the neutral position (Fig. 16 (2)). The two fundamental causes of muscle

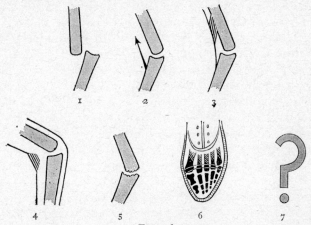

FIG. 16
Seven causes of deformity arising at a joint. 1. Dislocation.
2. Muscle imbalance. 3. Tethering of muscle or tendon.
4. Soft-tissue contracture. 5. Arthritis. 6. Posture.
7. Idiopathic (cause unknown).

imbalance are : 1) weakness or paralysis of muscles ; and 2) spasticity of muscles. Thus equinus deformity at the ankle may follow paralysis of the dorsiflexor muscles (for instance, in poliomyelitis) because the action of the plantarflexors and of gravity is unopposed. Or a similar deformity may be caused by spasticity of the calf muscles, which overpower their antagonists. This occurs commonly in cerebral palsy (p. 137).

Tethering or contracture of muscles or tendons. If something happens to muscles or tendons that prevents their normal to-and-fro gliding, or their elongation and retraction, the joint may be held in a position of deformity. Thus a muscle or tendon may be tethered to the surrounding tissues in consequence of local infection or injury (Fig. 16 (3)). An example is the anchoring of a flexor tendon of a finger within its fibrous sheath as a result of suppurative tenosynovitis, with consequent flexion deformity at the interphalangeal joints. Or a muscle may lose its elasticity and contractile power from impairment of its blood supply. An important example is Volkmann's ischaemic contracture of the forearm flexor muscles (p. 271) from occlusion of the brachial artery, with consequent flexion deformity of the wrist and fingers.

Contracture of soft tissues. Apart from any disturbance of the muscles, contracture of soft tissues alone can account for joint deformity. An example is the common condition of Dupuytren's contracture (p. 298), in which the thickened and contracted palmar aponeurosis pulls the metacarpo-phalangeal and proximal interphalangeal joints of one or more fingers into flexion. Similarly, a flexion deformity of the knee or elbow may occur from contracture of the scarred skin after burns of the flexor surface of the limb (Fig. 16 (4)).

Arthritis. The various types of arthritis will be discussed in a later section of this chapter. Any type of arthritis may lead to joint deformity. In some cases the joint is firmly fixed in a deformed position by bony or fibrous ankylosis. In other instances the joint retains some movement but is prevented from reaching the neutral position. Thus flexion and adduction deformity is common in osteoarthritis of the hip, flexion deformity is common in arthritis of the knee, and the deformity of ulnar deviation of the fingers (Fig. 186, p. 279) is a well known feature of rheumatoid arthritis of the metacarpo-phalangeal joints.

Posture. The habitual adoption of a deformed position of a joint often leads in time to permanent deformity. A common example is the lateral deviation of the great toe at the metatarso-phalangeal joint—hallux valgus—so common in women who cramp their feet into narrow pointed shoes (Fig. 16 (6)). Another postural deformity that is still seen—though it should never be allowed to occur—is fixed flexion of the knees in a patient confined to bed for a long time with the knees bent over a pillow.

Unknown causes. In some cases deformity occurs at a joint for no apparent reason. Thus many children develop knock-knee deformity between the ages of 3 and 5 years without demonstrable cause. It is usually unimportant because it tends to correct itself spontaneously. A more sinister deformity that is equally ill-explained is the idiopathic scoliosis of adolescents (p. 181).

DEFORMITY ARISING IN A BONE

Deformity exists in a bone when it is out of its normal anatomical alignment.

Causes

There are three causes of deformity arising in bone: 1) fracture; 2) bending; and 3) uneven epiphysial growth (Figs. 17-19).

Fracture. This is by far the most common cause. Unless a fracture is reduced so that the fragments are perfectly aligned deformity will result. Examples are the genu valgum (knock-knee) that is often the consequence of compression fractures of the lateral condyle of the tibia, the cubitus valgus that may follow displaced fractures of the lateral condyle of the humerus, and the common ' dinner-fork ' deformity of an unreduced fracture of the lower end of the radius.

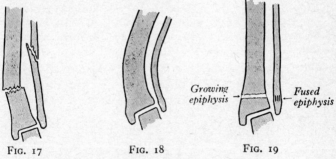

Growing epiphysis → ← *Fused epiphysis*

Fig. 17   Fig. 18   Fig. 19

Three causes of deformity arising in a bone.
Figure 17—Fracture. Figure 18—Bending of softened bone.
Figure 19—Uneven epiphysial growth.

Bending of softened bone. Many unrelated conditions can cause softening of bone, with liability to bending and consequent deformity. They are mostly generalised disorders in which several or all of the bones are affected. The following are examples. *Metabolic disorders :* rickets, osteomalacia. *Endocrine disturbances :* parathyroid osteodystrophy, Cushing's syndrome. *Affections of unknown cause :* osteitis deformans (Paget's disease), fibrous dysplasia of bone, senile osteoporosis. The main features of these disorders will be described later in this chapter.

Uneven growth of bone. In children any disturbance of the growing epiphysial cartilage may lead to uneven growth and consequent deformity.   The usual effect of interference with a growing epiphysial cartilage is that its growth is retarded ; occasionally it is accelerated.   Deformity will follow only if the growing cartilage is affected more in one part than another, or if the interference with growth affects only one bone of a pair, as in the forearm or leg (Fig. 19).   The most frequent causes of retarded epiphysial growth are : 1) fracture through the epiphysial cartilage ; 2) infection of the cartilage, usually from adjacent osteomyelitis or joint infection ; 3) enchondroma (a benign tumour) adjacent to the cartilage.   In the relatively uncommon cases in which epiphysial growth is accelerated the usual cause is local hyperaemia induced by an adjacent focus of infection or by a vascular tumour such as a haemangioma.

Treatment of Deformities

Each deformity must be considered as an individual problem. Many do not require treatment, or are not amenable to it.   In other cases an attempt may be made to correct or improve the deformity. One or more of the following methods may be used in appropriate cases : 1) manipulative correction and retention in a plaster or splint ; 2) gradual correction by prolonged traction ; 3) division or excision of contracted or tethered soft tissues ; 4) osteotomy or osteoclasis ; 5) arthrodesis ; 6) selective retardation of epiphysial growth (in children).

ARTHRITIS

The term arthritis is used here to include both inflammatory and degenerative lesions of a joint.[1]   It implies a diffuse lesion affecting the joint as a whole.   It does not include localised mechanical disorders such as loose body formation or tears of the menisci of the knee, which are better designated as internal derangements.   Nor should it embrace acute injuries of joints.

Clinically, arthritis is generally characterised by pain and restriction of movement at a joint, arising spontaneously ; in superficial joints these features are usually accompanied by obvious swelling or thickening.   If a joint is not swollen and if it moves freely and painlessly through its normal range it is very unlikely that it is affected by arthritis.

---

[1] The term *arthrosis* is sometimes used to denote a degenerative lesion of a joint.   In this sense it is strictly more accurate than *arthritis*, but the latter is established by long usage.

Types of Arthritis

If rare variations are excluded, there are nine types of arthritis to be described : 1) pyogenic arthritis ; 2) rheumatoid arthritis ; 3) tuberculous arthritis ; 4) osteoarthritis ; 5) gouty arthritis ; 6) haemophilic arthritis ; 7) neuropathic arthritis (Charcot's osteoarthropathy) ; 8) the arthritis of rheumatic fever ; and 9) ankylosing spondylitis. Of these, osteoarthritis and then rheumatoid arthritis are the most common.

PYOGENIC ARTHRITIS
(Infective arthritis ; septic arthritis)

In this form of arthritis a joint is infected by bacteria of one of the pyogenic groups. Typically there is acute joint infection of rapid development, but the infection may be subacute or even chronic. When pus is formed within the joint the condition is sometimes termed *suppurative arthritis*.

Cause. The staphylococcus, streptococcus or pneumococcus is usually responsible—occasionally the gonococcus or other organisms.

Pathology. The organisms may reach the joint by three routes : 1) through the blood stream (haematogenous infection) ; 2) through a penetrating wound ; or 3) by extension from an adjacent focus of osteomyelitis—especially when the infected metaphysis is wholly or partly within the joint cavity (as are the upper humeral metaphysis, all the metaphyses at the elbow, and the upper and lower metaphyses of the femur (Fig. 37, p. 71)).

The infection causes an acute or subacute inflammatory reaction in the joint tissues. There is exudation of fluid within the joint : the fluid is turbid or frankly purulent according to the severity of the infection. The outcome varies from complete resolution, with normal function, to total destruction of the joint and fibrous or bony ankylosis (Fig. 20).

Clinical features. The onset is acute or subacute, with pain and swelling of the joint. There is constitutional illness, with pyrexia. *On examination* the joint is swollen, partly from fluid effusion and partly from thickening of the synovial membrane. When the affected joint is superficial, the overlying skin is warmer than normal and it is often reddened. All movements are restricted ; in severe cases they are almost totally prevented by protective muscle spasm. Attempted or forced movement increases the pain. A boil or other primary focus of infection is often to be found elsewhere in the body. *Radiographs* in the early stages do not show any alteration from the normal (Fig. 21). Later, if the

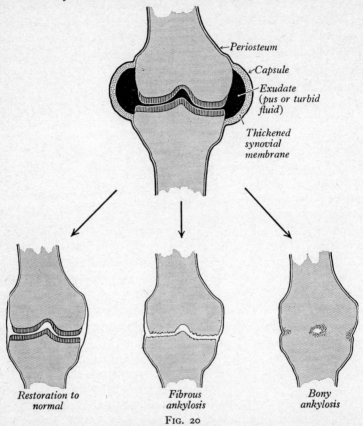

FIG. 20

Pyogenic arthritis, with possible results. In the active phase the joint is distended with pus or turbid fluid; the synovial membrane is inflamed and moderately thickened. The outcome varies with the intensity of the infection and the response to treatment. There may be: 1) restoration to normal; 2) fibrous ankylosis; or 3) bony ankylosis.

infection persists, there may be diffuse rarefaction, loss of cartilage space, and possibly destruction of bone (Fig. 22). *Investigations:* There is a polymorphonuclear leucocytosis. The erythrocyte sedimentation rate is raised. Bacteriological examination of aspirated joint fluid usually reveals the identity of the causative organism.

Diagnosis. This is from other forms of arthritis (especially tuberculous arthritis, gouty arthritis, and haemophilic arthritis), and from infections near the joint (especially acute osteomyelitis). The rapid onset, pyrexia, leucocytosis, and the character of the aspirated fluid are important diagnostic features.

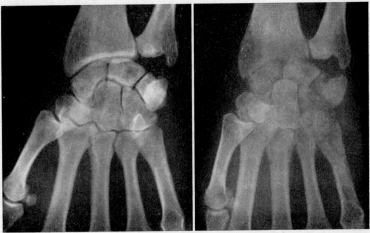

FIG. 21   FIG. 22

Pyogenic arthritis of the wrist. Figure 21—Initial radiograph, with no apparent abnormality. Figure 22—Four weeks after onset. Note the rarefaction and the slight but significant narrowing of the cartilage space, indicating destruction of articular cartilage. (See also Figure 41, p. 73.)

Prognosis. This varies widely according to the severity of the infection, the organism responsible, and the promptness with which efficient treatment is begun. Many joints can be saved intact, but many are destroyed more or less completely, with fibrous or bony ankylosis (Fig. 20).

Treatment. Early treatment is absolutely essential if there is to be a reasonable prospect of preserving normal joint function. *Constitutional treatment :* This is by rest in bed and appropriate antibiotic drugs. Whenever possible the causative organism must be identified and its sensitivity to antibiotics determined, so that the most effective drug may be given. Until that information is available treatment should be begun with a ' broad spectrum ' antibiotic or with a combination of two bactericidal antibiotics such as ampicillin and cloxacillin. *Local treatment :* The joint is rested, usually in a plaster splint. In the case of the hip or knee, sustained weight traction is useful in relieving spasm and pain. The fluid exudate, which is often purulent, is removed by aspiration or, if necessary, by incision. At the same time a solution of the appropriate antibiotic drug is injected into the joint. Aspiration and injection of antibiotic solutions are repeated daily so long as the exudate continues to form. Rest is enforced until the infection is overcome, as shown by the subsidence of pyrexia and retrogression of the local signs. Thereafter active movements are encouraged in order to restore the greatest possible function to the joint.

RHEUMATOID ARTHRITIS
(Rheumatoid polyarthritis)

Rheumatoid arthritis is a chronic non-bacterial inflammation of joints, often associated with mild constitutional symptoms. It nearly always affects several joints at the same time (polyarthritis). Joint changes of a similar nature also occur in a number of other conditions such as Still's disease of children, Reiter's syndrome and other connective tissue or collagen diseases.

Cause. The cause is unknown. At present only two possibilities attract serious consideration: 1) that the disease is due to autoimmunity; and 2) that it is caused by infection. The hypothesis of autoimmunity is based mainly on the observation that the blood of many patients with rheumatoid arthritis contains an antibody known as rheumatoid factor, which reacts with the body protein gamma globulin. The source of the antigen, and many other details of the mechanism by which rheumatoid factor is formed, are unknown. The hypothesis of infection is likewise without sure foundation. Organisms of the mycoplasma group have been incriminated, but preliminary observations concerning them have not been confirmed. The same applies to certain diphtheroid organisms. Two facts are, however, of interest: 1) that rheumatoid factor has been found in the blood of patients with many types of infection, including endocarditis, leprosy, syphilis and viral infections; and 2) that the arthritis of swine caused by Erysipelothrix infection presents pathological and clinical features that closely resemble those of rheumatoid arthritis in man: moreover

infected animals have a high concentration of rheumatoid factor
in their blood.

Pathology. The synovial membrane is thickened by chronic
inflammatory changes (Fig. 23). Much later the articular cartilage

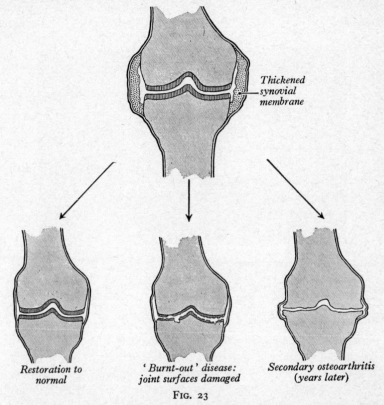

*Thickened
synovial
membrane*

*Restoration to
normal*

*'Burnt-out' disease:
joint surfaces damaged*

*Secondary osteoarthritis
(years later)*

FIG. 23

Rheumatoid arthritis, with possible results. In the active phase there is marked
thickening of the synovial membrane. Later, the articular cartilage is often
eroded and in severe cases there may be some destruction of bone. The possible
results are : 1) restoration to normal (only after mild disease of short duration) ;
2) 'burnt out' disease with permanently damaged joint surfaces and restricted
movement ; and 3) secondary osteoarthritis from wear-and-tear degeneration
of the damaged joint surfaces.

is softened and eroded, and in long-established cases there may
be small erosions of the bone ends. After months or years of
activity the disease 'burns itself out,' leaving a joint that is
usually permanently damaged. In the hands, tendons may become

softened and may rupture, aggravating the deformity of the fingers. Inflammatory nodules may form in the soft tissues.

Clinical features. The patient is usually a young or middle-aged adult. Any joint may be affected, but the incidence is higher in the more peripheral joints such as the hands, wrists, feet, knees, and elbows than in the spine, shoulders, or hips. The onset

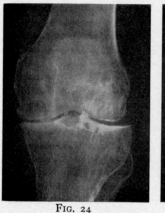 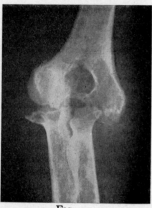

FIG. 24   FIG. 25

Figure 24—Long-established rheumatoid arthritis of the knee. Note the rarefaction and loss of cartilage space. Figure 25— Destruction of the elbow in a case of severe rheumatoid arthritis of long duration.

is gradual, with increasing pain and swelling of a joint. Soon a number of other joints are similarly affected. Pain and stiffness are often worst when activity is resumed after resting. *On examination* the affected joints are swollen from synovial thickening. The overlying skin is warmer than normal. The range of joint movements is limited, and movement causes pain, especially at the extremes. *Radiographic examination :* At first there is no alteration from the normal. Later, there is diffuse rarefaction in the area of the joint. Eventually destruction of joint cartilage may lead to narrowing of the cartilage space (Fig. 24) and, in severe cases, to localised erosion of the bone ends (Fig. 25). *Investigations :* The erythrocyte sedimentation rate is raised during the active phase. The Rose-Waaler sheep-cell agglutination test and the latex fixation test for rheumatoid factor are often positive.

Diagnosis. The clue to the diagnosis is the simultaneous involvement of several joints, with raised sedimentation rate. The presence of rheumatoid factor in the blood is highly suggestive, though the tests are not specific for rheumatoid arthritis; and rheumatoid factor may be absent even in well established rheumatoid arthritis. A search should always be made for evidence of one of the distinct medical entities that may be associated with joint changes of a rheumatoid type. The most important of such conditions are: 1) Still's disease (confined to children; spleen and lymphatic glands enlarged); 2) Reiter's syndrome (urethritis, arthritis, conjunctivitis, and hyperkeratotic eruptions on the skin); 3) lupus erythematosus (scaly erythema of face or other parts); 4) scleroderma ; and 5) psoriasis.

Course. There is a tendency for rheumatoid arthritis to become quiescent after remaining active for months or years. In most cases there is permanent impairment of joint function. In certain joints—especially the knees—osteoarthritis is often superimposed upon the 'burnt out' rheumatoid condition, and leads to increasingly severe disability even though the original rheumatoid affection is no longer active.

Treatment. The treatment of rheumatoid arthritis is unsatisfactory. No specific cure has been found. Innumerable drugs have been tried and many are in use; yet it is by no means certain—opinions differ on this point—that any of them has an influence on the duration of the disease or on its eventual outcome in a particular case. Undoubtedly some drugs can mitigate the symptoms—if only by an analgesic effect—but this may well be the sole extent of their benefit.

Methods of treatment may be classified into the following categories: 1) rest and constitutional treatment; 2) drugs; 3) physiotherapy; 4) intra-articular injections; and 5) operation.

Rest and constitutional treatment. Rest is thought to be beneficial, especially in the early stages of the disease and during an exacerbation. At many centres patients are admitted to hospital at the outset for a period of rest lasting one or two months, and sometimes this temporary removal from the home environment, with skilled nursing, regular food and proper sleep, has a remarkably good effect on the general health, which is often impaired in these cases. Rest for individual joints is also helpful during the initial active stage of inflammation, provided it is not enforced for too long. Convenient light splints for this purpose may be made from expanded polystyrene, or plaster-of-

Paris may be used. Splintage is seldom required for more than two months, and should be followed by graduated exercises under the supervision of a physiotherapist.

Drugs. Drugs used in rheumatoid arthritis fall mainly into the categories of analgesics, mild anti-inflammatory drugs, and the potent anti-inflammatory agents grouped under the heading corticosteroids. A logical plan is to use aspirin or a related salicylate as the first-line drug and to follow with other drugs if the response is unsatisfactory. Aspirin has both analgesic and mild anti-inflammatory properties but to be effective it may have to be given in fairly large doses. The second-line drug, after aspirin, is probably phenylbutazone, which also combines analgesic and anti-inflammatory effects. Next comes indomethacin, which is comparable in its effects with phenylbutazone but may in different patients prove more or less harmful in its side effects. More recent drugs in this group of reasonably safe analgesic and anti-inflammatory drugs are ibrufen and flufenamic acid, each of which may have its place.

In a different class of anti-rheumatic agents is the potentially toxic group of drugs containing gold salts. These must be used with care, but their use is thought to be sometimes beneficial and therefore justified in severely afflicted patients who have failed to respond to the first and second line drugs.

The place of corticosteroids in rheumatoid arthritis is still controversial. There can be little doubt, however, that because of their serious side effects they should be avoided altogether in the great majority of patients. Otherwise there is a real risk that the ill effects of treatment may be actually worse than those of the disease. It has been said that the use of corticosteroids may be justified in about 20 per cent of patients who have steadily worsening disease unrelieved by simpler measures, but even this is probably far too high a proportion. Only in very few patients indeed do the advantages seem to outweigh the hazards.

Physiotherapy. Physiotherapy is widely used and generally beneficial, even though some of the benefit may result from suggestion or ' placebo effect ' rather than from a direct effect on the disease process. Heat in the form of infra-red radiation, short-wave diathermy or paraffin-wax arm baths is commonly used, but probably the most useful contribution of physiotherapy is active exercises, designed both to keep joints as mobile as possible and to strengthen the muscles that control them.

Intra-articular injections. Injections of corticosteroids (usually hydrocortisone) into an affected joint can produce worth-while relief, but their disadvantages have prevented their widespread use. The main disadvantages are : 1) risk of infection, especially with repeated injections ; 2) risk of accelerating a degenerative reaction, the mechanism of which is not yet clear ; 3) the short duration of the relief obtained ;

and 4) the multiplicity of joint involvement, necessitating perhaps repeated injections at several sites which may become so irksome to the patient as to be unacceptable.

Operation : Operation has an important place in treatment, but each operation must be considered as a component in the overall plan of management and not as a substitute for other measures. Operation may be applicable to the early stage of the disease, or it may be used in the later stages to salvage a joint that has been permanently damaged and remains a source of persistent pain. In the early stages the operation most commonly used is synovectomy—excision of thickened and inflamed synovial membrane from joint or tendon sheath. As well as relieving pain, this may possibly slow down the inflammatory process and so help to preserve articular cartilage in an affected joint. It is undertaken mainly in the knee and wrist, and in the small joints and tendon sheaths of the hand.

Operations used in the later stages are osteotomy, arthroplasty, and arthrodesis. *Osteotomy* is applied chiefly to the upper end of the tibia, and sometimes to the upper end of the femur : it is valuable particularly in correcting varus or valgus deformity at the knee. *Arthroplasty* is applicable particularly to the hip, but sometimes also to the knee or elbow, and to the joints of the fingers and toes. *Arthrodesis* is usually the operation of choice for the joints of the spine, the shoulder joint, the wrist and the ankle, and often for the elbow and the knee.

Operation may also be required in the hand for repair or replacement of ruptured tendons, or for correction of finger deformities.

TUBERCULOUS ARTHRITIS

In Great Britain the incidence of tuberculous arthritis has decreased in recent years, probably because of the general improvement in living standards. Pasteurisation of milk and elimination of infected cattle have virtually abolished bovine infection. In most juvenile cases there is a history of contact with open pulmonary tuberculosis, often in a parent. In some Asiatic and African countries tuberculous infection is still common.

Since the second world war there have also been important developments in treatment, chief among which has been the use of streptomycin and other antibiotic drugs. Whereas formerly a joint affected by tuberculosis was nearly always destroyed, full recovery of function may now be hoped for in a reasonable proportion of cases.

Cause. Tuberculous arthritis is caused by infection of a joint with tubercle bacilli, human or (rarely) bovine.

Pathology. No joint is immune, but the joints most often

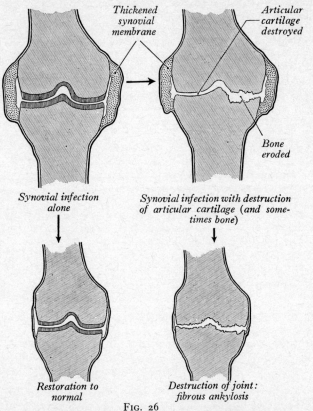

Synovial infection alone

Synovial infection with destruction of articular cartilage (and sometimes bone)

Restoration to normal

Destruction of joint: fibrous ankylosis

FIG. 26

Tuberculous arthritis, with possible results. When infection is purely synovial there is marked thickening of the synovial membrane but the articular cartilage is intact (note similarity to early rheumatoid arthritis). With efficient treatment begun at this stage restoration to normal is possible. But often the disease progresses to involve the articular cartilage and bone : the joint is destroyed, and fibrous ankylosis is the natural outcome.

affected are the large joints such as the hip and knee, and the symphysial joints between the vertebral bodies. The organisms reach the joint through the blood stream from a focus elsewhere. The synovial membrane is much thickened (Fig. 26) by the tuberculous inflammatory reaction which is of characteristic type, with round-cell infiltration and giant-cell systems. Unless the disease is arrested the articular cartilage is soon destroyed and the underlying bone is eroded. Sometimes the infection begins in bone adjacent to a joint rather than in the joint itself : thence it extends into the joint by direct continuity. The formation of an abscess—a ' cold ' abscess—is a common feature. The abscess often makes its way towards the skin surface and may

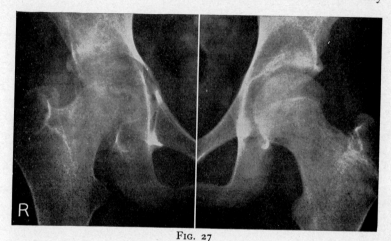

FIG. 27

Tuberculous arthritis of right hip. Note the rarefaction, loss of joint cartilage, and erosion of bone surfaces. The normal side is shown for comparison.

rupture, giving rise to a chronic tuberculous sinus. This may provide a route for the entry of secondary infecting organisms.

Healing is by fibrosis. If it occurs before the articular cartilage and bone have been damaged the function of the joint is restored virtually to normal. But if cartilage or bone is damaged before healing is secured permanent impairment—often complete loss of function—is inevitable (Fig. 26).

Clinical features. Children and young adults are most commonly affected. There is often a history of contact with a patient with active pulmonary tuberculosis. In general, the predominant symptoms are pain, swelling, and impairment of function of the affected joint. *On examination* the characteristic features are increased warmth of the overlying skin, swelling from synovial thickening, and limitation of movement in all directions. Forced movement causes sharp pain and induces protective muscle spasm. The muscles controlling the joint are usually wasted. An abscess or sinus is often apparent. A tuberculous lesion may be found elsewhere in the body. *Radiographic examination :* The earliest change in tuberculous arthritis is diffuse rarefaction throughout a fairly wide area of bone adjacent to the joint. If the disease is arrested early there may be no further change. But if the infection progresses the cartilage space is narrowed and the underlying bone is eroded (Fig. 27). As the disease heals the bones ' harden up ' again—that is, the rarefaction becomes gradually less apparent until the bone density is restored to normal. *Investigations :* The erythrocyte sedimentation rate is raised in the active stage. Its gradual decrease is an indication of healing. The Mantoux test is positive. Aspiration of the joint may yield a little turbid fluid, in which organisms can seldom be demonstrated, but its inoculation into a guinea-pig may prove its tuberculous nature. Examination of pus withdrawn from an abscess often reveals tubercle bacilli. Biopsy of thickened synovial membrane shows the typical histological features of tuberculosis.

Complications. These are : 1) sinus formation ; 2) secondary infection through a sinus track ; 3) spread of disease to another part of the body. Other complications are peculiar to special regions—for example, compression of the spinal cord by an abscess in tuberculosis of an intervertebral joint.

Course. Under favourable conditions there is a tendency towards slow healing by fibrosis. With early treatment a movable or even a normal joint is sometimes preserved, especially in children. But in many cases the joint is largely or totally destroyed.

Treatment. The principles of treatment are the same no matter which joint is affected ; variations in detail will be discussed in the sections on the individual joints. *Constitutional treatment :* This is by rest, fresh air, adequate diet, and systemic chemotherapy. It is recommended that streptomycin, para-amino-salicylic acid[1] (PAS), and isonicotinic acid hydrazide (INAH) be given together in a course of treatment extending over six months, if there is no toxic reaction. Thereafter para-amino-salicylic acid and isonico-tinic acid hydrazide, without streptomycin, may be continued for a further six to twelve months. *Local treatment :* At first the joint should be rested in a splint or plaster for three to six months,

---

[1] Given as sodium amino-salicylate.

depending on the severity of the disease. Meanwhile abscesses should be aspirated or drained surgically. The subsequent management depends upon the state of the joint and the response to treatment, which should be assessed at the end of the first six months. If at that time the articular cartilage and bone are still intact, if the general health is good and the local signs have sub-sided, and if the erythrocyte sedimentation rate has shown a steady improvement, there is a good prospect that the disease has been aborted. In that event active joint movements are encouraged and gradually increased, under supervision, until adequate function is restored.

On the other hand, if the review at the end of the first six months' treatment shows that articular cartilage or bone has been destroyed, the joint must be ' written off ' as a functional unit, and in the case of most joints a sound bony fusion should be the ultimate objective. To this end immobilisation is continued—if necessary for many months—until the disease is quiescent. Thereupon arthrodesis is undertaken if required.

OSTEOARTHRITIS
(Hypertrophic arthritis ; degenerative arthritis ; arthrosis ; osteoarthrosis ; post-traumatic arthritis)

Osteoarthritis is a degenerative wear-and-tear process occurring in joints that are impaired by congenital defect, age, vascular insufficiency, or previous disease or injury. It is by far the commonest variety of arthritis.

Cause. It is caused by wear and tear. If a joint were never put under stress it would never become osteoarthritic. Hence the relatively lightly stressed joints of the upper limb are, in general, less prone to osteoarthritis than the heavily stressed joints of the lower limb. Nearly always, however, there is a predisposing cause that accelerates the wear-and-tear process. Almost any abnormality of a joint may be responsible, indirectly, for the development of osteoarthritis—often many years later. The main predisposing factors are : 1) congenital ill-development ; 2) senility—that is, an impaired capacity for tissue repair inherent in the process of ageing ; 3) irregularity of joint surfaces from previous fracture ; 4) internal derangements, such as a loose body or a torn meniscus ; 5) previous disease, leaving a damaged articular cartilage (for example, rheumatoid arthritis or haemophilia) ; 6) mal-alignment of a joint from any cause (for example, bow-leg) ; 7) obesity and overweight.

Pathology.   Any joint may be affected, the lower limb joints more often than the upper.   The articular cartilage is slowly worn away until eventually the underlying bone is exposed (Fig. 28).   This subchondral bone becomes hard and glossy (' eburnation ').   Meanwhile the bone at the margins of the joint hypertrophies to form a rim of projecting spurs known as osteophytes.   There is no primary change in the capsule or synovial membrane, but the recurrent strains to which an osteoarthritic joint is subject often lead to slight thickening and fibrosis.

Clinical features.   Most patients with osteoarthritis are past middle age.   When it occurs in younger patients there is usually a clear predisposing cause such as previous injury or disease of the joint.   The onset is very gradual, with pain that increases almost imperceptibly over months and years. Movements slowly become more and more restricted. In some joints (notably the hip) deformity is a common feature in the later stages.   *On examination* slight thickening is often found on palpation ; it is mainly a bony thickening caused by the marginal osteophytes.   There is no increased warmth.   Movements are impaired slightly or markedly according to the degree of arthritis ; in most joints move-

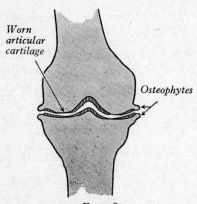

Worn articular cartilage

Osteophytes

FIG. 28

Osteoarthritis.   The main changes are in the articular cartilage and underlying bone.   The cartilage is gradually worn away, disappearing first at the points of greatest pressure.   The subchondral bone becomes sclerotic, and at the joint margins it hypertrophies to form osteophytes.

ment is accompanied by palpable or audible crepitation of a rather coarse type.   Fixed deformity (that is, inability of the joint to assume the neutral anatomical position) is often found in the hip, and sometimes in other joints.

Radiographic examination : The characteristic features of osteo-arthritis are : 1) diminution of cartilage space ; 2) subchondral sclerosis ; and 3) spurring or ' lipping ' of the joint margins from the formation of osteophytes (Fig. 29).

Diagnosis. This is usually made clear by the history, clinical findings, and radiographic features. Osteoarthritis is not easily confused with inflammatory forms of arthritis, because there is no synovial thickening, no increased local warmth, and no muscle

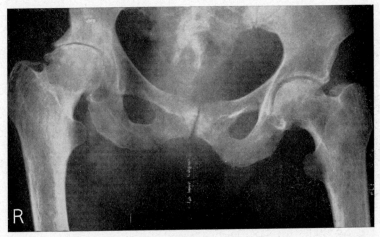

FIG. 29

Osteoarthritis of the right hip, with the sound hip shown for comparison. Note the narrowing of the cartilage space, the subchondral sclerosis, and the marginal osteophytes. Note also the adduction deformity : this is a common feature.

spasm ; radiographs show sclerosis rather than rarefaction, and the erythrocyte sedimentation rate is not increased.

Course. Osteoarthritis usually increases slowly year by year. In many cases the disability never reaches the stage at which treatment is required. In others increasing pain, stiffness, or deformity drives the patient to demand measures for its relief.

Treatment. The management of osteoarthritis exemplifies well the three categories of treatment that should be considered in every orthopaedic problem—namely, 1) no treatment ; 2) conservative treatment ; and 3) operative treatment (p. 17).

In many cases treatment is not required. The patient may have sought advice only because of anxiety lest some grave disease be present. Reassurance, with advice to restrict the wear and tear on the affected joint, is all that is required.

3

When more active treatment is called for, conservative measures should usually be tried first. The methods available include physiotherapy (local heat and muscle-strengthening exercises), analgesic drugs such as phenylbutazone or indomethacin, local injections of hydrocortisone, and supportive bandages or appliances.

When severe disability is unrelieved by conservative treatment operation may be justified. Chief among the operations available are arthroplasty (the construction of a new joint) (p. 28) and arthrodesis (elimination of the joint by fusion of the bone ends) (p. 26). Arthroplasty is applicable only to a few joints, particularly the hip, elbow, certain joints of the hand, and the metatarso-phalangeal joints. For most other joints arthrodesis is the operation of choice. Further details of treatment will be given in the sections on individual joints.

GOUTY ARTHRITIS

(Podagra ; urate crystal synovitis)

Gout is the clinical manifestation of a disturbed purine metabolism. It is characterised by deposition of uric-acid salts—especially sodium biurate—in connective tissues such as cartilage (of joints, or of the ear), the walls of bursae, and ligaments.

Cause. The precise cause of the disturbance of metabolism is unknown. There is an inherited predisposition to the disease. In susceptible persons an attack may be induced by excessive consumption of beer or heavy wines, or by recent injury or operation.

Pathology. The primary fault is an impaired excretion of uric acid by the kidneys. In consequence the level of uric acid in the blood is increased, sometimes to 6 mg. per 100 ml. or more (normal=3·5 mg. per 100 ml. by Folin method). In the blood the uric acid is in solution in a loose combination with proteins ; it readily comes out of solution as a sodium salt (sodium biurate) to be deposited in the form of crystals in certain connective tissues, especially those that have been injured or those that have a sluggish blood supply, such as the articular cartilage of the joints of the foot. The deposited crystals set up an inflammatory reaction. In acute gout the deposit is microscopic in amount and is soon reabsorbed, with restoration of the tissue to normal. In chronic gout, however, widespread deposits of sodium biurate in joint cartilages, ligaments, and the articular ends of bones lead to considerable disorganisation of the joint. Gouty deposits (tophi) are also common at other sites, notably in the olecranon bursa and in the cartilage of the ear.

Clinical features. The patient is nearly always over 40, and more often a man than a woman. The chief clinical manifestations are arthritis and bursitis. *Arthritis :* Gout affects principally the peripheral joints such as the joints of the toes, tarsus, and ankle, and the small joints of the hands. It occurs in recurrent attacks. The first attack is usually in the great toe ; later attacks may affect other joints. In an acute attack the onset is sudden—often during the night. The affected joint is swollen, red, shiny, and very painful. Movements are greatly restricted because of the pain. The attack subsides after a few days and the joint is normal between attacks. In chronic gout several joints are affected together. They are thickened and nodular, and painful on movement. *Bursitis :* The bursa most commonly affected by gout is the olecranon bursa. It becomes distended with fluid, and there may be palpable deposits of uric acid salts. *Other manifestations :* Deposits of uric acid salts (tophi) are common in the ear cartilages. They may also occur at other sites. *Radiographic examination :* In acute attacks of articular gout the joints show no radiographic abnormality. In chronic gout the deposits of uric acid salts in the bone ends show as clear-cut erosions adjacent to the joint, for the deposits are transradiant. *Investigations:* There is sometimes a mild leucocytosis and the erythrocyte sedimentation rate may be increased. The blood uric acid content is raised. Aspiration of swollen joints may yield a small quantity of turbid fluid, but never organisms. Polarised light microscopy of synovial fluid usually reveals birefringent crystals.

Diagnosis. Acute gout has to be distinguished from other forms of arthritis of sudden onset, especially from acute pyogenic arthritis, haemophilic arthritis, and rheumatic fever. Features suggestive of gout are : a history of previous attacks, with symptom-free intervals ; a raised blood uric acid content ; the presence of tophi in the ears or elsewhere; detection of crystals in synovial fluid; and a favourable response to treatment. Chronic gout involving several joints may simulate rheumatoid arthritis.

Course. Gout usually occurs in recurrent attacks. Early attacks subside in a few days, leaving the joint clinically normal. In chronic gout the affected joints are gradually disorganised and permanent disability is inevitable.

Treatment. For acute attacks a reliable remedy is phenylbutazone, given in high doses for the first few days and then in reduced doses. Colchicine is also effective. The affected joint should be rested until the attack has subsided. For patients with frequent attacks or with chronic gout, especially if the plasma urate level is persistently very high, long-term drug therapy to reduce the plasma urate level may be required. The two types of drug available are represented by 1) probenemid, which paralyses renal tubular reabsorption of urates and thus increases their excretion in the urine; and 2) allopurinol, which reduces the formation of uric acid by inhibiting the enzyme xanthine oxydase. Provided its long-term use is not associated with toxic reactions, allopurinol is probably to be preferred because it does not increase the load of urate in the urine, with its hazard of stone formation.

OTHER FORMS OF CRYSTAL SYNOVITIS

With the general acceptance of the idea that joint manifestations in gout are caused by the presence of urate crystals, it has recently come to be appreciated that similar manifestations may be induced by the crystals of other salts. In most such cases the crystals are composed of calcium pyrophosphate, and characteristically calcification of articular cartilage or of menisci is demonstrable radiologically. Arthritis of this type, due to crystals other than urate crystals, has been termed ' pseudogout '. It seems better, however, to include it under the general term ' crystal synovitis,' which embraces also the joint manifestations of classical gout. Treatment should be by rest, aspiration of joint fluid, and phenylbutazone.

HAEMOPHILIC ARTHRITIS

Joint manifestations are common in haemophilia, but examples are seen only infrequently because haemophilia is itself an uncommon disease.

Pathology. The term ' haemophilia ' is used loosely to embrace a group of different defects in the process of coagulation of the blood. Classical haemophilia, the commonest of the group, occurs only in males but is transmitted by females. There is a deficiency of a specific clotting factor known as antihaemophilic factor (factor VIII). In consequence the clotting time of the blood is prolonged and there is a tendency to undue bleeding when even quite small vessels are cut or torn. Joint manifestations are caused by haemorrhage into a joint, occurring after a minor strain or even without any known injury. The joints most commonly affected are those most vulnerable to strain—especially the knee, elbow, and ankle. The joint cavity is distended with blood (haemarthrosis), which is later slowly reabsorbed if the joint is rested. Recurrent haemarthroses lead eventually to degenerative change in the articular cartilage and to fibrosis of the synovial membrane.

Clinical features. The boy is often a known sufferer from haemophilia or can recall previous episodes of bleeding. He suddenly finds that a joint has become painful and swollen. *On examination* the findings vary according to the phase and duration of the arthritis. In the absence of specific treatment the joint remains swollen for several weeks after the acute onset—partly from effused blood and partly from the synovial thickening that results from interstitial extravasation. The overlying skin is abnormally warm. Joint movements are restricted and very painful. In the quiescent phase between attacks of haemarthrosis there is moderate thickening of the joint from synovial fibrosis, movements are slightly impaired, and often there is some degree of fixed deformity.

Diagnosis. Because of the synovial thickening, increased warmth of the skin, and restriction of joint movements, haemophilic arthritis is easily mistaken for acute or chronic inflammatory arthritis. The history of previous episodes of bleeding, the sudden onset, and the recurrent nature of the attacks are important diagnostic features ; and the prolonged clotting time of the blood is confirmatory evidence.

Treatment. When the necessary facilities are available, the correct treatment for a recent acute incident is to promote coagulability of the blood by the administration of concentrated antihaemophilic factor in the form of cryoprecipitate, and then to treat the joint as for ordinary traumatic haemarthrosis by aspiration and firm bandaging. Failing adequate supplies of antihaemophilic factor, resort must be had to firm bandaging and prolonged splintage. In the chronic degenerative phase that follows repeated haemarthroses it is often necessary to give permanent support to the joint by means of a moulded plastic splint or other appliance. Operation must be avoided whenever possible.

NEUROPATHIC ARTHRITIS
(Charcot's osteoarthropathy)

In neuropathic arthritis a joint is disorganised by repeated minor injuries because it is insensitive to pain.

Cause. The underlying cause is a neurological disorder interfering with the deep pain impulses. In patients with involvement of joints of the lower limb the commonest causes are tabes dorsalis, diabetic neuropathy, cauda equina lesion, and in some countries leprosy. In those with upper limb involvement the usual cause is syringomyelia.

Pathology. Any of the large joints may be affected, including the joints of the spine. The knee, ankle and subtalar joint are most commonly affected in the lower limb, and the elbow in the upper limb. In a normal joint harmful strains are prevented by a protective reflex whereby muscle contraction is evoked by incipient pain. When joint sensibility is destroyed the protective function of pain is lost. Strains are unrecognised and, cumulatively, they lead to severe degeneration of the joint. The changes may be regarded as a much exaggerated form of osteoarthritis. The articular cartilage is worn away, but at the same time there is sometimes massive hypertrophy of bone at the joint margins. The ligaments become lax and the joint is unstable. Indeed it is often subluxated or even dislocated.

Clinical features. The patient is usually in adult life. The main symptoms are swelling and instability of the affected joint. Since the joint is insensitive pain is slight or absent. *On examination* the joint is thickened, mostly from irregular hypertrophy of the bone ends. The range of movement is moderately restricted, and there is marked lateral laxity. In extreme cases the joint may be dislocated. Further examination will reveal evidence of the underlying neurological disorder. *Radiographs* show severe disorganisation of the joint. The changes are basically those of osteoarthritis, but enormously exaggerated. There are loss of cartilage space and some absorption of the bone ends, often with considerable hypertrophy of bone at the joint margins (Fig. 172, p. 257, and Fig. 270, p. 373).

Treatment. In most instances the best treatment is simply to provide support for the joint by a suitable appliance. Sometimes operation may be undertaken to fuse the joint. The primary neurological disorder will usually demand appropriate treatment.

ARTHRITIS OF RHEUMATIC FEVER

In adolescent children and young adults arthritic manifestations are a prominent feature of rheumatic fever.

Cause. Rheumatic fever is ascribed to a sensitivity reaction associated with infection by a haemolytic streptococcus. There may be an inherited predisposition to the disease.

Pathology. Any joint may be affected. The synovial membrane is acutely inflamed, but there is no suppuration. Clear fluid is effused into the joint.

Clinical features. The patient is usually a child over 10, or a young adult. There is constitutional illness, with malaise and pyrexia. A joint becomes painful and swollen, and soon afterwards other joints are likewise affected. *On examination* an affected joint is swollen, partly from contained fluid and partly from synovial thickening. The overlying skin is warmer than normal. Movements are markedly restricted, and painful if forced. Other features of rheumatic fever, such as carditis and chorea, should be looked for. *Radiographs* of affected joints do not show any alteration from the normal. *Investigations:* There is a mild leucocytosis. The erythrocyte sedimentation rate is increased.

Diagnosis. Arthritis of rheumatic fever has to be distinguished from other forms of arthritis—especially from acute pyogenic arthritis, rheumatoid arthritis, gout, and haemophilic arthritis—and from acute osteomyelitis. Features suggestive of rheumatic fever are : onset in adolescence ; affection of several joints together or in succession ; severe pain with signs of acute inflammation, but without suppuration ; a mild rather than a marked leucocytosis ; and a rapid favourable response to salicylates.

Treatment. For joint involvement alone salicylates are adequate, but prednisone or a related steroid may be required if the heart is affected. A therapeutic course of penicillin should also be given to eliminate streptococci, and thereafter twice-daily oral penicillin should be continued well into adult life to reduce the risk of recurrent attacks.

ANKYLOSING SPONDYLITIS
(Spondylitis ankylopoietica; Marie-Strümpell arthritis)

As the name implies, ankylosing spondylitis is primarily a disease of the spine, though in a few cases the arthritic changes involve also the proximal joints of the limbs, especially the hips.

Briefly, it is a chronic inflammatory affection of the joints and ligaments of the spine, beginning in the sacro-iliac joints. It progresses slowly, the changes gradually creeping up the spinal column from below. The natural outcome is bony ankylosis of the affected joints, but the disease may be arrested at any stage short of this.

Typically, ankylosing spondylitis affects men in early adult life. After remaining active for several years it ' burns itself out,' always leaving some degree of permanent stiffness of the spine. A fuller description is given in Chapter IV (p. 195).

DISLOCATION AND SUBLUXATION OF JOINTS

A joint is dislocated or luxated when its articular surfaces are wholly displaced one from the other, so that all apposition between them is lost. A joint is subluxated when its surfaces are partly displaced but retain some contact one with the other (Fig. 30).

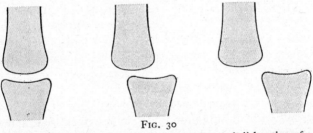

FIG. 30

To show the difference between subluxation and dislocation of a joint. *Left*—The normal state : joint surfaces congruous. *Middle*—Subluxation : incomplete loss of contact between the joint surfaces. *Right*—Dislocation : total loss of contact between the joint surfaces.

Dislocation or subluxation may be congenital, spontaneous, traumatic, or recurrent.

CONGENITAL DISLOCATION OR SUBLUXATION

The most important representative of this group is congenital dislocation of the hip (p. 321). Congenital club foot (talipes equino-varus) (p. 409) may be regarded as congenital subluxation of the talo-navicular joint. Congenital displacement of other joints is rare.

SPONTANEOUS (PATHOLOGICAL) DISLOCATION OR SUBLUXATION

Displacement may occur spontaneously at any joint in consequence of a structural defect or of destructive disease. It is encountered frequently in the spine, where the stability of the intervertebral joints may be impaired by structural defects, by previous injury, or by destructive arthritis (spondylolisthesis, pp. 168 and 209). It is common for a phalanx to become dislocated dorsally at the metatarso-phalangeal joint in cases of severe clawing of the toes. Another example is the dislocation of the hip that sometimes complicates severe tuberculous arthritis or pyogenic arthritis. Subluxation or dislocation is also a common feature of neuropathic arthritis (p. 62).

TRAUMATIC DISLOCATION OR SUBLUXATION

Injury is by far the commonest cause of dislocations. Traumatic dislocations are described in textbooks of fractures and joint injuries, and they will not be considered further here.

RECURRENT DISLOCATION OR SUBLUXATION

Certain joints are liable to repeated dislocation or subluxation. Usually, but not always, there has been an initial violent dislocation which causes permanent damage to the ligaments or articular surfaces. The joints most often affected are the shoulder (p. 230), the patello-femoral joint (p. 383), and the ankle (p. 407).

INTERNAL DERANGEMENTS OF JOINTS

The term internal derangement implies a localised mechanical fault which interferes with the smooth action of a joint. An internal derangement is distinct from arthritis, which is nearly always a diffuse lesion involving the joint as a whole.

Internal derangements will be considered in three groups : 1) interposition of soft tissue ; 2) loose body formation ; and 3) osteochondritis dissecans.

INTERPOSITION OF SOFT TISSUE IN JOINTS

The smooth action of a joint may be obstructed by a displaced mass of soft tissue within it. The soft tissue most often responsible is an intra-articular fibrocartilage, especially a meniscus in the

3*

knee (p. 374). As a rule a fibrocartilage can be displaced only when it is torn. Other soft tissues that are occasionally interposed are synovial fringes and ligamentous tags.

Clinical features. Disorders of this type are common only in the knee. The characteristic features are recurrent sudden ' locking ' or giving way of the joint, with later an effusion of clear fluid within it.

LOOSE BODIES IN JOINTS

Intra-articular loose bodies may be derived from bone, cartilage, or synovial membrane. They may be entirely free within the joint or they may retain a pedicle of soft tissue.

Causes. The commonest causes of loose bodies are : 1) osteochondritis dissecans (one to three loose bodies) ; 2) osteoarthritis (one to ten loose bodies) ; 3) chip fracture of the articular end of a bone (one to three loose bodies) ; and 4) synovial chondromatosis (fifty to five hundred loose bodies).

Pathology. *Osteochondritis dissecans* (p. 67) : The loose body is derived from a part of the articular surface that undergoes necrosis and separates. *Osteoarthritis :* The bodies may be derived from marginal osteophytes, in which case they often retain firm soft-tissue attachments and may cause little trouble. Free bodies may be derived from shed flakes of articular cartilage. *Fracture of articular margin :* Fractures only occasionally cause intra-articular loose bodies. A well recognised example is a fractured medial epicondyle which may be sucked into the elbow joint while still retaining its muscle attachments. *Synovial chondromatosis* (osteochondromatosis) : This is a rare disease of synovial membrane. A large number of villous folds become pedunculated and their bulbous extremities undergo metaplasia to cartilage. Eventually they separate from their pedicles to become free mobile bodies, and many of them become calcified. The disease may affect any joint.

Clinical features. Loose bodies do not necessarily cause symptoms unless they become jammed between the joint surfaces. The characteristic feature is sudden and usually momentary locking of the joint, succeeded by an effusion of clear fluid within it.

Treatment. When a loose body causes trouble it should be removed.

OSTEOCHONDRITIS DISSECANS

Osteochondritis dissecans is a localised disorder of convex joint surfaces in which a segment of subchondral bone becomes avascular and, with the articular cartilage that covers it, may slowly separate from the surrounding bone to form a loose body.

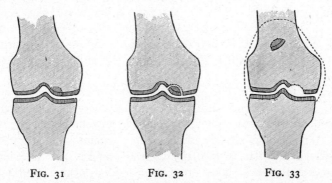

FIG. 31   FIG. 32   FIG. 33

Evolution of osteochondritis dissecans. Figure 31—Segment of articular surface deprived of blood supply. Figure 32—A line of demarcation has formed and the avascular fragment is separating from the surrounding healthy bone. Figure 33—Fragment loose in joint. A cavity remains in the articular surface.

Common sites. The only joints commonly affected are the knee and the elbow. In the knee the site of the lesion is nearly always the medial femoral condyle, and in the elbow, the capitulum of the humerus. Occasionally the hip joint (femoral head) and the ankle joint (talus) are affected.[1]

Cause. The precise cause is unknown. Impairment of blood supply to the affected segment of bone and cartilage—possibly by thrombosis of an end-artery—has been suggested. The significance of injury is uncertain. There is probably an inborn susceptibility to the disease, for it may occur in several joints of the same patient, or in several members of a family.

Pathology. A segment of the articular surface of a bone becomes avascular (Fig. 31), and a line of demarcation slowly forms between

---

[1] The disorder of the metatarsal head known as Freiberg's disease (p. 441) is thought by some to be an example of osteochondritis dissecans and by others to represent osteochondritis juvenilis. It shows some features common to both conditions.

the avascular segment and the surrounding normal bone (Fig. 32). The affected segment varies in size : in the knee it often measures about one to three centimetres in diameter and half a centimetre in depth. It is always on the convex joint surface. If the segment is small it is sometimes re-attached spontaneously, especially in adolescents ; but in most cases it finally separates to form a loose body in the joint, still covered by its articular cartilage (Fig. 33). The resulting cavity in the articular surface of the bone fills with fibrous tissue, but there is inevitably some irregularity of the joint surface which predisposes to the later development of osteoarthritis.

Clinical features.   The patient is an adolescent or a young adult. The early symptoms and signs are those of a mild mechanical irritation of the joint—namely a tendency to aching after use, with recurrent effusion of clear fluid. After separation of a fragment from the articular surface the clinical features are those of an intra-articular loose body—recurrent sudden locking of the joint accompanied by sharp pain and followed by effusion. *Radiographs* show a clearly defined shallow excavation into the articular surface of the bone, with a discrete bone fragment lying either within the cavity or elsewhere in the joint.

Treatment.   Until a loose body has separated or appears ' ripe ' for separation treatment should be expectant. In the case of a small lesion rest in plaster for two months may help to allow spontaneous re-attachment of the fragment. When a fragment has separated it should usually be removed. Further details will be found in the appropriate sections on the knee (p. 379), the elbow (p. 258), and the foot (p. 441).

INFECTIONS OF BONE

Infection of bone by pyogenic organisms is termed osteomyelitis.[1] It occurs in acute and chronic forms. The only other infections of bone with which the student in Western countries need concern himself are tuberculous infection and syphilitic infection.

---

[1] There is nothing to be gained by distinguishing between *osteitis* (inflammation of bone) and *osteomyelitis* (inflammation of bone and bone marrow). For practical purposes the two terms may be regarded as synonymous.

ACUTE OSTEOMYELITIS
(Acute pyogenic infection of bone; acute osteitis)

Acute osteomyelitis is one of the important diseases of childhood ; it may also occur in adults. Early diagnosis is especially important because a satisfactory outcome depends to a great extent upon prompt and efficient treatment.

Cause. It is caused by infection of the bone with pyogenic organisms—usually the staphylococcus, less commonly the streptococcus or pneumococcus. A minor injury to a bone renders it vulnerable to infection by organisms circulating in the blood.

Pathology. The organisms usually reach the bone through the blood stream from a septic focus elsewhere in the body (haematogenous osteomyelitis). Less commonly they are introduced from outside, through the wound of an open fracture.

Haematogenous osteomyelitis. In the usual haematogenous type the infection begins in the metaphysis of a long bone (Fig. 34) ; thence it may spread to involve a large part of the bone. The organisms induce an acute inflammatory reaction, but the marshalling of the body's defensive forces is greatly handicapped in bone because its rigid structure does not allow of swelling. Pus is formed and soon finds its way to the surface of the bone where it forms a subperiosteal abscess (Fig. 35) ; later the abscess may burst into the soft tissues.

Often the blood supply to a part of the bone is cut off by septic thrombosis of the vessels (Fig. 35). The ischaemic bone dies and eventually separates from the surrounding living bone as a sequestrum (Fig. 36). Meanwhile new bone is laid down beneath the stripped-up periosteum, forming an investing layer known as the involucrum (Fig. 36).

The epiphysial cartilage plate is a barrier to the spread of infection, but if the affected metaphysis lies partly within a joint cavity the joint is liable to become infected (acute pyogenic arthritis). Metaphyses that lie wholly or partly within a joint cavity include the upper metaphysis of the humerus, all the metaphyses at the elbow, and the upper and lower metaphyses of the femur (Fig. 37). Even when the joint is not infected it may swell from an effusion of clear fluid (sympathetic effusion).

With efficient treatment, the infection may be aborted in its earliest phase. But when it has progressed to the stage of septic thrombosis and death of bone it almost inevitably passes into a state of chronic osteomyelitis.

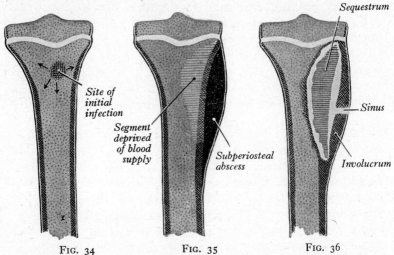

FIG. 34   FIG. 35   FIG. 36

The natural evolution of a focus of osteomyelitis. Figure 34—Initial lesion in the metaphysis. Figure 35—Pus has escaped to the surface of the bone and formed a subperiosteal abscess. Part of the bone has lost its blood supply from septic thrombosis of vessels. Figure 36—The devitalised area eventually separates as a sequestrum. Meanwhile new bone (involucrum) is formed beneath the stripped-up periosteum ; it is perforated by sinuses through which pus escapes. This is the stage of chronic osteomyelitis. With prompt treatment the disease can often be arrested at the stage shown in Figure 34.

Osteomyelitis complicating open fracture. The organisms are introduced directly through the wound. Any part of the bone may be affected, depending upon the site of injury. Suppuration and necrosis occur as in haematogenous osteomyelitis, but the pus discharges through the primary wound rather than collecting under the periosteum. The infection often becomes chronic.

Clinical features. The haematogenous type of osteomyelitis usually occurs in children, especially boys. The bones most commonly affected are the tibia, the femur and the humerus. The onset is rapid. The child complains of feeling ill, and of pain over the affected bone. There may be a history of recent boils or of a minor injury.

On examination there is obvious constitutional illness with pyrexia. Locally there is exquisite tenderness over the affected bone. The area of tenderness is clearly circumscribed ; it is usually near the end of the bone in the metaphysial region. The overlying skin is warmer than normal, and often the soft tissues are indurated; later a fluctuant abscess may be present. The neighbouring joint is often distended with clear fluid, but a good range of movement is retained. (In the event of associated septic arthritis movement would be greatly restricted.) *Radiographic examination :* In the early stages the radiographs do not show any alteration from the normal (Fig. 39). Only after two or three weeks do visible changes appear, and they may never do so if efficient treatment is started very early. The important changes are diffuse rarefaction of the metaphysial area, and new bone outlining the raised periosteum (Figs. 38 and 40). *Investigations :* Blood culture is sometimes positive in the incipient stage. There is a marked polymorphonuclear leucocytosis. The erythrocyte sedimentation rate is increased.

In osteomyelitis complicating an open fracture the temperature fails to settle after the primary treatment of the wound or rises a few days later. Pain is not a prominent feature. Re-examination of the wound reveals a purulent discharge.

Diagnosis. Acute osteomyelitis is to be distinguished from pyogenic arthritis of the adjacent joint by the following features : 1) the point of greatest tenderness is over the bone rather than the joint ; 2) a good range

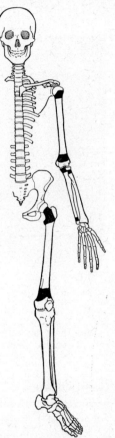

FIG. 37

The metaphyses shown in black are wholly or partly intracapsular. Infection at one of these sites is liable to involve the adjacent joint.

of joint movement is retained ; and 3) although the joint may be distended with fluid it does not contain pus (this may be confirmed by aspiration). Acute osteomyelitis may also be confused with poliomyelitis (which in the early stages is associated with limb pain), with rheumatic fever, and, in infants, with scurvy (p. 115) or syphilitic metaphysitis (p. 79). Whenever possible the causative organism must be identified bacteriologically.

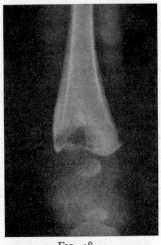

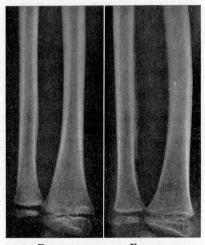

| FIG. 38 | FIG. 39 | FIG. 40 |

Acute osteomyelitis of the femur in an infant, three weeks after onset. Note new bone outlining the raised periosteum and area of rarefaction in lower metaphysis and epiphysis. The infection spread to the knee joint.

Acute osteomyelitis of the ulna in a child. The initial film taken two days after the onset (Fig. 39) shows no abnormality. Two weeks later (Fig. 40) a faint shadow along the radial side of the ulna denotes new bone formation beneath the raised periosteum.

Complications. The important complications are : 1) septicaemia or pyaemia ; 2) extension of infection to the adjacent joint with consequent pyogenic arthritis (Fig. 41) ; and 3) retardation of growth from damage to the epiphysial cartilage (Fig. 42). Acute osteomyelitis often passes into a state of chronic infection.

Treatment. *Haematogenous osteomyelitis.* Efficient treatment must be begun at the earliest possible moment. *General treatment :* This is by rest in bed and systemic antibiotic therapy. Initially, reliance must be placed upon a ' broad spectrum ' antibiotic or a combination of two bactericidal antibiotics such as ampicillin and cloxacillin, but as soon as the causative organism has been identified the antibiotic to which it is most sensitive should be ordered. Antibiotics should be continued for at least four weeks, even when the response has been rapid. *Local treatment:* The question of operation and its timing is still controversial. Operation may be unnecessary if effective antibiotic treatment can be

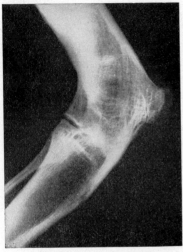

FIG. 41

Two complications of osteomyelitis. Figure 41—Pyogenic arthritis, which led in this case to bony ankylosis. Figure 42—Arrest of epiphysial growth, with consequent shortening. The normal arm is shown for comparison.

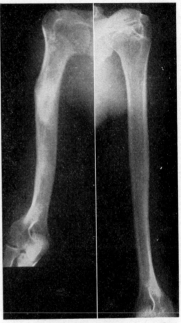

FIG. 42

begun within twenty-four hours of the onset of symptoms. But in practice it seems wiser to undertake immediate operation, in order to release pus under tension and thus to minimise the risk of bone necrosis from interference with its blood supply. Operation also facilitates identification of the organism, and determination by sensitivity tests of the most appropriate antibiotic. An incision is made down to the bone and subperiosteal pus is evacuated. It is advisable—though not always essential—to make one or two drill holes in the bone to improve drainage. In most cases the wound may safely be sutured. Thereafter the limb is splinted until the infection is overcome.

Osteomyelitis complicating open fracture. The main principle of treatment is to secure free drainage through the wound, which may be enlarged if necessary for the purpose. Appropriate antibiotic drugs should be ordered. Later, any bone fragments that have sequestrated should be removed.

CHRONIC OSTEOMYELITIS
(Chronic pyogenic osteomyelitis)

Chronic osteomyelitis is nearly always a sequel to acute osteomyelitis. Occasionally infection is subacute or chronic from the beginning.

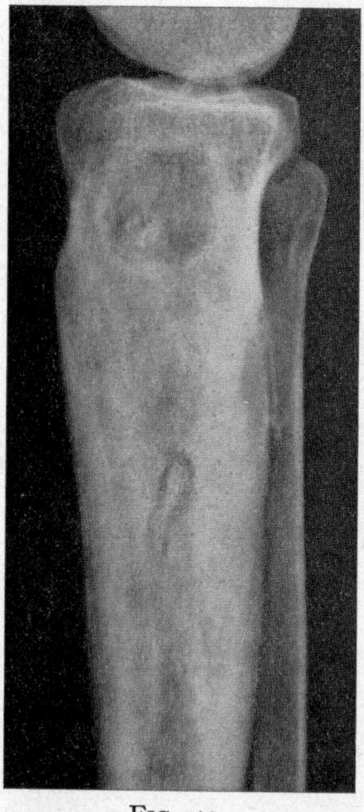

FIG. 43

Extensive chronic osteomyelitis of the tibia. The upper part of the shaft is thickened and shows patchy sclerosis. Two cavities are evident, each containing a sequestrum.

Cause. As with acute osteomyelitis, the staphylococcus is the usual causative organism, but streptococci, pneumococci, typhoid bacilli, or other bacteria may be responsible.

Pathology. It is commonest in the long bones. It is often confined to one end of the bone, but it may affect the whole length. The bone is thickened and generally denser than normal, though often honeycombed with granulation tissue, fibrous tissue or pus. Sequestra are commonly present within cavities in the bone. Often a sinus track leads to the skin surface : the sinus tends to heal and break down recurrently, but if a sequestrum is present it never heals permanently.

Clinical features. The main symptom is usually a purulent discharge from a sinus over the affected bone. In other cases pain is the predominant feature which brings the patient to the doctor. Discharge of pus may be continuous or intermittent. Reappearance of a sinus that has been healed for some time is heralded by local pain, pyrexia, and the formation of an abscess. This is termed a ' flare-up,' or ' flare,' of infection. *On examination* the bone is palpably thickened, and there are nearly always a number of overlying scars or sinuses. *Radiographic examination :* The bone is thickened and shows irregular and patchy sclerosis which may give a honeycombed appearance. If a sequestrum is present it is seen as a dense loose fragment, with irregular but sharply demarcated edges, lying within a cavity in the bone (Fig. 43).

Complications. Rarely, amyloid disease may complicate long-continued chronic osteomyelitis with persistent discharge of pus.

Treatment. An acute flare-up of chronic osteomyelitis often subsides with rest and antibiotics. If an abscess forms outside the bone it must be drained. If there is a persistent and profuse discharge of pus a more extensive operation is advised. The aim should be to remove fragments of infected dead bone (sequestra) and to open up abscess cavities by chiselling away the overlying bone. Sometimes it is possible to obliterate a cavity with a flap of muscle, or to exteriorise it and line its walls directly with split-skin grafts.

BRODIE'S ABSCESS (Chronic bone abscess)

This is a special form of chronic osteomyelitis which arises insidiously, without a preceding acute attack. There is a localised abscess within the bone, often near the site of the metaphysis. A deep ' boring ' pain is the predominant symptom. *Radiographically*, the lesion is seen as a circular or oval cavity surrounded by a zone of sclerosis (Fig. 44). The rest of the bone is normal. *Treatment* is by operation. The cavity is de-roofed and the pus evacuated. Whenever possible the cavity should be filled with a muscle flap to obliterate the dead space.

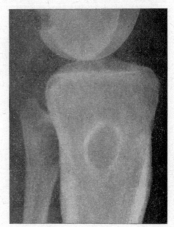

FIG. 44

Brodie's abscess. The cavity in the tibia is surrounded by a zone of sclerosis.

FIG. 44

TUBERCULOUS INFECTION OF BONE

Tuberculous infection of bone is uncommon except in the vertebral bodies and in association with tuberculous infection of joints. Occasionally it occurs as an isolated lesion of a long bone or of a bone of the hand or foot.

Pathology. Tubercle bacilli reach the bone either through the blood stream or by direct extension from an adjacent focus in joint or soft tissue. There is a typical tuberculous inflammatory reaction. Part of the bone is destroyed and replaced by granulation tissue. A tuberculous abscess is commonly formed ; it tracks beneath the soft tissues or towards the surface of the body. With treatment there is a tendency to healing, with fibrosis.

Tuberculosis of a vertebra. The infection typically affects the vertebral body. It may arise initially in the bone (Fig. 45) or it may spread to the vertebra from the adjacent intervertebral disc. Tuberculous vertebral bodies collapse anteriorly but retain their full depth behind, thereby becoming wedge-shaped (Fig. 46). An abscess usually tracks downwards along the vertebral column ; it may also extend backwards to the spinal canal, where it may interfere with the spinal cord.

Juxta-articular tuberculosis. The articular ends of bones are frequently eroded by tuberculosis beginning primarily in the joint. Less often there is an isolated focus of infection within the bone (Fig. 47). From such a lesion the infection may spread eventually to the neighbouring joint.

Bony tuberculosis in the hand or foot. The metacarpals or phalanges are the bones most commonly affected (tuberculous dactylitis). Characteristically the bone is enlarged by a fusiform swelling which at first represents thickened and raised periosteum. Later, much of the original bone is destroyed, but at the same time new bone is laid down beneath the expanded periosteum, giving the affected metacarpal or phalanx a ' distended ' appearance (Fig. 48). Similar changes may affect the bones of the feet, or occasionally a long bone.

Clinical features. There is usually evidence of constitutional ill health. The symptoms and signs depend upon the site of the infection. In general, pain is the initial symptom ; and at most sites it is associated with obvious swelling and often with the formation of a ' cold ' abscess. When the bone lesion is associated

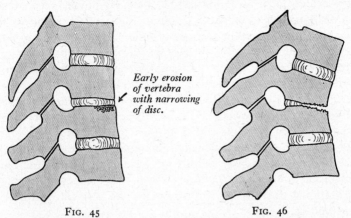

*Early erosion
of vertebra
with narrowing
of disc.*

FIG. 45   FIG. 46

Tuberculosis beginning in a vertebral body. The infection starts
close to the anterior border and adjacent to an intervertebral disc
(Fig. 45). It soon involves the disc and may spread to adjoining
vertebrae. The bone destruction is most marked anteriorly; so the
affected vertebral bodies become wedge-shaped (Fig. 46).

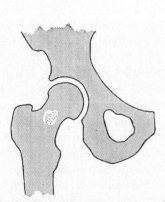

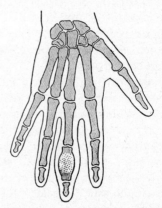

FIG. 47   FIG. 48

Juxta-articular tuberculous
focus in the neck of the femur.
There is no sclerosis of the
surrounding bone. If un-
checked by treatment, such a
focus of infection may spread
eventually to involve the joint.

Tuberculous dactylitis. The
affected phalanx has been ' distended ' by destruction of the
original cortex and the
laying down of new cortical
bone beneath the expanded
periosteum.

with tuberculous joint disease the joint symptoms predominate (see sections on the individual joints). *Radiographic examination :* The typical radiographic features of tuberculous infection of bone are : 1) diffuse rarefaction around the site of infection ; 2) erosion or ' eating away ' of bone, leaving a fluffy, ill-defined outline with no suggestion of a surrounding zone of sclerosis ; and 3) in many cases a shadow in the soft tissues, denoting abscess formation. *Investigations :* The erythrocyte sedimentation rate is raised. The Mantoux test is positive. Aspirated pus is yellow and creamy : only occasionally can organisms be identified by direct examination, but culture or guinea-pig inoculation may prove its tuberculous nature. Biopsy of affected bone or surrounding soft tissue will show the histological features of tuberculosis.

Diagnosis. The diagnosis can often be presumed with fair certainty from a consideration of the history, clinical features, and radiographic findings. Features that lend support are a history of contact with tuberculosis, a positive Mantoux test (particularly in children), a raised erythrocyte sedimentation rate, and evidence of a tuberculous lesion elsewhere. The diagnosis can be proved only by identifying the causative organism or by demonstration of the typical histological features in excised fragments of tissue.

Treatment. In most instances tuberculosis of bone is associated with infection of a joint, and the treatment is mainly that of the joint lesion (tuberculous arthritis, p. 51). The treatment of an isolated tuberculous focus in bone is along similar lines. *Constitutional treatment :* This consists of rest in good surroundings, adequate diet, and systemic chemotherapy. The recommended programme of chemotherapy is to give streptomycin, para-amino-salicylic acid (PAS), and isonicotinic acid hydrazide (INAH) together in standard doses for a six months' course, provided no toxic reaction occurs. Thereafter para-amino-salicylic acid and isonicotinic acid hydrazide, without streptomycin, may be continued for a further six to twelve months. *Local treatment :* The principles are to provide prolonged rest or immobilisation for the affected part, and to remove collections of pus by aspiration or, sometimes, by operative drainage followed by immediate suture of the wound. Rest is continued until the disease becomes quiescent, as judged from improvement in the general health and weight, decrease of erythrocyte sedimentation rate, and improved radiographic appearance.

SYPHILITIC INFECTION OF BONE

In Western countries syphilitic infection of bone is uncommon. But it is still common in some parts of the world, and it is important that the possibility of its occurrence should be borne constantly in mind. Bone changes are a late manifestation of acquired syphilis, but they may appear early in life in patients with congenital syphilis. Syphilis of bone can take many forms. Only two will be described here: 1) syphilitic metaphysitis of infants; and 2) osteo-periostitis (combined osteitis and periostitis) in children or adults.

SYPHILITIC METAPHYSITIS

This is an affection of young infants with congenital syphilis. **Pathology.** Several metaphyses are affected. The zone of temporary calcification next to the epiphysial cartilage—normally seen in section as a thin grey line—is widened and yellowish. The adjacent part of the metaphysis is partly replaced by granulation tissue.

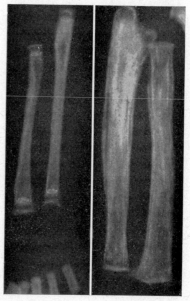

Clinical features. The condition affects infants in the first six months of life. There may be severe local pain, in consequence of which the child refuses to use the affected limb (pseudoparalysis): there is no actual loss of muscle power. *On examination* the metaphysial region is thickened and tender.

FIGS. 49 and 50

Two examples of congenital syphilis of bone. Figure 49—Metaphysitis in an infant. Note white lines at ends of metaphyses, with adjacent zones of rarefaction. Figure 50—Osteoperiostitis in a child. New bone has been laid down in layers under the periosteum.

FIG. 49   FIG. 50

Radiographs are characteristic.   The part of the metaphysis adjacent to the epiphysial cartilage shows a zone of sclerosis whereas the rest of the metaphysis is rarefied (Fig. 49).   Often there is also evidence of periostitis in the form of subperiosteal new bone in the metaphysis and adjacent part of the shaft.   *Investigations :* The Wassermann reaction is positive.

Diagnosis.   The condition may be confused with acute osteomyelitis, but the absence of leucocytosis and the positive Wassermann reaction help to distinguish the two.   Metaphysitis may also be confused with scurvy, but the other features of scurvy (haemorrhage from the gums and elsewhere) are absent.   Moreover, scurvy occurs in the second six months of life rather than the first.

Treatment.   Intensive antisyphilitic measures are rapidly effective.

Syphilitic Osteo-periostitis

When the diaphysis or body of a bone is infected by syphilis there is usually a combination of osteitis and periostitis, although one or other may predominate.   Osteo-periostitis often occurs with metaphysitis in infants ; it may occur separately in older children with congenital syphilis (Fig. 50), or in adults with acquired syphilis.

Pathology.   Of the long bones, the tibia is most commonly affected.

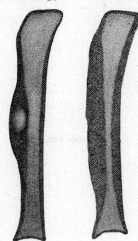

Other bones sometimes involved are the femur, the skull, the clavicle, and the bones of the hand or foot (syphilitic dactylitis).   The bone is infiltrated with syphilitic granulation tissue, which may undergo central necrosis. The extent of the lesion varies from case to case.   There may be no more than a localised thickening, or there may be diffuse infiltration of the whole of the bone (Fig. 51).   The texture of

FIG. 51

FIG. 51

Acquired syphilis of bone.   Two examples of osteo-periostitis seen in diagrammatic section. *Left*—Zone of destruction surrounded by localised area of thickening.   *Right*—Diffuse sclerotic thickening of the whole shaft.

the diseased bone also varies : the bone structure may be partly replaced by granulation tissue, or the formation of much new bone may lead to well marked sclerosis.

Clinical features. Deep boring pain, worse at night, and swelling are the predominant symptoms. *On examination* there is either a localised fusiform swelling over the shaft of the bone or a diffuse thickening of the whole length of the bone. *Radiographic examination :* Syphilitic bone disease is represented by a variety of radiographic changes ranging from severe osteoporosis to dense sclerosis. The commonest appearances are : 1) widespread sub-periosteal new bone (Fig. 50) ; 2) a localised area of destruction or rarefaction, with dense thickening of the overlying cortex ; and 3) diffuse sclerotic thickening of the whole bone. Occasionally the predominant change is bone destruction without new bone formation. *Investigations :* The Wassermann reaction is positive.

Diagnosis. Syphilis of bone or periosteum is easily confused with a malignant bone tumour. Mistakes will be avoided if syphilis is considered as a possibility in every case of localised swelling in a limb. A positive Wassermann reaction lends support to the possibility, and the diagnosis is confirmed if there is rapid improvement under antisyphilitic treatment. This therapeutic test may eliminate the need for biopsy in cases of limb swellings of doubtful nature.

Treatment. The bone lesions usually respond well to intensive antisyphilitic measures.

TUMOURS OF BONE

Bone tumours are subdivided into benign or malignant types, and malignant tumours are further classified as primary or secondary (metastatic). It is necessary here to consider only four types of benign bone tumour and six types of malignant tumour.

BENIGN TUMOURS OF BONE

The following types will be described : 1) osteoma ; 2) chondroma ; 3) osteochondroma ; 4) giant-cell tumour.

OSTEOMA

This forms a smooth rounded prominence upon the surface of a long or a flat bone, or of a skull bone (Fig. 52). It may be composed of hard compact bone (ivory osteoma) or of spongy bone (cancellous osteoma). Apart from visible or palpable swelling there are usually no symptoms.

Treatment. It may either be left alone or excised, according to the circumstances of each case.

CHONDROMA

Pathology. There are two forms of chondroma : in one the tumour grows outwards from a bone (ecchondroma) ; in the other it grows within a bone (enchondroma) (Fig. 53). Most *ecchondromata* arise in the hands or feet, or from flat bones such as the scapula or ilium. They often reach a large size. *Enchondromata* are fairly common in the bones of the hands and feet : the affected bone is expanded by the tumour and its cortex is much thinned ; so pathological fracture is common. Chondromata of the major long bones occur mainly in the distinct clinical condition known as dyschondroplasia (multiple chondromatosis or Ollier's disease) (p. 106). In this disorder, which begins in childhood, enchondromata arise in the region of the growing epiphysial cartilages of several bones : they interfere with normal growth at the epiphysial plate and consequently may lead to shortening or deformity. Occasionally a chondroma undergoes malignant change, becoming a chondrosarcoma : when this occurs it is usually in one of the major bones rather than in the small bones of the hands or feet.

Treatment. A chondroma is often best left alone. When a tumour causes trouble or is unsightly it should be removed if removal is practicable.

OSTEOCHONDROMA

This is the commonest benign tumour of bone.

Pathology. It originates from the growing epiphysial cartilage plate, but as the bone grows in length the tumour gets ' left behind ' and thus appears to migrate along the shaft towards its centre. It grows outwards from the bone like a mushroom (Fig. 54). The stalk and part of the head of the tumour are of bone, but it is capped by cartilage. The tumour continues to enlarge until the cessation of skeletal growth, and even thereafter

BENIGN TUMOURS
OF BONE

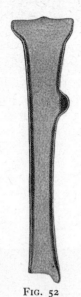

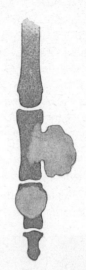

FIG. 52

Osteoma. It may occur on any bone, including those of the skull.

FIG. 53

Two types of chondroma : ecchondroma on proximal phalanx ; enchondroma in middle phalanx. (See also Figures 74 and 75.)

FIG. 52

FIG. 53

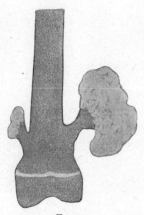

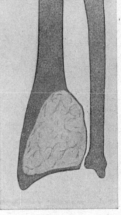

FIG. 54

A small and a large osteochondroma. They have originated at the growth cartilage but have ' migrated ' away from it with growth of the bone. Each is capped by cartilage. (See also Figure 73.)

FIG. 55

Giant-cell tumour (osteoclastoma). Note expansion of cortex and scanty fine trabeculae within the tumour. The tumour extends close up to the articular surface. (See also Figure 56.)

the cap of cartilage may persist. The ordinary osteochondroma is single ; but in the condition known as diaphysial aclasis (multiple exostoses) (p. 104) the tumours affect several or many bones. Rarely, malignant change occurs in one of the tumours.

Clinical features. The tumour is noticed as a circumscribed hard swelling near a joint. In severe examples of diaphysial aclasis there is interference with skeletal growth and the patient may be deformed or dwarfed. *Radiographs* show the mushroom-like bony tumour but not the cartilaginous cap. The stalk is often narrow.

Treatment. When necessary, the tumour should be excised.

GIANT-CELL TUMOUR (Osteoclastoma)

This is an important tumour because, though generally classed as benign, it tends to recur after local removal and sometimes

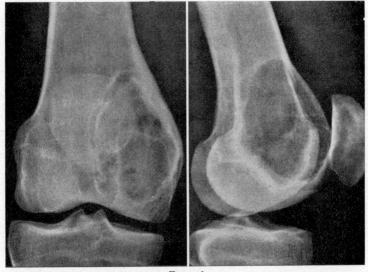

FIG. 56

Giant-cell tumour of bone at a common site. The tumour, faintly loculated, has destroyed most of one femoral condyle. It extends close up to the articular surface.

behaves as a frankly malignant tumour, metastasising through the blood stream. It occurs most commonly in young adults.

Pathology. The commonest sites are the lower end of the femur, the upper end of the tibia, the lower end of the radius, and the upper end of the humerus. Beginning in what was the metaphysial region, it extends across the former site of the epiphysial cartilage into the end of the bone, often reaching almost to the joint surface (Figs. 55 and 56). It destroys the bone substance, but new bone

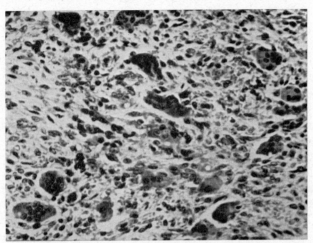

FIG. 57

A typical giant-cell tumour of bone, showing abundant oval and spindle-shaped cells with many multinucleated giant cells scattered among them. (Haematoxylin and eosin. × 150.)

forms beneath the raised periosteum, so that the bone end becomes expanded. A few bone trabeculae may remain within the tumour, giving it a faintly loculated appearance. Pathological fracture is common.

Histologically the tumour consists of abundant oval or spindle-shaped cells profusely interspersed with giant cells that may contain as many as fifty nuclei (Fig. 57). The giant cells possibly represent fused conglomerations of the oval or spindle-shaped cells. They do not resemble osteoclasts closely, nor do they behave like them: hence the name ' giant-cell tumour ' is preferred to ' osteoclastoma '. The actual cell of origin is uncertain.

A giant-cell tumour often recurs after incomplete removal. When it is malignant it metastasises readily, especially to the lungs.

Clinical features. The symptoms are pain at the site of the tumour and a gradually increasing local swelling. Sometimes the patient is made suddenly aware that something is wrong by the occurrence of a pathological fracture. Examination reveals a bony swelling which may be tender on firm palpation. *Radiographs* show destruction of the bone substance, with expansion of the cortex (Fig. 56). The tumour tends to grow eccentrically, and often extends as far as the articular end of the bone.

Treatment. This depends upon the site of the tumour. If the affected bone is one that can be reasonably dispensed with, such as the clavicle or fibula, excision of part of the bone or even the whole bone is recommended, to ensure complete removal of the tumour. But if the affected bone is one whose removal would cause severe disability, such as the femur, the problem is much more difficult. Curettage followed by packing with bone grafts is attended by a high rate of recurrence, which may then necessitate amputation. Probably the wisest course, therefore, is to advise wide local excision, even if this entails sacrifice of a major joint such as the knee or shoulder, which may have to be fused or replaced by a metal prosthesis. Radiotherapy is capable sometimes of bringing about permanent cure, but there is a risk that it may induce malignant change. It should therefore be confined to tumours at sites that are inaccessible to surgery.

MALIGNANT TUMOURS OF BONE

Classification. In the past there has been some confusion in the nomenclature and classification of primary malignant tumours of bone, largely because of difficulties in the interpretation of their histological and radiological features. One difficulty is that tumours of different origin sometimes appear very much alike. For instance, a tumour derived from primitive bone cells (osteosarcoma) may consist predominantly of fibroblasts and may thus resemble a fibrosarcoma ; or the predominant tissue may be cartilaginous and thus suggest a chondrosarcoma. Sometimes it is even difficult to distinguish between a primary and a metastatic tumour : a Ewing's sarcoma, for example, may resemble very closely a metastatic neuroblastoma. The fact that the radiological features of many of these tumours are also variable has added to the difficulties of classification. It will be clear from this that the differential diagnosis of a malignant bone tumour may be exceptionally difficult. A careful assessment of all the features—

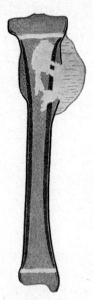

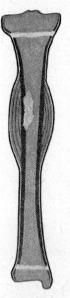

FOUR MALIGNANT TUMOURS OF BONE

FIG. 58

Osteosarcoma. It arises in the metaphysis. Note the destruction of bone, the raising of the periosteum with new bone formed beneath it, and disruption of the cortex by the tumour. The appearance is variable, and the formation of neoplastic bone by the tumour may be profuse or scanty.

FIG. 59

Ewing's tumour. It arises in the diaphysis. Note the central area of destruction and concentric layers of subperiosteal new bone giving an 'onion-peel' appearance.

FIG. 58

FIG. 59

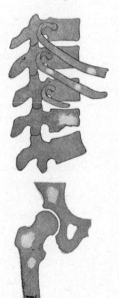

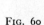

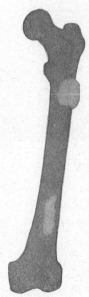

FIG. 60

Multiple myeloma. Small 'punched out' osteolytic tumours are scattered throughout the skeleton, especially in bones containing abundant red marrow.

FIG. 61

Metastatic tumours in bone, as found in disseminated carcinoma. Note the circumscribed destruction of bone without any periosteal reaction. Metastatic tumours in bone are very much more common than primary malignant bone tumours.

FIG. 60

FIG. 61

clinical, radiological, histological and biochemical—is always required.

In this brief review malignant tumours of bone will be classified and described under the following headings (the first five being primary tumours): 1) osteosarcoma (osteogenic sarcoma); 2) fibrosarcoma of bone [1]; 3) chondrosarcoma of bone; 4) Ewing's tumour; 5) multiple myeloma (plasmacytoma); 6) secondary (metastatic) tumours.

OSTEOSARCOMA (Osteogenic sarcoma)

This is predominantly a tumour of childhood or early adult life. When it occurs in later life it is often a complication of osteitis deformans (Paget's disease).

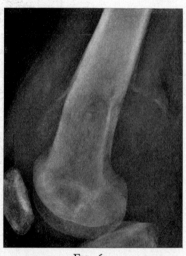

FIG. 62

An osteosarcoma at the commonest site. The tumour has destroyed much of the lower end of the femur and has burst through the cortex into the soft tissues. Though profuse new bone formation is a feature of some of these tumours, in this case (as in many others) the tumour is mainly osteolytic and there is evidence of neoplastic bone only in small scattered patches.

Pathology. An osteosarcoma arises from primitive bone-forming cells. The commonest sites are the lower end of the femur, the upper end of the tibia, and the upper end of the humerus. The tumour begins in the metaphysis. It destroys the bone substance and eventually bursts into the surrounding tissues, though it seldom crosses the epiphysial cartilage into the epiphysis (Fig. 58). The histological appearance varies widely, because any type of connective tissue may be represented. Thus the tumour may be composed largely of fibrous tissue, of cartilage or of myxomatous tissue; but characteristically there will always be found, in some parts of the tumour, areas

[1] Fibrosarcoma of soft tissue must be considered separately: it is described on page 131.

of neoplastic new bone or osteoid tissue that indicate the true nature of the lesion, and in some cases newly formed bone is abundant (Fig. 63). The tumour metastasises early by the blood stream, especially to the lungs and to other bones.

Clinical features. There are local pain and swelling, which gradually increase. Examination reveals a diffuse firm thickening

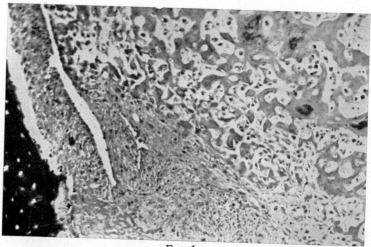

FIG. 63

Section illustrating the varied histological appearance that may be presented by an osteosarcoma. At the extreme left is a darkly-stained remnant of old mature bone. Adjacent to this is an area of fibroblastic tumour tissue. Above this and to the right is atypical immature bone produced by the tumour. (Azan stain. ×100.)

near the end of a bone, close to the joint. The overlying skin is warmer than normal because of the vascularity of the tumour. *Radiographs* show irregular destruction of the metaphysis. Later the cortex appears to have been 'burst open' at one or more places, but there are always vestiges of the original cortex. There is usually evidence of new bone formation under the corners of the raised periosteum (Codman's triangle) (Fig. 62). Occasionally well marked radiating spicules of new bone are seen within the tumour ('sun-ray' appearance). A chest radiograph may show pulmonary metastases (Fig. 64).

4

Diagnosis. In atypical cases an osteosarcoma may be confused with subacute osteomyelitis, with syphilis of bone, or with other bone tumours such as chondrosarcoma, fibrosarcoma, giant-cell tumour, Ewing's tumour, or a metastatic tumour. A representative piece of the tumour should be removed for histological examination.

Prognosis. The mortality—usually from pulmonary metastases —is in the region of 85 per cent even after amputation.

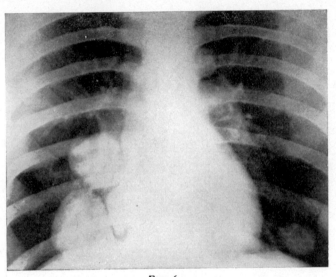

FIG. 64

Pulmonary metastases in a case of osteosarcoma of the tibia. Such metastases are the usual cause of death.

Treatment. The accepted method of treatment is by amputation through a site well clear of the tumour. However, the policy of immediate amputation has been challenged by some authorities, who believe 1) that metastases are usually already seeded by the time the diagnosis is made ; 2) that therefore amputation, however prompt, will very often be too late ; and 3) that by high-voltage radiotherapy the tumour cells can be 'sterilised' for many months, if not permanently. They therefore advocate early radiotherapy in heavy dosage, followed by a period of observation. If lung metastases have already been seeded before treatment they are likely to become manifest within six months or a year, and in that event a fruitless amputation, with its psychological trauma, will be avoided. On the other hand, if after six months or a year there is no evidence of metastases the limb may then be amputated with a reasonable hope of permanent cure. The results of this semi-conservative plan of treatment seem to be at least as good as those of immediate amputation; so at many centres it has become the method of choice.

CHONDROSARCOMA OF BONE

A chondrosarcoma is a malignant tumour derived from cartilage cells and it tends to maintain its cartilaginous character throughout its evolution.

Pathology. It may develop in the interior of the bone (central chondrosarcoma) or upon its surface (peripheral chondrosarcoma). A *central chondrosarcoma* occurs most commonly in the femur, the tibia or the humerus. It may arise *de novo*, without there having been a pre-existing lesion, or it may arise from malignant transformation of a previously existing enchondroma (especially in the condition known as dyschondroplasia or multiple chondromatosis (p. 106)). A *peripheral chondrosarcoma*, on the other hand, tends usually to affect a flat bone such as the innominate bone, the sacrum or the scapula, and it generally arises from malignant transformation of a previously existing osteochondroma (especially in the condition of diaphysial aclasis or multiple exostoses (p. 104)). Histologically, a chondrosarcoma may be highly cellular ; the cartilage cell nuclei tend to be swollen, and double nuclei may be seen. These features, suggestive of malignancy, may be found in only a few microscopic fields, the remainder of the tissue appearing relatively benign.

Clinical features. The patient is usually a person of middle age, who complains of pain and local swelling. The tumour grows slowly and may attain a large size. *Radiographically*, a central chondrosarcoma is seen to grow at the expense of the bone and may burst through the cortex, whereas a peripheral chondrosarcoma shows as a soft-tissue shadow growing outwards from the surface of the bone. Both types characteristically show blotchy areas of calcification within the tumour mass.

A chondrosarcoma grows slowly and does not metastasise early ; so the prognosis is considerably more favourable than it is in osteosarcoma.

Treatment. Amputation well above the tumour gives a reasonable prospect of permanent cure.

FIBROSARCOMA OF BONE

Fibrosarcoma of bone is uncommon. It is a fibroblastic connective-tissue tumour which arises within a bone, and is therefore distinct from a fibrosarcoma of soft tissue that has invaded the bone from outside. It occurs mainly in young adults and, as with osteosarcoma, the femur and the tibia are the commonest sites. Pale and fleshy, the tumour grows at the expense of the bone and eventually bursts through the cortex. Histologically, it is composed of rather large fibroblasts which may be well differentiated or poorly differentiated according to the malignancy of the tumour. *Radiographically* the tumour is osteolytic (bone-destroying), and evidence of neoplastic new bone formation is absent.

The prognosis is poor, but in the case of a well differentiated tumour it is certainly more favourable than that of osteosarcoma. **Treatment.** Amputation is usually to be advised. If biopsy shows a tumour that appears to be of low malignancy wide local excision may sometimes be considered if it is technically feasible. The tumour responds poorly to irradiation.

EWING'S TUMOUR (Endothelial sarcoma of bone)

Ewing's tumour is an uncommon but highly malignant sarcoma that arises in bone marrow.
Pathology. The tumour is commonest in the shaft of the femur, tibia, or humerus ; it arises in the diaphysis rather than the metaphysis of a bone. It probably develops from endothelial elements within the bone marrow. The tumour tissue is soft and vascular. As it expands it gradually destroys the bone substance. There is a striking reaction beneath the periosteum, where abundant new bone is formed in successive layers (Fig. 59). Histologically the tumour consists of sheets of uniform small round cells. The tumour metastasises early through the blood stream, especially to the lungs, and sometimes to other bones.
Clinical features. Children are the usual victims. Typically, there are local pain and swelling over one of the long bones, usually about the middle of the shaft (contrast osteosarcoma,

which arises at the metaphysis). *On examination* the swelling is diffuse or fusiform, and of firm consistence. The overlying skin is warmer than normal owing to the vascularity of the tumour. *Radiographs* show destruction of bone substance and concentric layers of subperiosteal new bone (' onion-peel ' appearance) (Fig. 59). A chest radiograph may show pulmonary metastases.

Diagnosis. In atypical cases there may be confusion with sub-acute osteomyelitis, with syphilitic osteo-periostitis, or with other tumours. In particular, it may be confused histologically with a metastasis from a suprarenal neuroblastoma ; indeed some authorities have denied the existence of Ewing's tumour, believing that every such alleged tumour is in fact derived from a neuroblastoma. Biopsy should be undertaken when the tumour is suspected.

Prognosis. The tumour is nearly always fatal—usually from pulmonary metastases—though death is sometimes averted for several years by treatment.

Treatment. The choice lies between amputation and radio-therapy. In many centres amputation is the accepted method if there are no demonstrable metastases. But it has been claimed that very high voltage x-ray therapy or radiation from the cobalt unit is as often effective as amputation. If this is sub-stantiated, radiotherapy should be preferred because it obviates the psychological trauma of an amputation in a young person.

Multiple Myeloma (Myelomatosis ; plasmacytoma)

This is a uniformly fatal tumour of bone marrow, occurring in adults.

Pathology. It probably arises from plasma cells. It is dissemin-ated to many parts of the skeleton through the blood stream, so that by the time the patient seeks advice the tumour foci are usually multiple, affecting chiefly the bones that contain abundant red marrow. The lesions are mostly small and circumscribed (Figs. 60 and 65) : the bone is simply replaced by tumour tissue and there is no reaction in the surrounding bone. Pathological fracture is common, especially in the spine (Fig. 66) Histologically the tumour consists of a mass of small round cells of plasma-cell type : the cells may be somewhat larger than normal plasma cells, and less uniform (Fig. 67).

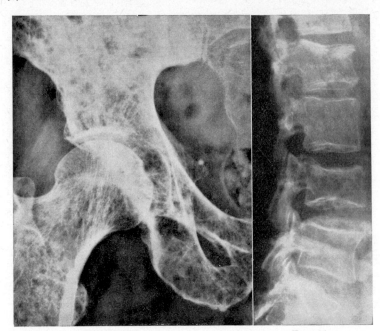

FIG. 65   FIG. 66

Multiple myeloma.   Figure 65—Part of pelvis and femur, showing numerous
small tumour foci.   Figure 66—Spine, showing diffuse rarefaction, with
collapse of the bodies of the second and fourth lumbar vertebrae.

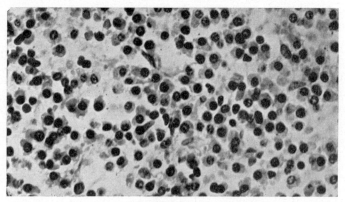

FIG. 67

Multiple myeloma.   Sheets of cells resembling plasma cells.
(Haematoxylin and eosin.   × 400.)

Clinical features. In most cases the tumour affects adults past middle age. There is general ill health, with local pain at one or more of the tumour sites. *On examination* the patient is pale. There is often local tenderness over the affected bones, but there may be no obvious swelling or deformity unless pathological fracture has occurred. *Radiographs* show multiple small areas of transradiance, especially in bones containing red marrow, such as ribs, vertebral bodies, pelvic bones, skull, and proximal ends of femur and humerus (Figs. 60, 65, 66). Sometimes there is diffuse rarefaction (Table III, p. 127). *Investigations :* There is microcytic anaemia. The erythrocyte sedimentation rate is increased. Bence-Jones proteose is present in the urine in more than half the cases. Serum globulin is increased, often so much that the albumin-globulin ratio (normally 2:1) is reversed. Marrow biopsy usually shows a profusion of plasma cells.

Diagnosis. Iliac or sternal marrow biopsy will often confirm the diagnosis when the clinical and radiographic features are equivocal.

Prognosis. The tumour is uniformly fatal, though its progress can often be checked for several years.

Treatment. The tumour foci respond to radiotherapy for a while. When the response is poor a trial may be made of cytotoxic substances such as nitrogen mustard.

SECONDARY (METASTATIC) TUMOURS IN BONE

Secondary malignant tumours in bone are much more common than primary tumours ; but whereas most primary malignant bone tumours occur in children or young adults, secondary tumours generally occur in later life.

Pathology. The tumours that metastasise most readily to bone are carcinomas of the lung, breast, prostate, thyroid, and kidney (hypernephroma). Metastases occur most commonly in the parts of the skeleton that contain vascular marrow, especially the vertebral bodies, ribs, pelvis, and upper ends of the femur and humerus. The bone structure is simply destroyed and replaced by tumour tissue (Fig. 61). Pathological fracture is common.

Clinical features. Pain is the usual main symptom, but sometimes the disability is insignificant until a pathological fracture occurs. The primary tumour can usually be demonstrated.

Radiographic examination : The bone appears to have been eaten away, so that there is a clear circumscribed area of transradiance, without any reaction in the surrounding bone (Fig. 68). Exceptionally, new bone is laid down within the metastasis, causing marked sclerosis—the exact opposite from the usual osteolytic lesion. This type is almost confined to the secondary deposits from prostatic carcinoma. In cases of diffuse infiltration there may be widespread osteoporosis (Table III, p. 127). *Investigations :* In prostatic metastases the content of acid phosphatase in the blood is usually increased above the normal level of 1-3 King-Armstrong units per 100 ml. The increase is specifically in the tartrate labile or ' prostatic ' phosphatase.

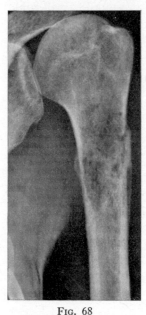

FIG. 68

Typical appearance of a metastatic carcinoma in the humerus. The primary tumour was in the lung.

Treatment. Radiotherapy is a valuable palliative. Radio-active iodine is valuable for metastases from carcinoma of the thyroid. Hormone therapy (stilboestrol or testosterone according to circumstances) is worth trying in metastases from the breast or prostate, and in selected cases adrenalectomy has proved worth while in slowing the progress of the disease when other measures have failed. Local splintage or internal fixation may be required for a pathological fracture, which may or may not unite. Analgesics and sedatives may be given as required, and cordotomy or selective leucotomy is sometimes justified for severe intractable pain.

BONE CHANGES IN LEUKAEMIA AND HODGKIN'S DISEASE

This is a convenient place to note that changes may occur in the skeleton in leukaemia and in Hodgkin's disease or related reticuloses. In *leukaemia* the changes are due to infiltration of bone by proliferating white cells, and they are seen most commonly in subacute lymphatic leukaemia in children. Characteristically there are zones of rarefaction with delicate subperiosteal new bone formation in the metaphysial regions of the femur or humerus, or in the spine or pelvis. Leukaemia is also an occasional cause of diffuse widespread rarefaction of the skeleton (Table III, p. 127).

In *Hodgkin's disease* or the related reticuloses there may be osteolytic lesions in the proximal limb bones or in the spine or pelvis, denoting destruction and replacement by tumour tissue.

OTHER LOCAL AFFECTIONS OF BONE

There is a miscellaneous group of solitary lesions of bone that do not fall into the category of infection or tumour. The most important members of the group are osteochondritis juvenilis, solitary bone cyst, localised fibrous dysplasia of bone, and osteoid osteoma.

OSTEOCHONDRITIS JUVENILIS
(Osteochondrosis)

The term osteochondritis [1] juvenilis, or simply osteochondritis, is used to describe certain obscure affections of developing bony nuclei in children and adolescents. The term has also been used, wrongly, for some other affections of epiphyses or apophyses that are more likely traumatic in origin. Typically, a bony centre affected by osteochondritis becomes temporarily softened, and while in the softened state it is liable to deformation by pressure. The disease runs a course of variable length (often about two years), but eventually spontaneous rehardening occurs. The precise cause of the disease is unknown. It should be noted that osteochondritis juvenilis is distinct from osteochondritis dissecans.

Sites. Osteochondritis juvenilis is well recognised at the following sites (Fig. 69): 1) the 'ring' epiphyses of the vertebral bodies (Scheuermann's disease or adolescent kyphosis,[2] p. 198); 2) the central epiphysis of a vertebral body (Calvé's disease, p. 201); 3) the upper epiphysis of the femur (Perthes' or Legg-Perthes' disease, p. 342); 4) the nucleus of the navicular bone (Köhler's disease, p. 421). Kienböck's disease of the lunate bone (p. 284)

---

[1] The term osteochondritis is misleading because it implies inflammation of bone and cartilage, whereas in fact the important change is necrosis followed by regeneration. 'Osteochondrosis' is preferable, but 'osteochondritis' is established by long usage.

[2] This disorder presents atypical features which suggest that it is not homologous with other examples of osteochondritis.

4*

presents similar features and may be included in this group despite the fact that it occurs in fully developed adult bone.   The

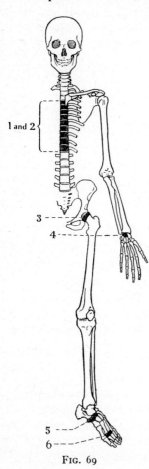

disorder of the head of the second or third metatarsal known as Freiberg's disease (p. 441) may possibly fall into the category of osteochondritis juvenilis, but there is a tendency now to ascribe it instead to osteochondritis dissecans.

Radiological appearances that bear some resemblance to the changes of osteochondritis are also seen in cases of pain at the apophysis of the tibial tubercle (Osgood-Schlatter's disease, p. 388) and at the apophysis of the calcaneus (Sever's disease, p. 425).   These conditions were formerly classified as examples of osteochondritis, but it is now recognised that their pathology is not in fact that of true osteochondritis. Probably they should be regarded as traumatic in nature : that is to say there is a chronic strain of the affected apophysis, caused by the pull of the tendon that is inserted into it.   This type of lesion is now usually termed apophysitis.

FIG. 69

Common sites of osteochondritis.   1. Ring epiphyses of vertebral bodies (multiple) (Scheuermann). 2. Central epiphysis of vertebral body (Calvé). 3. Capital epiphysis of femur (Perthes).   4. Lunate bone (Kienböck).   5. Navicular bone (Köhler).   6. Head of second or third metatarsal (Freiberg).

FIG. 69

Pathology. In a typical example of osteochondritis the histological and radiological evidence suggests that the affected bony centre undergoes partial necrosis, possibly from interference with its blood supply. The necrotic bone is invaded by granulation tissue, broken up, and eventually removed by osteoclasts. During the stage of fragmentation the centre is liable to deformation if subjected to pressure (Fig. 70). The dead tissue is gradually replaced by new living bone trabeculae and eventually the bone texture is restored to normal; but if deformation has been allowed to take place there is permanent alteration of shape.

Clinical features. The age at which the condition arises varies according to the particular bone affected. In general, it occurs

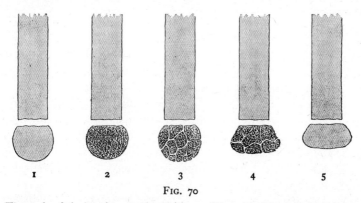

FIG. 70

The cycle of changes in osteochondritis. 1. Normal epiphysis before onset. 2. The bony nucleus undergoes necrosis, loses its normal texture, and becomes granular. 3. The bone becomes fragmented. 4. If subjected to pressure the softened epiphysis is flattened. 5. Normal bone texture restored, but deformity persists. The cycle occupies about two years.

during the stage of active development of the bony nucleus. The main symptom is local pain. If the affected epiphysis forms part of a joint, the function of the joint is disturbed and joint movement aggravates the pain. The general health is not impaired. *Radiographic examination :* The cycle of changes can be followed in serial radiographs taken at intervals of a few months. First there is a slight and often patchy increase in density of the bony nucleus. Next the patchy appearance passes to one of fragmentation, and the increased density is more pronounced. At this stage some flattening of the nucleus may be apparent by comparison with the normal side. Later there is a gradual return to normal bone texture, but any flattening that has occurred will remain.

Prognosis. Osteochondritis in itself is harmless, but if it leads to distortion of a joint surface it predisposes to osteoarthritis which, in the case of a large joint such as the hip, may cause serious disability.

Treatment. The treatment depends largely upon the site of the affection. When the bony nucleus is relatively unimportant (as for instance that of the navicular bone) treatment may be unnecessary, or it may be sufficient to protect the part in a plaster for a month or two while the pain is severe. The same applies to cases of apophysitis.

But in the case of osteochondritis involving such an important joint as the hip every effort must be made to prevent distortion of the softened epiphysis. There is at present no unanimity on the best method of doing this. Some surgeons recommend protecting the bone from the pressure of weight-bearing, either by prolonged recumbency or by means of a weight-relieving caliper, whereas others advise operation to centre the softened femoral head snugly in the hemispherical socket, which serves as a mould to preserve the shape of the head until it re-hardens (see p. 342).

In Kienböck's disease of the lunate bone it is probably best to excise the bone entire.

Further details of these disorders will be found in the chapters dealing with individual regions.

SOLITARY BONE CYST
(Simple bone cyst ; unicameral bone cyst)

Solitary bone cysts occur mostly in the long bones of children or adolescents, and especially near the proximal end of the humerus. They also occur occasionally in the small bones of the adult carpus, especially in the scaphoid or lunate bone.

Pathology. The cyst begins as a spherical lesion, but as it enlarges it tends to become oblong with its long diameter in the axis of the bone. In the long bones it tends to lie centrally in the shaft rather than to grow eccentrically, and the remaining cortex may appear expanded equally in all directions. The cyst contains clear fluid. It weakens the bone and often leads to pathological fracture. It is often taught that after a fracture through the wall of a cyst spontaneous filling in of the cyst may occur, but in fact this is unusual.

Histologically, a bone cyst has only a very thin connective-tissue lining. Its wall contains abundant osteoclasts, a fact that has led to confusion with giant-cell tumour.

Clinical features. Single bone cysts often cause no symptoms unless a pathological fracture occurs. *Radiographs* show a circumscribed area of transradiance without a surrounding zone of sclerosis (Fig. 71). The cyst may appear faintly loculated and the overlying cortex may be distended or fractured.

Diagnosis. A cyst must be differentiated from other osteolytic lesions. It may be confused with a bone abscess, with a lipoid or eosinophilic granulomatous deposit, with localised fibrous dysplasia, or occasionally with a tumour.

Treatment. Small uncomplicated cysts do not require treatment, but they should be kept under periodic observation. A large cyst should be curetted and packed with bone chips. If fracture occurs each case must be treated on its merits : bone grafting, preferably combined with rigid internal fixation, will sometimes be required.

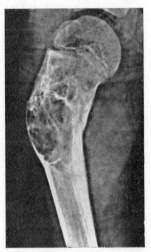

FIG. 71

Simple cyst in upper metaphysis of humerus in a child. There has been a pathological fracture, now united with moderate angulation. The cyst has a faintly loculated appearance.

FIG. 71

ANEURYSMAL BONE CYST

Aneurysmal bone cysts also occur in children or young adults, but they are distinct from the solitary bone cysts described above. Their origin is unknown : the term ' aneurysmal ' signifies no more than a seeming ' blown-out ' distension of one surface of the bone. The cyst may bulge into the soft tissues, contained only by periosteum and a thin shell of newly formed cortex. The lining consists of connective tissue with numerous vascular spaces and some giant cells ; the cyst contains fluid blood. Radiographically the cyst is seen to be situated eccentrically in the bone and presents the characteristic ' blown-out ' appearance already mentioned. These features distinguish it from the ordinary solitary bone cyst, which is placed centrally in the shaft and expands the bone uniformly. *Treatment* of accessible cysts is by curettage and filling with bone chips.

LOCALISED FIBROUS DYSPLASIA OF BONE
(Monostotic fibrous dysplasia)

In this condition a solitary area of bone is partly replaced by fibrous tissue, in which scanty bone trabeculae may persist. The cause is unknown, as also is its relationship to polyostotic fibrous dysplasia (p. 109). It is not related to the fibrous dysplasia of hyperparathyroidism.

Pathology. One of the limb bones is usually the site affected. The fibrous lesion expands at the expense of the bone, which is much weakened and may fracture.

Clinical features. There may be local pain in the affected bone. *Radiographs* show a clear zone of transradiance within the bone. The area has a homogeneous ' ground-glass ' appearance.

Treatment. If the lesion is seen to be extending, the affected segment of bone should be excised and replaced by a bone graft.

OSTEOID OSTEOMA

Osteoid osteoma is a benign circumscribed lesion of bone, of uncertain nature. It has been regarded variously as a benign tumour and as an infective lesion.

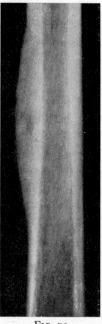

Pathology. The characteristic feature is the formation of a small nidus of osteoid tissue, seldom more than half a centimetre in diameter, usually in the cortex of a long bone but occasionally in cancellous bone. In the long bones the central nidus of osteoid tissue is surrounded by a zone of dense sclerotic bone which causes localised thickening of the shaft. Sclerosis is slight or absent when the lesion occurs in cancellous bone.

Clinical features. The only symptom is a severe deep ' boring ' pain, which is ill localised and worst at night. The pain is often eased by aspirin or its derivatives. There may be thickening and local tenderness at the site of the lesion. *Radiographs* typically show local sclerotic thickening of the shaft (Fig. 72), with a small central area of rarefaction which, however, may be visible only in radiographs of very good quality, or in tomographs.

Diagnosis. This is mainly from low-grade osteomyelitis, and especially from Brodie's chronic bone abscess.

FIG. 72

Osteoid osteoma of femur. Note the localised thickening of the cortex with small central nidus.

Treatment. The nidus of osteoid tissue should be excised together with a margin of surrounding bone. This operation gives immediate and dramatic relief of pain.

GENERAL AFFECTIONS OF THE SKELETON

A large number of general affections of the skeleton have been described. Many of them are so rare that it is unnecessary for the student to concern himself with them. Most of the others require only brief consideration.

Classification

The following classification is based on that of Fairbank (1951).

CONGENITAL DEVELOPMENTAL AFFECTIONS
        Osteogenesis imperfecta
        Diaphysial aclasis
        Dyschondroplasia
        Achondroplasia
        Myositis ossificans progressiva
        Multiple neurofibromatosis

ACQUIRED AFFECTIONS OF UNKNOWN ORIGIN
        Polyostotic fibrous dysplasia
        Osteitis deformans
        Senile osteoporosis

AFFECTIONS DUE TO ERRORS OF DIET AND METABOLISM
        Infantile scurvy
        Infantile rickets
        Other forms of rickets
        Osteomalacia
        Idiopathic steatorrhoea
        Granulomatosis (reticulosis)
            Eosinophilic granuloma
            Hand-Schüller-Christian disease
            Letterer-Siwe disease
            Gaucher's disease

AFFECTIONS DUE TO ENDOCRINE ERRORS
        Parathyroid osteodystrophy
        Hyperpituitarism
            Gigantism
            Acromegaly
            Cushing's syndrome
        Hypopituitarism
        Cretinism

References and bibliography, page 445.

CONGENITAL DEVELOPMENTAL AFFECTIONS

OSTEOGENESIS IMPERFECTA
(Fragilitas ossium)

Osteogenesis imperfecta is a congenital and inheritable affection in which the bones are abnormally soft and brittle. It is transmitted by a dominant mutant gene.

Clinical features. In the worst cases the child is born with multiple fractures and does not survive. In the less severe examples fractures occur after birth, often from trivial violence. As many as fifty or more may be sustained in the first few years of life. The fractures unite readily, but in the more severe cases marked deformity often develops, either from malunion or from bending of the soft bones, and such patients may be badly crippled. In the milder cases there is a tendency for fractures to occur less frequently in later life.

Additional features, not always present, are a deep blue coloration of the sclerotics, deafness from otosclerosis (which becomes worse in later life), and ligamentous laxity.

Treatment. Fractures are generally treated in the ordinary way, but in a severe case intramedullary nailing of affected long bones should be considered as a means of preventing crippling deformity. Protective appliances, such as walking calipers, may be required in older children and adults.

DIAPHYSIAL ACLASIS
(Multiple exostoses)

This is a congenital affection characterised by the formation of multiple exostoses (osteochondromata) at the metaphysial regions of the long bones. It is transmitted by a dominant mutant gene.

Pathology. The fault is in the epiphysial cartilage plate. Nests of cartilage cells become displaced and give rise to bony outgrowths, which are capped by proliferating cartilage. The cartilaginous caps may persist after the general cessation of skeletal growth, despite statements that have been made to the contrary. These exostoses, or osteochondromata, constitute one type of benign bone tumour (p. 82). The number of outgrowths

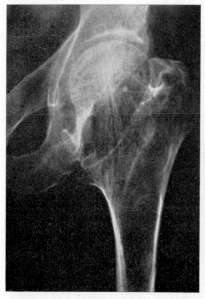 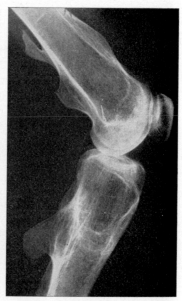

FIG. 73   FIG. 74

Diaphysial aclasis (multiple exostoses). Figure 73 shows stunting of the upper end of the femur due to failure of the remodelling process that accompanies normal growth. Defective remodelling is a characteristic feature of the disease in its more severe forms. Figure 74 shows typical exostoses (osteochondromata) projecting from femur and tibia. Such outgrowths are always directed away from the end of the bone.

varies; often there are between ten and twenty. In severe cases the process of remodelling by which a bone attains its normal adult shape is impaired, and there may be marked deformity, with reduction of longitudinal growth. Rarely, malignant change in the cartilaginous cap of one of the tumours leads to the development of a chondrosarcoma (p. 91).

Clinical features. Usually the only symptoms and signs are those caused by the local swellings, or by their pressure effects. The patient is of short stature, and there may be marked deformity of the limbs. Malignant change is suggested by rapid enlargement of one of the swellings.

Radiographs show the bony outgrowths. In severe cases the bones are broad and ill modelled (Figs. 73 and 74).

Treatment. An outgrowth that is causing trouble should be excised.

DYSCHONDROPLASIA

(Multiple chondromatosis; Ollier's disease)

In dyschondroplasia masses of unossified cartilage persist within the metaphyses of certain long bones, and the growth of the bone is retarded. The condition is congenital, but the cause is unknown. Heredity plays no part.

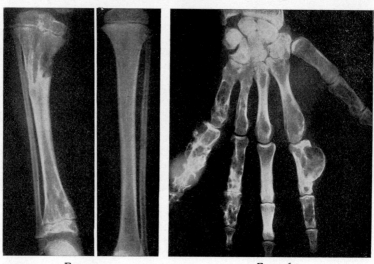

FIG. 75   FIG. 76

Dyschondroplasia (multiple chondromata). Figure 75—Masses of proliferating cartilage occupy the metaphyses of one tibia. Growth is retarded and uneven. The normal tibia is shown for comparison. Figure 76—Multiple enchondromata in the metacarpals and phalanges.

Pathology. The fault is in the epiphysial cartilage plate. In this respect dyschondroplasia resembles diaphysial aclasis, but the two conditions are otherwise distinct. Nests of cartilage cells are displaced from the epiphysial plate into the metaphysis, where they persist as enchondromata. These masses of cartilage have been regarded as a type of benign bone tumour (p. 82), although it is doubtful whether they are true neoplasms.[1]

Any bone formed in cartilage may be affected. The more rapidly growing ends of the femur and tibia (that is, the ends near the knee) and the small long bones of the hands and feet are particularly common sites. There is a tendency for the disorder

[1] It is impossible to give a precise definition of a benign tumour.

to be unilateral. When a major long bone is affected interference with growth at the epiphysial cartilage adjacent to the lesion may lead to serious shortening and distortion of the bone (Fig. 75). When skeletal growth ceases the masses of cartilage may ossify. Occasionally one of the tumours undergoes malignant change, to become a chondrosarcoma (p. 91).

Clinical features. A limb affected by dyschondroplasia is usually short and may be markedly deformed. The hands may be grotesquely enlarged by multiple cartilaginous swellings. *Radiographs* show multiple areas of transradiance in the affected bones (Figs. 75 and 76).

Treatment. Osteotomy may be required to correct deformities resulting from uneven growth of bone. If there is marked discrepancy in the length of the lower limbs a leg equalisation procedure (p. 33) may be advisable.

ACHONDROPLASIA

Achondroplasia is a congenital inheritable affection in which there is marked shortness of the limbs, with consequent dwarfing. It is ascribed to a dominant mutant gene.

Pathology. There is a failure of normal ossification in the long bones, which may be only half their normal length. Growth of the trunk is only slightly impaired.

Clinical features. Achondroplasia is apparent at birth, the child being strikingly dwarfed, with very short limbs that are out of proportion to the trunk (Fig. 77). Adult achondroplasiacs are seldom more than four feet in height. The hands are short and broad, the central three digits being divergent and of almost equal length (' trident ' hand). The head is slightly larger than normal, but there is no mental impairment.

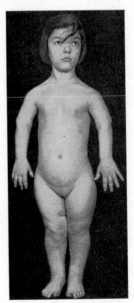

FIG. 77

Achondroplasia, showing the typical features in a child. The dwarfing is due to shortness of the limbs ; development of the trunk is but little impaired.

FIG. 77

MYOSITIS OSSIFICANS PROGRESSIVA

Myositis ossificans progressiva[1] is a congenital affection characterised by the formation of masses of bone in the soft tissues, with consequent limitation of movement. It is often associated with shortness of the great toe or of other digits (microdactyly). Heredity plays only a small part.

Pathology. The bone is formed by metaplasia of connective-tissue cells, not from displaced osteoblasts.

Clinical features. Changes usually appear first in early childhood. Swellings develop in the region of the neck and trunk. At first soft and perhaps transient, they later give place to hard masses of bone which lie in the course of muscles, ligaments, and fasciae. Movements of the spine and ribs are reduced progressively until in the worst cases there may be total immobility. In most cases the great toe is congenitally short; the thumbs or other digits may also be short. *Radiographs* show the plates of bone in the soft tissues.

Progress. After many years increasing rigidity renders the patient bedridden. No effective treatment is known.

NEUROFIBROMATOSIS
(von Recklinghausen's disease)

This is a congenital inheritable affection characterised by pigmented areas on the skin, cutaneous fibromata, and multiple neurofibromata in the course of the cranial or peripheral nerves. It is ascribed to a dominant mutant gene.

Pathology. The neurofibromata consist of connective tissue arranged in whorls, with a few nerve fibres.

Clinical features. Skin lesions may be present at birth or develop later. They consist of small ' *café au lait* ' areas, and of small fibromata which may be flat or raised. Neurofibromata may occur on any of the cranial or peripheral nerves. Occasionally a neurofibroma may undergo malignant change.

---

[1] Myositis ossificans progressiva must not be confused with post-traumatic myositis ossificans. The two conditions are entirely distinct. Post-traumatic ' myositis ossificans ' is misnamed : it is nothing more than ossification within a subperiosteal haematoma.

The orthopaedic significance of neurofibromatosis lies mainly in the liability to scoliosis and to neurological disturbances in the limbs.

Scoliosis. Why scoliosis should occur is unknown : but it is a common complication and it sometimes progresses to an angulation so severe that the function of the spinal cord is impaired.

Neurological disturbances. These are the consequence of neurofibromata lying in the course of nerve trunks. Various manifestations are observed, depending upon the site of the tumour. For instance, a tumour of a nerve root within the spinal canal may compress the spinal cord and give the typical picture of a spinal cord tumour. Or it may compress the cauda equina or an individual nerve trunk, with consequent radiating pain and impairment of function of the involved nerve. Thus neurofibromatosis enters into the differential diagnosis of brachial pain and sciatica. *Radiographs* may show erosion of a bone where a neurofibroma lies in contact with it.

Diagnosis. The pigmented spots or areas and cutaneous fibromata afford important clues to the diagnosis. A positive family history is important corroborative evidence.

Treatment. A neurofibroma that is causing trouble should be excised.

ACQUIRED AFFECTIONS OF UNKNOWN ORIGIN

POLYOSTOTIC FIBROUS DYSPLASIA

Replacement of bone by fibrous tissue forms a conspicuous part of several unrelated bone diseases. In two conditions in particular, fibrous replacement is the predominant change. In one of these—parathyroid osteodystrophy—the changes are associated with hyperparathyroidism (p. 124). In the other, now to be described, there is fibrous replacement without any evidence of excessive parathyroid secretion.

Polyostotic fibrous dysplasia, then, is a condition in which parts of several bones are replaced by masses of fibrous tissue, but in which there is no evidence of hyperparathyroidism. The cause is unknown.

Pathology. The number of bones involved varies from two or three to twelve or more. The major long bones are those mainly affected—especially the femur. The skull is also commonly involved. Affected bones are liable to bend or break.

Clinical features. The onset is in childhood but the condition is often not recognised until adult life. The main features are

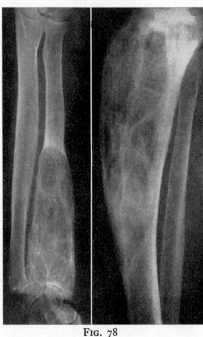

deformity, from bending or local enlargement of bone, and pathological fracture. The disease progresses for years and may lead to severe crippling. *Radiographs* of the affected bones show well defined transradiant areas which often have a characteristic homogeneous or ' ground-glass' appearance. The lesions are in the shaft and metaphyses rather than the epiphyses. When the lesion is extensive the cortex is expanded and thin, and the bone is bent. Sometimes the lesion has a honey-combed appearance (Fig. 78). *Investigations :* Biochemical examination of the blood does not show any alteration from the normal.

FIG. 78

Polyostotic fibrous dysplasia affecting the radius (*left*) and the tibia (*right*). Parts of the skeleton are replaced by fibrous tissue. Unlike parathyroid osteodystrophy, this disorder is not associated with any known endocrine dysfunction.

The bone lesions of polyostotic fibrous dysplasia sometimes occur in association with pigmentation of the skin and, in females, sexual precocity. This combination of clinical features is known as Albright's syndrome.

OSTEITIS DEFORMANS
(Paget's disease)

Osteitis deformans is a slowly progressive disorder of one or several bones. Affected bones are thickened and spongy,

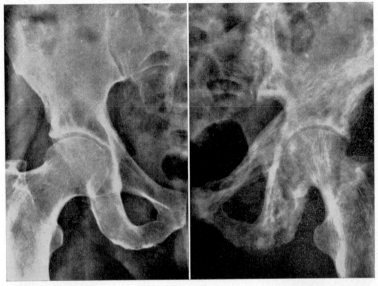

FIG. 79

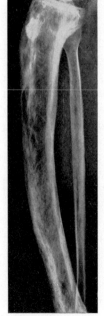

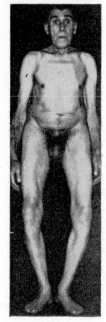

FIG. 79

Paget's disease. Half-pelvis, side by side with the normal for comparison. Note the coarse trabeculae and slight distortion of the pelvic ring.

FIG. 80

Paget's disease. Tibia, showing bending, coarsening of trabeculae, and thickened cortex which, however, is not sharply demarcated from the medulla.

FIG. 81

Typical appearance of a patient with widespread Paget's disease. Note the bowing of the legs, and the shortened trunk, due to collapse of softened vertebrae.

FIG. 80   FIG. 81

and show a tendency to bend. The disease is one of the commonest general affections of the skeleton. The cause is unknown.

Pathology. The bones most commonly affected are the pelvis, vertebrae, femur, tibia, and skull. The disease may be confined to a single bone at first, but it often spreads to involve other bones later. The cortex of the bone loses its normal compact density and becomes spongy. At the same time it is widened by the formation of new bone on both its outer and inner surfaces. The whole bone is thus thickened, but the usual sharp distinction between cortex and medulla is lost. The marrow spaces are filled with fibrous tissue. In the later stages there is a tendency for the affected bones to become gradually denser.

In the spongy state the bones are softer than normal and are liable to bend. Pathological fracture may occur. In rare instances osteosarcoma develops in the diseased bone.

Clinical features. The affection seldom begins before the age of 40. Often there are no symptoms, the condition being discovered incidentally during routine radiographic examination. When long bones are affected pain is sometimes complained of, but it is by no means an invariable feature. The only other symptoms arise from the bony thickening and the deformity. Thickening may be obvious clinically, especially in the case of the tibia or the skull. Thus the patient may notice that he requires progressively larger hats. Bending of the softened long bones leads to deformity, usually in the form of anterior and lateral bowing of the femur or tibia (Fig. 81). *Radiographic examination* (Figs. 79-80) : The main radiographic features are : 1) thickening of the bone, mainly from widening of the cortex ; 2) diminished density of the cortex, which loses its compact appearance and assumes a spongy or honeycombed texture ; 3) marked coarsening of the bone trabeculae ; 4) in the later stages a general increase of density of the affected bones. The long bones are often shown to be bowed, the pelvis may be deformed, and the vertebrae may be compressed. *Investigations :* The alkaline phosphatase content of the serum is increased, often to a high level if several bones are affected.

Complications. The important complications are pathological fracture and, occasionally, osteosarcoma.

Treatment. Treatment is usually unnecessary, except when complications arise. If local pain is particularly severe and inadequately controlled by analgesics radiotherapy may afford relief.

SENILE OSTEOPOROSIS
(Idiopathic osteoporosis)

This condition is characterised by diffuse osteoporosis of unknown cause. It affects the elderly, especially women, but it may be seen also in patients of middle age. It may possibly have an endocrine basis.

Pathology. The whole skeleton is affected, but the changes in the spine are more obvious than those elsewhere. The cortices of the vertebrae are thinner than normal, and the bone is rarefied throughout from thinning of the individual trabeculae and widening of the vascular canals. In other words there is a reduction of total bone mass. Compression fracture of one or more of the vertebral bodies is liable to occur from only trivial violence. Even without fracture the thoracic vertebrae tend gradually to become wedge-shaped so that the spine bends forward to produce a rounded kyphosis. The long bones are also prone to fracture easily.

Clinical features. The patient is often a woman of over 60. The osteoporosis may be symptomless and may be found only by chance. In other cases there is pain in the back. The pain occurs in two forms—a mild generalised ache, and a sharper pain of sudden onset, denoting a compression fracture. Examination reveals a rounded kyphosis in the thoracic region. If a vertebral body has collapsed there may be a more angular kyphosis with prominence of a spinous process in the thoracic or thoraco-lumbar region. The trunk is shortened and there is a transverse furrow across the abdomen (Fig. 82). *Radiographic examination :* The striking feature is the reduced density of the vertebral bodies, which become concave at their upper and lower surfaces from pressure of the intervertebral discs. Often there is wedging of one or more of the vertebral bodies from compression fracture (Fig. 83). Other parts of the skeleton may be rarefied, but in less degree. *Investigations:* The biochemistry of the blood is normal. Metabolic balance studies may show a negative calcium balance.

Diagnosis. Senile osteoporosis may be confused with other forms of diffuse rarefaction of bone, especially that caused by parathyroid osteodystrophy, Cushing's syndrome, osteomalacia of various types, carcinomatosis, multiple myelomatosis, or

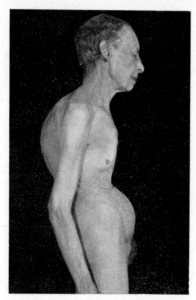

FIG. 82

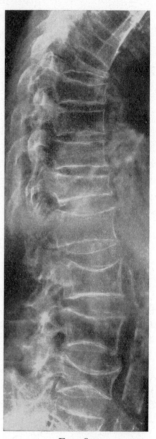

Senile osteoporosis. Note in Figure 82 the rounded kyphosis and the shortened trunk. The radiograph (Fig. 83) shows marked loss of density, with thinning of the cortices. The intervertebral disc spaces are ballooned into the concave vertebral surfaces. Several vertebral bodies have collapsed. Differential diagnosis was from parathyroid osteodystrophy, osteomalacia, multiple myelomatosis, diffuse carcinomatous deposits, and leukaemia.

FIG. 83

leukaemia (Table III, p. 127). Diagnosis rests largely on the exclusion of these specific disorders.

Treatment. Treatment is rather unsatisfactory. It may be possible to restore the patient to positive calcium balance by calcium supplements to the diet, but the gain is usually small and a dramatic improvement in the radiographic appearance cannot be expected. In the belief that the disorder has an endocrine basis oestrogen and androgen therapy has been used, but with doubtful benefit. If back pain is troublesome a light spinal brace should be prescribed.

AFFECTIONS DUE TO ERRORS OF DIET AND METABOLISM

INFANTILE SCURVY

Scurvy is a haemorrhagic disease caused by a deficiency of vitamin C in the diet.

Pathology. The most striking changes are in the long bones. There is a lack of osteoblastic activity in the epiphysial growth cartilage. Haemorrhage, beginning at the epiphysial cartilage, extends beneath the periosteum, which may be raised from the bone throughout its whole length. Haemorrhages also occur from other sites, especially from the gums or within the orbit.

Clinical features. Scurvy affects infants during the second six months of life if the diet is deficient in fresh milk or other sources of vitamin C. The onset is rapid, with loss of use of a limb because of pain (pseudoparalysis). The limb is swollen and exquisitely tender over the affected bone or bones. The gums are often spongy and bleed, and there may be a ' black ' eye.

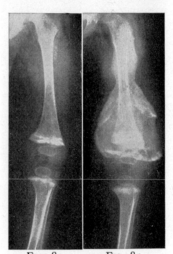

FIG. 84   FIG. 85

Infantile scurvy. Figure 84—Early active stage. Note the clear zone in the metaphysis, indicating arrest of osteoblastic activity. Figure 85—Later stage, showing well marked ossification in the subperiosteal haematoma.

Radiographs show a dense line at the junction between metaphysis and epiphysial cartilage, with a clear band of rarefaction on the diaphysial side (Fig. 84). Later there is ossification in the subperiosteal haematoma, as a result of which the bone is often markedly thickened (Fig. 85). *Investigations :* Ascorbic acid is absent from the plasma.

Diagnosis. The skeletal features of scurvy are similar to those of syphilitic metaphysitis, which, however, occurs at an earlier age—namely during the first six months of life. Other distinctive features are the positive Wassermann reaction in syphilis and bleeding from the gums in scurvy. Scurvy may also be confused with acute osteomyelitis.

Treatment. The disease responds readily to the administration of vitamin C.

NUTRITIONAL RICKETS

In rickets there is defective calcification of *growing* bone[1] in consequence of a disturbed calcium-phosphorus metabolism. With the general improvement in economic conditions infantile rickets has become rare in Western countries. There is, however, a relatively higher incidence among immigrants from the West Indies and from Asia.

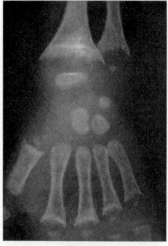

FIG. 86

Rickets. Note the typical widening and 'cupping' of the metaphyses. The depth of the epiphysial cartilage is increased, and the general density of the bones is reduced.

Cause. Nutritional rickets is caused by a deficiency of vitamin D in the diet and by inadequate exposure to sunlight, which promotes the synthesis of vitamin D in the body.

Pathology. Vitamin D promotes the absorption of calcium and phosphorus from the intestine. Its deficiency therefore leads to inadequate absorption of calcium and phosphorus. The level of calcium in the blood can then be maintained only at the expense of the skeletal calcium. Proliferating osteoid tissue in the growing epiphyses thus remains uncalcified, and there is a general softening of the bones already formed.

[1] When similar influences act on mature adult bone the condition is known as osteomalacia.

Clinical features. The ordinary nutritional rickets usually occurs in children about one year old. The general health is impaired. The predominant signs are a large head, retarded skeletal growth, enlarged epiphyses, curvature of long bones, and deformity of the chest, which may show a transverse sulcus. In a typical case these signs produce an easily recognised clinical picture. *Radiographs* show a general loss of density of the skeleton. The most striking changes, however, are in the growing epiphyses. The vertical depth of the epiphysial lines is increased, the epiphyses are widened laterally, and the ends of the shafts are hollowed out or ' cupped ' (Fig. 86). Bending of the bones may be obvious. *Investigations :* The serum phosphate level is usually decreased. The serum calcium is normal. The alkaline phosphatase is increased, often markedly : its level gives some indication of the severity of the disease and of the response to treatment.

Diagnosis. If rickets is suspected an antero-posterior radiograph of a wrist should be obtained. The radiographic features are diagnostic of rickets, but biochemical examinations are required to indicate its type (Table II, p. 121).

Treatment. Nutritional rickets responds well to vitamin D in ordinary doses. In cases of severe bony deformity osteotomy or osteoclasis may be required for its correction.

OTHER FORMS OF RICKETS

The characteristic epiphysial changes seen in nutritional rickets occur in a number of other diseases, the primary factor responsible for the disordered calcium-phosphate metabolism being different in each type. Four types will be described : vitamin-resistant rickets, the Fanconi syndrome, renal (glomerular) rickets, and coeliac (gluten-induced) rickets.

VITAMIN-RESISTANT RICKETS
(Chronic phosphate diabetes)

Vitamin-resistant rickets is a hereditary disorder transmitted probably by a sex-linked dominant gene. The nature of the primary defect is uncertain : it may be a failure of normal reabsorption of phosphate by the renal tubules, or it may be a fault in the absorption of calcium from the intestine. Bone changes, which are like those of nutritional rickets, may become manifest soon after the first year of life. The characteristic biochemical features are : normal serum calcium, low serum phosphate level *not corrected by vitamin D*, increased alkaline phosphatase, and excess of phosphate in the urine (Table II, p. 121). Relatives who are clinically unaffected may nevertheless show hypophosphataemia.

Treatment. Vitamin D in massive doses corrects the bone changes but does not restore the serum phosphate to a normal level.

FANCONI SYNDROME
(Renal tubular rickets with glycosuria and amino-aciduria)

In the Fanconi syndrome rachitic changes in the bones are associated with renal glycosuria and amino-aciduria. The primary defect, a congenital fault transmitted by a recessive mutant gene, is a failure of the proximal renal tubules to reabsorb phosphate, glucose, and certain amino acids in the normal way. The excessive loss of phosphates in the urine leads to depletion of the bone phosphate. Onset may be later in childhood than that of nutritional rickets, but the bone changes are the same. The characteristic biochemical features are : normal serum calcium ; low serum phosphate ; increased alkaline phosphatase ; and excess of phosphate in the urine, which also contains glucose and certain amino acids (Table II, p. 121).

Treatment. The intake of calcium, phosphate, and vitamin D should be increased. Alkalis (sodium citrate) should be given to combat the associated acidosis.

Related Disorders

A number of similar disorders from renal tubular defects are recognised. In all of them there is deficient reabsorption of phosphate, but they differ in the extent to which other functions of the tubules are impaired.

RENAL (GLOMERULAR) RICKETS
(Renal osteodystrophy ; renal dwarfism ; renal infantilism)

In renal rickets general skeletal changes are associated with chronic renal impairment. The skeletal changes often become manifest between the ages of 5 and 10 years.

Pathology. The renal impairment may be due to congenital cystic changes, to ureteric obstruction with hydronephrosis, or to chronic nephritis. The mechanism by which the renal deficiency leads to rachitic changes in the skeleton is uncertain. Probably the essential factor is inadequate excretion of phosphorus by the kidneys. This leads to retention of phosphorus in the blood, and its excretion in the intestine. There it forms an insoluble compound with calcium, which in consequence is not absorbed in proper amounts. The skeletal changes consist in deficient epiphysial growth and multiple deformities from bone softening. The parathyroid glands are hypertrophied, probably as a secondary effect.

Clinical features. The child is dwarfed and deformed. There are symptoms of renal impairment, such as excessive thirst and sallow complexion. The common skeletal deformities are coxa vara, genu valgum, and severe valgus deformity of the feet. *Radiographs* show epiphysial changes that are generally similar to those of infantile rickets (Fig. 87). *Investigations:* The biochemical changes are characteristic (Table II, p. 121). The serum phosphate is markedly increased. The serum calcium is low. The blood urea is raised, often to a high figure. Albumin is usually present in the urine.

Treatment. This should be directed primarily against the underlying renal condition. The diet should be supplemented with calcium and vitamin D.

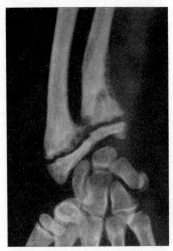

FIG. 87

Rachitic changes in the epiphyses of a renal dwarf aged 14 years. There was diffuse rarefaction of the skeleton, with multiple deformities from bending of softened bones.

FIG. 87

COELIAC (GLUTEN-INDUCED) RICKETS

Coeliac disease (gluten-induced enteropathy) is a digestive disorder characterised by malabsorption and consequently by an excess of fat in the stools. Before a knowledge was gained of how to control the disease it was often complicated by rachitic changes in the bones. Such changes will now be seen only in neglected cases. The primary fault is a susceptibility of the villi of the small intestine to atrophy under the influence of gluten, the protein fraction of flour. This villous atrophy leads to deficient absorption of fats and of fat-soluble vitamin D.

The disease begins in infancy or early childhood. The general features are wasting, impaired growth, failure to gain weight, muscular hypotonia, distended abdomen, and loose offensive stools containing 40 to 80 per cent fat after drying (normal = 25 per cent). The skeletal changes, which do not develop for several years, are like those of infantile rickets. *Investigations:* The biochemical changes in the blood differ from those of infantile rickets. The serum calcium is low. The serum phosphorus is normal or low (Table II, p. 121). Diagnosis may be confirmed by jejunal biopsy effected by a swallowed capsule with a special cutting device.

Treatment. There is steady improvement in the calcification of the skeleton as the primary disorder is brought under control. The diet should be free from gluten and should contain an abundant supply of calcium and vitamin D.

NUTRITIONAL OSTEOMALACIA

Nutritional osteomalacia [1] is the adult counterpart of infantile rickets. It is rare except in certain Asiatic countries. Nevertheless cases are encountered occasionally in Britain, chiefly in elderly women.

Cause and pathology. As in infantile rickets, there is a deficiency of vitamin D (and often of calcium) in the diet. In consequence the intestinal absorption of calcium and phosphorus is inadequate, and calcium is withdrawn from the bones to maintain a reasonable level in the blood. The trabeculae are not abnormally thin, but they are largely composed of poorly calcified osteoid tissue. There is an abundance of fibrous tissue in the marrow.

Clinical features. The main features are pain in the bones, and deformity. Fractures are common. *Radiographs* show rarefaction of the whole skeleton. The bone cortices are abnormally thin. The long bones may be curved and the pelvis triradiate. Multiple spontaneous fractures (Looser's zones), seemingly ununited though possibly bridged by unmineralised osteoid tissue, may be shown in ribs, pelvic rami, or elsewhere. These are characteristic of osteomalacia and are not seen in osteoporosis. *Investigations* (Table II, p. 121) : The serum calcium is normal or low. Serum phosphate is low. Alkaline phosphatase is increased. The calcium balance is negative.

Diagnosis. Nutritional osteomalacia must be distinguished from other causes of diffuse rarefaction of bone (Table III, p. 127). In the elderly it may be mistaken for senile osteoporosis.

Treatment. Recalcification of the skeleton is induced by adequate diet and administration of vitamin D. Osteotomy may be required to correct deformity.

OTHER FORMS OF OSTEOMALACIA

Just as in children rachitic changes in the bones may occur from a number of different metabolic faults, so in adults osteomalacia may arise from causes other than purely nutritional. Such causes include advanced renal disease, and mal-absorption syndromes such as chronic obstruction of the bile ducts, chronic pancreatic disease and idiopathic steatorrhoea. Of these, only idiopathic steatorrhoea will be described here, as an example.

[1] The essential distinction between *osteoporosis* and *osteomalacia* was made in a footnote on page 10

TABLE II

SUMMARY OF THE BIOCHEMICAL CHANGES IN THE VARIOUS FORMS
OF RICKETS AND OSTEOMALACIA

	Primary Fault and Mechanism	Serum Calcium	Serum Inorganic Phosphate	Urine	Stools
Nutritional rickets (children) Nutritional osteomalacia (adults)	Deficiency of vitamin D in diet——→impaired absorption of calcium and phosphorus	Normal	Low	Normal	Normal
Vitamin-resistant rickets	Congenital fault : impaired reabsorption of phosphates by renal tubules——→excessive excretion of phosphates	Normal	Low	Excess of phosphate	Normal
Fanconi syndrome . .	Impaired reabsorption of phosphates, glucose and some amino acids by renal tubules——→excessive excretion of phosphates, etc.	Normal	Low	Glucose Amino acids Excess of phosphate	Normal
Renal rickets . .	Impaired glomerular function——→retention of phosphorus——→excretion in bowel——→combination with calcium preventing its normal absorption	Low	High	Albumin	Normal
Coeliac rickets (children) Idiopathic steatorrhoea (adults)	Digestive deficiency——→impaired absorption of vitamin D and calcium	Low	Normal	Normal	Excess of fat

NOTE : The serum alkaline phosphatase is increased in all types of rickets in the active stage. It is an index of activity rather than of type.

5

IDIOPATHIC STEATORRHOEA

In most instances so-called idiopathic steatorrhoea is the adult counterpart of coeliac disease and may therefore be termed gluten-induced enteropathy. There is deficient absorption of fats, and

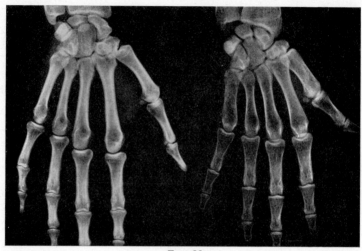

FIG. 88

Demonstration of generalised rarefaction by radiography of one of the patient's hands side by side with a hand of a normal person (*left*) of the same sex and age. Note the obvious difference in bone density. A case of idiopathic steatorrhoea.

consequently of the fat-soluble vitamin D and of calcium. Eventually, skeletal changes may occur which are identical with those of nutritional osteomalacia.

Clinical features. The disease may be unrecognised until a fracture occurs or a deformity becomes evident. *Radiographs* show rarefaction of bone (Fig. 88), with thinning of the cortices. *Investigations* (Table II, p. 121): The stools contain an excess of fat and of calcium. The serum calcium is low. The serum phosphorus is normal. The urinary excretion of calcium is low. Jejunal biopsy may show villous atrophy.

Treatment. In cases ascribed to the influence of gluten, a gluten-free diet, supplemented with calcium and vitamin D, should be ordered.

GRANULOMATOSIS AFFECTING THE SKELETON
(Skeletal reticulosis)

The general title skeletal granulomatosis or skeletal reticulosis includes a number of rather uncommon disorders of the reticulo-endothelial system, some possibly related, in which deposits of granulomatous tissue occur in the bones or elsewhere. In some examples the reticulo-endothelial cells contain lipoid: these are often referred to as the *lipoid granulomatoses*, as distinct from the *non-lipoid* forms for which the term histiocytosis X is also used.

Three members of the group of non-lipoid granulomatoses will be mentioned here: eosinophilic granuloma, Hand-Schüller-Christian disease, and Letterer-Siwe disease. Lipoid granulomatosis is represented here by Gaucher's disease. All occur mostly in children or young adults.

EOSINOPHILIC GRANULOMA

In eosinophilic granuloma the bone lesion is usually solitary. It consists of brownish granulation tissue containing abundant histiocytes and eosinophils, with leucocytes and giant cells. Often there are no symptoms, but there may be local pain, or occasionally a pathological fracture. Radiologically the lesion is seen as a clear-cut hole in the bone—usually a rib, skull bone, vertebra, pelvic bone, femur or humerus. An affected vertebral body may collapse, with consequent angular kyphosis. Investigations may show an excess of eosinophils in the blood. Eosinophilic granuloma may simulate a bone cyst, a primary or metastatic bone tumour, or tuberculosis. If multiple, it resembles Hand-Schüller-Christian disease.

Treatment. The lesion often heals spontaneously. Surgical curettage may accelerate healing. Radiotherapy has sometimes been given but it is now widely regarded as unnecessary.

HAND-SCHÜLLER-CHRISTIAN DISEASE

In this condition there is proliferation of reticulo-endothelial cells to form multiple lesions, chiefly in the skull but also in other bones. The deposits, yellowish in colour, consist of granulation tissue with abundant histiocytes, many of which contain cholesterol esters and from their vacuolated appearance are known as foam cells. The characteristic clinical features—diabetes insipidus and exophthalmos—are explained by the localisation of the lesions in the region of the hypophysis and orbits. There may be other manifestations of pituitary dysfunction, such as retarded growth. The disease progresses very slowly but is often fatal eventually.

Treatment. Radiotherapy may cause the lesions to regress.

LETTERER-SIWE DISEASE

This is the most serious form of non-lipoid granulomatosis or histiocytosis X. It begins in early childhood and progresses rapidly, usually with fatal outcome. Granulomatous deposits occur not only in bone but also in lymph glands, spleen and liver, which may show enlargement clinically. Radiographically, the skeletal lesions resemble those of Hand-Schüller-Christian disease.

GAUCHER'S DISEASE

Gaucher's disease is due to an inborn error of lipoid metabolism. There is deposition of the lipoid kerasin in the reticulum cells of the spleen, liver, bone marrow, and other tissues. The chief clinical manifestations are enlargement of the spleen and liver, and cyst-like changes in the bones due to deposits of kerasin-laden reticulum cells (Gaucher cells). The general health remains good. Radiographs show irregular cyst-like spaces in some of the bones, usually without enlargement of the bone. *Investigations :* Sternal puncture usually yields typical Gaucher cells.

Treatment. Splenectomy relieves local discomfort but does not cure the disease. Radiotherapy may cause the lesions to regress.

AFFECTIONS DUE TO ENDOCRINE ERRORS

PARATHYROID OSTEODYSTROPHY

(Hyperparathyroidism ; generalised osteitis fibrosa cystica; von Recklinghausen's disease)

The characteristic features of parathyroid osteodystrophy are lassitude, dyspepsia, generalised osteoporosis, and cystic changes in some of the bones.

Cause. It is caused by excessive parathyroid secretion, usually from an adenoma of one of the parathyroid glands.

Pathology. The excessive secretion of parathormone causes generalised absorption of bone, the calcium from which is liberated into the blood, whence it is excreted in excessive quantities in the urine. The bone becomes spongy and the cortices are thin. Cystic changes often develop in one or more of the long bones. The kidneys frequently contain calculi.

Clinical features. The patient is adult. There are pains in the bones, indigestion, and weakness. There may also be deformity from bending of softened bone, or a pathological fracture. *Radiographs* show rarefaction of the whole skeleton. The loss of density may be marked, and the cortices very thin. An early sign is irregular cortical erosion in the phalanges of the fingers. Scattered cystic changes may or may not be present in the long bones (Fig. 89). The skull shows a uniform fine granular mottling, sometimes with small translucent cyst-like areas. Radiographs of the renal tracts often show nephrolithiasis. *Investigations:* The

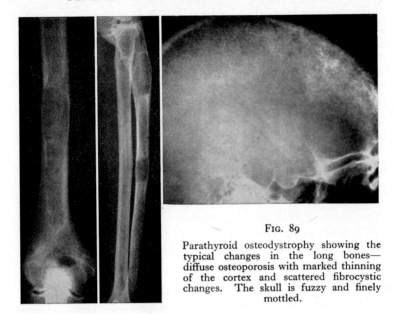

FIG. 89

Parathyroid osteodystrophy showing the typical changes in the long bones—diffuse osteoporosis with marked thinning of the cortex and scattered fibrocystic changes. The skull is fuzzy and finely mottled.

serum calcium is increased but the serum inorganic phosphate is diminished. The excretion of calcium and phosphate in the urine is increased.

Diagnosis. This is from other causes of diffuse or generalised rarefaction of bone. These are summarised in Table III (p. 127).

Treatment. The causative parathyroid tumour should be searched for and removed.

GIGANTISM

In gigantism (one form of hyperpituitarism) skeletal overgrowth is caused by an excess of anterior pituitary hormone occurring before the growth epiphyses have fused.

Pathology. There is an eosinophilic adenoma of the anterior lobe of the pituitary. Excessive growth occurs at the epiphysial cartilages. Despite this overactivity, epiphysial fusion occurs at about the normal time.

Clinical features. The patient, usually a boy, may grow to a height of seven feet or more, the main increase being in the limbs. Sexual development is often impaired and the mentality may be subnormal. Signs of acromegaly often develop later.

ACROMEGALY

The primary fault is the same as in gigantism—namely, an excessive secretion of anterior pituitary hormone—but it occurs after the epiphyses have fused. It is characterised by enlargement of the bones, especially of the hands, feet, skull, and mandible.

Pathology. As in gigantism, there is usually an eosinophilic adenoma of the anterior lobe of the pituitary. The enlargement of the bones is caused by deposition of new bone upon the surface of the original cortex.

Clinical features. The disease begins in early adult life. The physical features become coarse and heavy, the skin is thickened, and the hands and feet slowly enlarge. At first strong, the patient often becomes weak and sluggish later. *Radiographs* show marked enlargement of the bones of the hands and feet, and especially of the mandible. The vertebral bodies are also enlarged, especially in the antero-posterior plane.

CUSHING'S SYNDROME

This endocrine disorder is characterised by obesity, hyper-trichosis, hypertension, and, in women, amenorrhoea. It is induced by excessive secretion of adrenocortical hormones, caused either by a tumour of the adrenal cortex or by hyperplasia of the gland which may be secondary to a basophil adenoma of the pituitary. A similar condition may also be caused by prolonged administration of cortisone, prednisone, or related drugs.

The orthopaedic significance of Cushing's syndrome lies in the fact that it is accompanied by generalised rarefaction of the skeleton (Table III, p. 127). The bones become soft and may be fractured by trivial violence.

HYPOPITUITARISM

Deficient secretion of the anterior lobe of the pituitary leads to various types of physical and mental underdevelopment. In the **Lorain** type the main features are marked dwarfism and sexual infantilism, often with mental backwardness. In the **Fröhlich** type (dystrophia adiposo-genitalis) the predominant features are marked adiposity with impaired sexual development and sometimes with mental backwardness, but without marked dwarfism. Its importance in orthopaedic surgery arises from the fact that it predisposes to slipping of the upper femoral epiphysis (p. 346). About half the cases of slipped upper femoral epiphysis occur in patients of this type.

CRETINISM

Cretinism is characterised by dwarfism with sexual and mental retardation. It is caused by congenital deficiency of thyroid secretion. From the orthopaedic viewpoint the important features are retarded growth of the limb bones, kyphosis, and distortion of the joint surfaces. Early diagnosis is important because marked improvement follows treatment with thyroid extract.

TABLE III

TEN CAUSES OF DIFFUSE RAREFACTION OF BONE

Cause	Diagnostic Features
Osteoporosis	
Prolonged recumbency .	History of confinement to bed for months or years.
Senile (idiopathic) osteo-porosis	Spine predominantly affected. No biochemical change in blood.
Parathyroid osteodystrophy	Diagnostic biochemical changes in blood—serum calcium increased ; serum phosphate decreased.
Cushing's syndrome .	Characteristic clinical features—obesity, hypertrichosis, hypertension, amenorrhoea in women.
Osteomalacia	
Rickets (all types) . .	Rachitic changes at growing epiphyses. Biochemical changes depend on type of rickets (Table II, p. 121).
Nutritional osteomalacia .	Dietary deficiency apparent. Characteristic biochemical changes in blood — serum calcium normal (or decreased) ; serum phosphate decreased (Table II, p. 121).
Idiopathic steatorrhoea .	Excess of fat in faeces. Blood changes—serum calcium decreased ; serum phosphate normal (Table II, p. 121).
Tumour	
Multiple myelomatosis .	Usually multiple circumscribed lesions, but may be diffuse. Bence-Jones proteose often present in urine. Marrow biopsy shows excess of plasma cells.
Diffuse carcinomatosis .	Primary tumour demonstrable.
Leukaemia . . .	Blood examination and marrow biopsy show excess of immature white cells.

INFLAMMATORY LESIONS OF SOFT TISSUE

BURSITIS

Inflammation may occur in a normally situated bursa or in an adventitious bursa. It may arise from mechanical irritation or from bacterial infection.

IRRITATIVE BURSITIS

This is caused by excessive pressure or friction, occasionally by a gouty deposit. There is a mild inflammatory reaction in the wall of the bursa, and there is usually an effusion of clear fluid within the sac. Examples are the common bunion that forms over a prominent metatarsal head, prepatellar bursitis or ' housemaid's knee,' olecranon bursitis (sometimes caused by gout), and subacromial bursitis.

Treatment. In many cases the inflammation subsides with rest if continued pressure or friction is prevented. If the sac is distended the fluid may be aspirated, and the instillation of hydrocortisone through the aspiration needle may help to prevent recurrence. In resistant cases cure can be effected only by operative excision of the bursa.

INFECTIVE BURSITIS

There may be acute inflammation from infection with an organism of the pyogenic group, or chronic inflammation as in tuberculous bursitis. Examples of acute pyogenic bursitis are infected bunion and infected prepatellar bursitis. A bursa that is sometimes affected by tuberculosis is the trochanteric bursa.

Treatment. Treatment of acute suppurative bursitis is by surgical drainage and antibiotic drugs. In chronic bursitis excision of the bursa is required.

TENOSYNOVITIS

The term tenosynovitis implies inflammation of the thin synovial lining of a tendon sheath as distinct from its outer fibrous sheath. Like bursitis, tenosynovitis may be caused by mechanical irritation or by bacterial infection.

IRRITATIVE (FRICTIONAL) TENOSYNOVITIS

This is caused by excessive friction from over-use. The synovial sheath is mildly inflamed and there is an exudate of watery fluid within it. A similar traumatic inflammation may affect the flimsy paratenon surrounding those tendons that are devoid of synovial sheaths. This is termed paratendinitis (p. 275).

INFECTIVE TENOSYNOVITIS

Bacterial infection of a tendon sheath may be acute or chronic. Acute infective (suppurative) tenosynovitis is caused by an organism of the pyogenic group. There is an acute inflammatory reaction in the wall of the sheath, with a purulent exudate from it. It is an uncommon condition, but it is well recognised in the flexor tendon sheaths in the hand (p. 292).

In chronic bacterial tenosynovitis, also an uncommon lesion, the infection is often tuberculous. The synovial wall is much thickened and there is a fibrinous exudate. The flexor sheaths of the forearm and hand are the usual sites (compound palmar ganglion, p. 293).

TENOVAGINITIS

In tenovaginitis there is a mild chronic inflammation or thickening of the fibrous wall of a tendon sheath as distinct from the synovial lining. The cause is unknown : it is not due to bacterial infection. The only common sites are the mouths of the fibrous flexor sheaths in the fingers or thumb (' trigger ' finger, p. 305), and the sheaths of the extensor pollicis brevis and abductor pollicis longus tendons at the radial side of the wrist (de Quervain's syndrome, p. 304).

FIBROSITIS

Fibrositis is a clinical rather than a pathological entity. Some deny its existence. Certainly its nature is obscure. Nevertheless the term is a useful label for a clinical condition that at present lacks a complete explanation. The main features are pain in certain muscles, with tenderness when they are gripped or squeezed. Small firm nodules may be felt. Joint movements are full and there are no other objective signs. The condition is commonest in the muscles of the back, especially in the trapezius area (p. 171).

5*

TUMOURS OF SOFT TISSUE

The soft-tissue tumours that are met with in orthopaedic practice arise from the connective tissues or blood-vessels of the limbs or trunk. They may be benign or malignant.

BENIGN TUMOURS OF SOFT TISSUE

In the soft tissues of the limbs and trunk benign tumours are much more common than malignant tumours. Five types will be described: 1) neurofibroma; 2) fibroma; 3) lipoma; 4) haemangioma; 5) giant-cell tumour of tendon sheath.

NEUROFIBROMA

A neurofibroma forms a rather soft, circumscribed, rounded and slightly tender swelling in the skin or deeper tissues. It arises from the interstitial tissue of a peripheral nerve. Histologically it is composed of cellular fibrous tissue arranged in whorls. The tumour may be solitary; but in the condition known as multiple neurofibromatosis (von Recklinghausen's disease) (p. 108) numerous tumours are associated with pigmented areas on the skin. A neurofibroma growing within the spinal canal is an important cause of compression of the spinal cord or cauda equina.

FIBROMA

This is rather uncommon in the extremities. It is a firm, rounded, painless nodule, usually connected with a fascial or aponeurotic structure such as a digital flexor sheath.

LIPOMA

A common tumour that may arise in almost any part of the body, a lipoma forms a soft, lobulated mass enclosed within a thin capsule. It consists of fat, usually with little connective-tissue stroma. Less often it contains an abundance of fibrous tissue, which gives it a firm consistence (fibrolipoma).

HAEMANGIOMA

Haemangioma is a benign tumour of blood vessels. A **capillary haemangioma** forms a dark red, irregular, slightly raised blotch on the skin. It is usually congenital. A **cavernous haemangioma** is composed of widely dilated vascular channels with intervening connective tissue. It forms a localised or diffuse tumour within the skin, subcutaneous tissue or muscle. A characteristic feature of diagnostic importance is that the tumour is compressible.

Treatment. Superficial capillary haemangiomata fall within the province of the plastic surgeon. A localised deep cavernous haemangioma is usually amenable to excision. Extensive diffuse tumours cannot be eradicated, and in the worst cases amputation may be required.

Giant-cell Tumour of Tendon Sheath

This tumour occurs almost exclusively in the hand. It is described on page 296.

MALIGNANT TUMOURS OF SOFT TISSUE

Malignant tumours of soft tissue are uncommon. Of mesenchymal origin, they arise from connective tissues such as fascia, aponeurosis, tendon sheath, intermuscular septa, voluntary muscle, and synovial membrane. The following varieties will be considered : 1) fibrosarcoma ; 2) synovial sarcoma (malignant synovioma) ; 3) liposarcoma ; 4) rhabdomyosarcoma.

Fibrosarcoma

Fibrosarcoma is the commonest of the malignant connective tissue tumours arising from soft tissue. Derived from fibroblasts, it may arise in any fibrous connective tissue.

Pathology. The tumour consists of a firm rounded mass of pale pinkish tissue. It appears to be encapsulated, but the capsule forms no barrier to the spread of the tumour. Histologically it is composed of spindle cells with elongated nuclei. Metastases occur chiefly in the lungs.

Clinical features. The tumour occurs at any age. The complaint is of a progressively enlarging painless swelling. *On examination* the tumour is of firm consistence. A deep tumour is often attached to the underlying bone. Apart from the swelling, there is little interference with function until the late stages.

Course. Many fibrosarcomata grow slowly and are of relatively low malignancy. The prognosis is hopeful if efficient treatment is carried out at an early stage.

Treatment. Local excision, with a wide margin of healthy tissue, should be undertaken whenever practicable. Operation should be preceded and followed by radiotherapy. If local excision is impracticable, amputation will be required. In inoperable cases radiotherapy is a useful palliative measure.

SYNOVIAL SARCOMA (Malignant synovioma)

This is a rare tumour which arises from the synovial lining of a joint, tendon sheath, or bursa. It is usually highly malignant.

Pathology. The tumour grows as a solid, whitish, fleshy mass which tends to follow the plane of least resistance. It invades the surrounding soft tissues, but when it arises in a joint it seldom penetrates the bone or the articular cartilage. Histologically, the tumour is composed of masses of fusiform cells, but the picture is characterised by the formation of spaces or clefts lined by cuboidal cells, suggesting a synovial cavity. Metastasis occurs early through the blood stream, chiefly to the lungs.

Clinical features. Synovial sarcoma may occur at any age. The main symptoms are pain and swelling in the region of the affected joint, bursa, or tendon sheath. They develop insidiously and increase relentlessly without remission. When the swelling is superficial the overlying skin is warmer than normal. The movement of an affected joint is generally impaired only slightly, if at all. *Radiographic examination :* The tumour may be seen as a soft-tissue shadow, but there is seldom any alteration of bone texture or joint outline. Rather typically, flecks of calcification are seen scattered through the area of the tumour. Radiographs of the chest may show pulmonary metastases. *Investigations :* Biopsy reveals the characteristic histological appearance.

Diagnosis. A synovial sarcoma arising in a joint may be confused with chronic inflammatory arthritis, which may be associated with considerable thickening of the synovial membrane. A progressively increasing synovial swelling, with relatively little impairment of movement and normal radiographic findings, should always arouse suspicion of a synovial sarcoma. Biopsy should then be undertaken without delay.

Prognosis. The outlook is much worse than that for fibrosarcoma. The tumour is nearly always fatal from pulmonary metastases.

Treatment. If the anatomical relations of the tumour allow it, wide local excision, with pre-operative and post-operative radio-therapy, is recommended. When the tumour involves a joint amputation offers the best hope of cure. But if pulmonary metastases are already demonstrable amputation should usually be avoided and reliance placed upon palliative radiotherapy.

LIPOSARCOMA

This is a rare tumour whose characteristic histological feature is the presence of foamy embryonal cells containing intracellular fat. It grows as a multilobulated mass, usually in the buttock or thigh, and it often attains an enormous size. Metastases occur mainly in the lungs.

RHABDOMYOSARCOMA

This rare variety of soft-tissue sarcoma arises in skeletal muscle. It is characterised by cells with longitudinal and cross striation, or by primitive myoblasts. Highly malignant, it grows rapidly and metastasises early, mainly to the lungs.

NEUROLOGICAL DISORDERS
POLIOMYELITIS
(Infantile paralysis)

Poliomyelitis is a virus infection of nerve cells in the anterior grey matter of the spinal cord, leading in many cases to temporary or permanent paralysis of the muscles that they activate. In Great Britain the incidence of the disease increased so much in the years succeeding the second world war that its management—or rather the management of the paralytic disabilities that it produces—became one of the foremost problems of orthopaedic surgery. In recent years the incidence has decreased markedly, probably in consequence of the nation-wide programme of prophylactic vaccination.

Cause. It is caused by infection with an ultra-microscopic filterable virus, of which at least three types have been identified.

Pathology. The route of infection is uncertain. Probably the virus can gain access either through the nasopharynx or through the gastro-intestinal tract. Once in the body it finds its way to anterior horn cells of the spinal cord (Fig. 90) and sometimes to nerve cells in the brain stem. According to the virulence of the infection the cells may escape serious harm, or they may be damaged or killed.   If cells are damaged there is paralysis of the corresponding muscles but recovery is possible ; if the cells are killed paralysis is permanent.   The extent and distribution of the lesions vary widely from case to case.

Clinical features.   Although it is still commonest in children, poliomyelitis often attacks young adults.   For descriptive purposes the disease is conveniently divided into five stages.

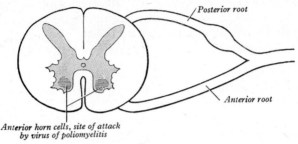

Posterior root

Anterior root

Anterior horn cells, site of attack by virus of poliomyelitis

FIG. 90

Section of spinal cord.   The virus of poliomyelitis attacks the anterior horn cells.   If the cells are killed there is permanent paralysis of the corresponding muscle fibres.   If the cells are damaged but not killed the paralysis is recoverable.

Stage of incubation.   This is the interval between infection and onset of symptoms.   It lasts about two weeks.   There are no symptoms.

Stage of onset.   This lasts about two days.   The symptoms are like those of influenza : headache, pains in the back and limbs, and general malaise.   *On examination* there is mild pyrexia, often with neck rigidity if flexion is attempted, and tenderness of muscles.   At this stage poliomyelitis may be confused with influenza or, on account of the limb pain, with acute osteomyelitis or pyogenic arthritis.   *Investigations :* Lumbar puncture usually reveals an increase of round cells in the cerebrospinal fluid.

In many cases the disease does not progress beyond this stage, the patient making a rapid and complete recovery.

Stage of greatest paralysis.   This stage, when it occurs, lasts about two months.   Paralysis develops rapidly and is usually at its greatest within a few hours, thereafter remaining unchanged throughout this stage.   The extent and distribution of the paralysis vary enormously. There may be no paralysis at all, or it may be total. In this stage muscle pain continues, and unparalysed muscles are often painful if stretched. If the respiratory muscles are paralysed preservation of life will be dependent upon the use of a mechanical respirator.

Stage of recovery. When any recovery of power occurs it may continue for about two years.[1] The degree of recovery varies within the widest limits. There may be complete recovery or there may be none.

Stage of residual paralysis. Paralysis or weakness persisting after two years is permanent. Its degree and extent vary from insignificant local weakness to almost total paralysis of the trunk and all four limbs.

Prognosis. In round figures, it may be stated that half of all patients clinically infected with poliomyelitis have no paralysis at any time. Of those with paralysis, 10 per cent die (usually from respiratory paralysis) ; 30 per cent recover fully ; 30 per cent have moderate permanent paralysis ; and 30 per cent have severe permanent paralysis.

Prophylaxis. In Britain prophylactic vaccination is by an attenuated living virus, taken by mouth.

Treatment. No specific treatment is available. In few diseases is the doctor so powerless to influence recovery : the patient either will or will not recover his muscle power, depending upon the severity of the neurological damage ; and there is very little that the doctor can do about it. The main duties of the orthopaedic surgeon are to prevent deformity, to assist returning muscle power by graduated exercises, and to reduce residual disability by the provision of appropriate appliances or by operations on joints or muscles. The treatment appropriate to each stage of the disease is best considered separately.

Stage of onset. The patient should rest in bed and may be given sedatives as required.

Stage of greatest paralysis. In this stage artificial respiration by a mechanical respirator may be necessary to preserve life if the respiratory muscles are paralysed. Paralysed limbs may have to be supported by splints in a neutral position to prevent the

---

[1] It will be observed that the figure 2 appears in the stated duration of each of the first four stages—2 weeks, 2 days, 2 months, 2 years. These are only very approximate figures, but they are easily memorised.

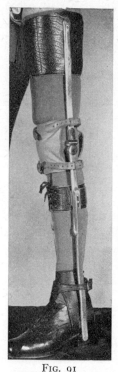

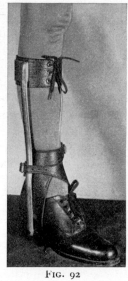

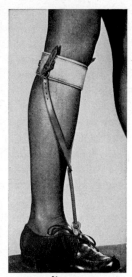

FIG. 92   FIG. 93

Three types of external supportive appliance for the
lower limb. Figure 91—Caliper to support the knee
after quadriceps paralysis. Figure 92—Below-knee
brace with T-strap for stabilising a weak ankle and
foot. Figure 93—Drop-foot spring used to maintain
dorsiflexion of the foot in paralysis of the anterior leg
muscles. This is only one of many types that
are available.

FIG. 91

development of contractures with consequent deformity. Fixed
equinus deformity of the ankle and foot is particularly liable to
develop in cases of paralysis of the anterior leg muscles unless
the foot is maintained at a right angle to the leg. Joints should
be put through a full range of movement daily, so far as pain
allows. Muscle pain may be eased by warmth, as from hot packs.
Whether or not the patient must remain in bed in this stage will
depend upon the degree and distribution of the paralysis.

Stage of recovery. The patient should be under the close supervision of a skilled physiotherapist. Any muscle that is seen to be
regaining power must be exercised, gently and patiently at first,
but later very strenuously, to encourage the greatest possible
redevelopment. It should be remembered that power may
improve partly as a result of recovery of the damaged nerve cells,
but partly also from hypertrophy of muscle fibres that have

escaped paralysis. When possible, walking should be resumed at this stage, if necessary with the aid of appliances, crutches, or sticks.

Stage of residual paralysis. The disability in this stage can often be reduced either by the provision of suitable external appliances, or by operation.

Appliances. The purpose of external appliances is to support joints that have lost their normal muscle control. They are required more often for the lower limbs and spine than for the upper limbs. The following are commonly prescribed : 1) spinal brace, to support a weakened spine ; 2) abdominal support, to check abdominal protrusion when the abdominal muscles are weak ; 3) knee caliper (Fig. 91), to hold the knee extended in cases of severe quadriceps paralysis ; 4) below-knee brace (Fig. 92), to stabilise a flail ankle or foot ; 5) single below-knee steel (lateral or medial) with ankle strap, to control varus or valgus deformity of the foot ; 6) drop-foot spring (Fig. 93), to hold the foot up when the dorsiflexor muscles are paralysed.

Operative treatment. Two main groups of operations are available : 1) arthrodesis of joints ; and 2) muscle or tendon transfers. *Arthrodesis* is a valuable method of stabilising joints that have lost their controlling muscles. It is particularly applicable to shoulder, elbow, wrist, spine, ankle, and foot. In *muscle or tendon transfer* operations the object is to use a healthy muscle to replace the function of one that is paralysed. The method finds its chief application in the upper limb. Examples are the transfer of part of the pectoralis major muscle to replace the function of paralysed elbow flexors, transfer of wrist flexors to serve as extensors of the fingers, and transfer of a flexor digitorum superficialis tendon to replace a paralysed opponens muscle.

CEREBRAL PALSY

(Spastic paralysis ; spastic paresis ; Little's disease)

The term cerebral palsy embraces a number of clinical disorders, mostly arising in childhood, the feature common to all of which is that the primary lesion is in the brain. The incidence of these disorders is such that cerebral palsy constitutes one of the country's major social and educational problems.

Cause. There is no single cause. Any event that results in damage to the brain may be responsible. Thus the causes may be classified into three groups : pre-natal, natal, and post-natal. *Pre-natal* causes include congenital defective development of the nervous system, and erythroblastosis leading to icterus gravis in the child, with consequent damage to the basal nuclei (kernicterus). *Natal* causes include damage to the brain from birth injury, and anoxaemia with consequent cerebral anoxia. Prematurity is believed to be an important factor. *Post-natal* causes include infections such as pertussis, encephalitis and meningitis, head injuries, and, in later life, cerebro-vascular accidents. In children it is not always easy to ascribe the fault in a given case, but probably the commonest causes are damage to the brain during difficult labour and cerebral anoxia during birth.

Types. A number of clinical types may be recognised, of which the most important are : 1) spastic paresis and 2) athetosis. Mixed types also occur.

SPASTIC PARESIS

Pathology. Part of the motor cortex is replaced by areas of gliosis. There is degeneration of the pyramidal tracts.

Clinical features. Usually within the first year it is noticed that the child has difficulty in controlling the movements of the affected limbs, and there is delay in sitting up, standing, and walking. Commonly the upper and lower limbs of one side are affected (hemiplegia). Less often there is involvement of a single limb (monoplegia), of both lower limbs (paraplegia), or of all four limbs (tetraplegia [1]). The trunk and face muscles may also be affected. *On examination* the features that are found constantly are weakness, spasticity, and imperfect voluntary control of movement. Usually there is also deformity, and in some cases there may be mental deficiency, impaired vision, or deafness. These various features are best considered separately.

Weakness. There is no true paralysis, but there may be fairly marked weakness of muscles. The weakness seldom affects all the muscles of a limb equally ; often there is marked muscle imbalance.

---

[1] Also termed (though less correctly) diplegia or quadriplegia.

Spasticity. The muscles are ' stiff ' : they resist passive movement of the joints, but when steady pressure is applied for some time they slowly relax, allowing the joint to be moved. When the pressure is released the spasm immediately returns. The tendon reflexes are exaggerated.

Lack of voluntary control. This is a striking feature, especially in severe cases. When the patient attempts to move a single group of muscles other groups contract at the same time.

Deformity. When spasm and muscle imbalance are pronounced they lead eventually to the development of fixed deformity. The stronger muscles hold the limb constantly in an unnatural position, and secondary adaptive changes take place in the muscles and periarticular tissues. The commonest deformities in the upper limb are flexion contracture of the elbow, pronation deformity of the forearm, flexion of the wrist, and adduction of the thumb. In the lower limb the common deformities are adduction of the hip, flexion of the knee, and equinus of the ankle.

Mental deficiency. Some impairment of mental capacity is often present, but by no means always. Lack of control of the facial and speech muscles makes the mental impairment seem worse than it actually is. *Defective vision* and *deafness* may also retard the child's progress.

The severity of the disability varies widely from case to case. In the mildest examples the child is able to lead a normal active life with very little handicap, whereas in a severe case the patient is almost helpless.

Prognosis. Since an essential part of the brain is destroyed and cannot be replaced complete cure is impossible. All that can be hoped for is improvement. To achieve even this requires endless patience on the part of the patient and the attendants. In many cases little or no real improvement is gained even after prolonged treatment, and the permanent shelter of a residential institution will be required. But in a small proportion gratifying improvement may be obtained, to the extent that a patient initially in need of institutional care is made independent and able to earn his own living.

Treatment. Up to the age of about 5 years treatment may be carried out at non-residential centres, but after the age of 5 a child who is considerably disabled should be admitted to a special residential school where adequate facilities and trained staff are available. During the first few months at the school a panel of specialists should decide whether or not the child is educable. If he is not, he should be returned to his own home, if suitable, or sent to a home for the helpless.

The methods of treatment available are muscle training, corrective splinting, speech therapy, and operations on tendons, bones, or nerves.

Muscle training. The principles of muscle training are to teach the child to relax spastic muscles, to develop the use of individual muscle groups, and to improve coordination. Repetitive rhythmic movements are valuable. Stage by stage the child is instructed in dressing, toilet, feeding, and walking.

Corrective splinting. Splints or plasters are especially useful in overcoming the deformities induced by spastic muscles. Deformity is first corrected by gradual stretching of the contracted muscles, if necessary under anaesthesia. The limb is held by plaster in the over-corrected position for three months. Thereafter removable braces or splints may be used indefinitely to prevent recurrence of the deformity.

Speech therapy. Many spastic children have a speech defect which, with constant grimacing and salivation, may lead one to suppose that there is mental deficiency when in fact this is not so. In these cases the speech therapist is sometimes able to achieve a marked improvement.

Operative treatment. Operations for spastic paralysis should be approached with caution, because the results are by no means uniformly satisfactory. Operation may be upon tendon, joint, or nerve.

Tendon division or elongation: Division or lengthening of the tendon of a spastic muscle reduces its mechanical advantage and improves muscle balance. Examples are lengthening of the tendo calcaneus in a case of spastic equinus deformity, and tenotomy of the adductors of the hip for adduction deformity. *Tendon transfer:* At certain sites transfer of the insertion of a muscle that is aggravating deformity may so modify the muscle's action that it serves as a correcting force instead of a deforming force. An example is the transfer of the insertion of the hamstring tendons from the tibia to the back of the femoral condyles : this eliminates the undesirable action of the spastic hamstrings in flexing the knee, while enhancing their desirable action as hip extensors. *Arthrodesis:* When skeletal growth is complete it is sometimes of benefit to fuse a joint in the position of function to overcome persistent deformity. *Neurectomy:* The principle is to divide part or the whole of a nerve that supplies an over-acting spastic muscle. An example is division of the anterior branch of the obturator nerve to overcome spastic adduction at the hip.

ATHETOSIS

Pathology. The main damage is in the basal nuclei.

Clinical features. The principal feature is the occurrence of generalised overlaid involuntary movements which have no pattern and which interfere with the performance of normal movements. Any part or the whole of the muscular system may be affected. In mild cases the child is able to lead a fairly normal life, but in the worst examples the patient may be unable to sit up, walk, feed himself, or express himself in words, even though the mental state may be good.

Treatment. In all except the mildest cases residential treatment is desirable, as for spastic paresis. The first essential in treatment is to teach the child general relaxation. Once this has been achieved, purposeful voluntary movements can be taught. Splints and appliances may be required, but in pure athetosis there is no place for operations on the limbs. Recently some successful results in cases of severe athetosis have been reported after surgical destruction of the globus pallidus.

SPINA BIFIDA

The neurological deficit that complicates the more severe cases of spina bifida leads to varying degrees of motor, sensory and visceral paralysis, and the consequent orthopaedic disability in the lower limbs may be complex. The number of children demanding orthopaedic care for such disabilities has greatly increased in recent years because a far higher proportion of children born with spina bifida survive now that the associated hydrocephalus can be controlled by a ventriculo-cardiac shunt. In fact spina bifida has become a combined neurological and orthopaedic problem second in importance only to that of cerebral palsy.

Pathology. The basic structural defect—failure of total closure of the embryonal neural tube or of mesodermal tissue to invest it—varies in degree. There may be no more than a dimple in the skin or a split spinous process, or at the other extreme there may be complete failure of closure of skin, vertebrae and dura, with failure of tubulation of part of the spinal cord.

It is important to distinguish between closed lesions, with intact skin, and open lesions in which skin is deficient and nerve tissue is exposed on the surface of the body. The distinction is important because open lesions demand urgent operation within a few hours of birth, to close the defect.

The neurological lesion. Neurological deficit may be primary or secondary. Primary paralysis is present at birth and implies failure of development of part of the spinal cord—myelodysplasia. This varies widely in degree. In a fairly common example there may be normal innervation down to the level of the fourth lumbar segment and failure of development below that level. But the lesion may be either less extensive or more extensive than this.

Secondary paralysis develops after birth, either from drying or infection of exposed nerve tissue when closure of an open lesion has been delayed, from stretching of tethered nerve fibres as growth occurs, or from compression of nerve tissue within the abnormal spinal canal.

Clinical assessment. It is difficult in small infants to assess accurately the extent of motor and of sensory paralysis, and particularly to determine the state of bladder function. Careful clinical assessment of muscle power may be aided when necessary by electrical tests.

Motor paralysis. Motor paralysis affects mainly the lower limbs and to some extent the trunk. The extent of limb paralysis corresponds to the degree of dysplasia or of secondary damage in the spinal cord. It varies from the very mild, in which there may be no more than minor weakness of a single muscle group, to the very severe in which there is total paralysis of the limbs. In the instance quoted above of normal cord function down to the fourth lumbar segment with loss of function below that, motor power is present only in the flexors and adductors of the hips, the quadriceps and the tibialis anterior: the remaining muscles are paralysed. This is a fairly common distribution but only one of an almost infinite variety. This uneven paralysis, with consequent muscle imbalance, leads commonly to secondary contractures with fixed deformity of hips, knees or feet. It may also lead to dislocation of the hip, a common sequel to gluteal and abductor paralysis in the presence of strong flexors and adductors.

Sensory paralysis. Motor paralysis is nearly always accompanied by sensory paralysis of approximately the same distribution. This makes treatment more difficult because the use of corrective splints is restricted by the risk of pressure sores on the insensitive skin.

Visceral paralysis. Incontinence of bladder and bowel is present in a high proportion of patients.

Hydrocephalus. Associated hydrocephalus, usually due to the Arnold-Chiari malformation of the hind-brain, is common and was formerly largely responsible for the poor rate of survival among children with severe spina bifida.

Treatment. No firm rules can be laid down because there is so much variation between individual cases. It is sufficient here to indicate the main principles of orthopaedic treatment. These have been well described by Sharrard (1969). They are: 1) to correct deformity; 2) to maintain correction; and 3) to promote the best possible function in the affected limbs. In general, orthopaedic treatment should be deferred until the age of one to three years, to ensure that the child is thriving well and is in a satisfactory state in so far as hydrocephalus and renal function are concerned: he may by then have had a ventriculo-cardiac shunt established and have undergone urinary diversion with the formation of an ileal conduit for reasons of hygiene.

Correction of deformity. There is only limited scope for non-operative correction of deformity because the insensitive skin will not tolerate well the pressure of splints or plasters. Nevertheless in a mild case daily manipulations by the parents may be of value. In most cases operation is required. This usually entails division or elongation of tight structures—tendon, muscle, ligament or joint capsule—in order to bring the limb into a neutral anatomical position. Occasionally corrective osteotomy may also be required. Dislocation of the hips can usually be reduced by manipulation after division of tight adductor muscles.

Maintenance of correction. To prevent recurrence of deformity, correct muscle balance must be established by appropriate tendon transfer operations (see p. 31) or by denervation of over-active muscles. At the hip, redislocation may be prevented by converting the ilio-psoas muscle, which in the absence of strong gluteal muscles tends to produce flexion and adduction contracture, into an abductor and extensor of the hip by transferring it through a window cut in the wing of the ilium to a new insertion at the back of the greater trochanter.

Development of limb function. Even when lower limb paralysis is severe it is nearly always possible to get the child walking with crutches once deformities have been overcome. In many cases external bracing in the form of limb calipers or other apparatus is essential, and prolonged training by a skilled physiotherapist is likely to be required if maximal function is to be achieved.

PERIPHERAL NERVE LESIONS

Disorders of the peripheral nerves come largely within the sphere of the neurologist, but the orthopaedic surgeon is concerned with lesions that have a mechanical basis and with those that lend themselves to reconstructive surgery.

Pathology. Nerves may be damaged by laceration, contusion, traction, compression, friction, or ischaemia. According to its severity, a nerve lesion may be classified as neurapraxia, axonotmesis, or neurotmesis (Seddon, 1942). In *neurapraxia* the damage is slight and it causes only a transient physiological block. Recovery occurs spontaneously within a few days or weeks. In *axonotmesis* the internal architecture of the nerve is preserved, but the axons are so badly damaged that peripheral degeneration occurs. Recovery can occur spontaneously, but it depends upon regeneration of the axons and may take many months (about 2·5 centimetres a month is the usual speed of regeneration). In *neurotmesis* the structure of the nerve is destroyed by actual division or by severe scarring. Recovery is possible only after excision of the damaged section and end-to-end suture of the stumps.

Clinical features. The effects of complete loss of conductivity of a nerve are motor, sensory, and autonomic. They are localised to the distribution of the nerve affected. *Motor changes :* The muscles are paralysed and wasted. Changes occur in the electrical

References and bibliography, page 445.

reactions, but they take between two and three weeks to develop. (These were described on p. 14.) *Sensory changes :* There is loss of cutaneous, deep, and postural sensibility. *Autonomic changes :* These include loss of sweating, loss of pilomotor response to cold (' goose-skin '), and temporary vasodilation with increased warmth, which, however, is followed later by vasoconstriction and coldness.

Complications. Injury to a peripheral nerve trunk is occasionally followed by severe burning pain in the distribution of the nerve. This is termed *causalgia*. It is a complication of incomplete rather than of complete lesions, and with few exceptions it is confined in the upper limb to the brachial plexus or the median nerve, and in the lower limb to the sciatic nerve or the tibial nerve. It may be a very disabling complication, the only effective treatment of which is by sympathetic denervation of the limb.

Treatment. *Severed nerve :* If a nerve is believed to be divided— for example, by a penetrating injury—the wound should be explored and the nerve identified. If the nerve is severed the ends should be examined carefully to determine the extent to which they have been damaged by laceration or bruising. Only in the case of a clean-cut division with minimal damage to the severed ends should primary suture be carried out. If these criteria are not satisfied it is better simply to tack the ends together with one or two sutures and to delay definitive repair until two or three weeks after the injury. At that time the extent of the scarring, and consequently the length of nerve to be resected, can be determined accurately, and thickening of the nerve sheath makes suture technically easier.

Closed injuries : In closed injuries complicated by nerve paralysis it is usually assumed that the nerve is in continuity, and expectant treatment is adopted at first. If signs of recovery are not observed within the expected time (calculated from the site of injury and length to be regenerated) exploration is advised. Such exploration should seldom be delayed for more than three or four months, because long delay prejudices successful repair if the nerve has been divided.

When a nerve lesion has been caused by stretching, compression, or ischaemia the essential principle of treatment is to ensure that the harmful conditions are relieved, if necessary by operation to free the nerve or to remove a compressing agent.

Irrecoverable lesions : The disability from permanent nerve paralysis can often be mitigated by tendon transfers or arthrodesis.

BRACHIAL PLEXUS INJURIES

Injuries of the brachial plexus are a major cause of partial or complete loss of function of the upper limb. Most of them are caused by forcible distraction of the upper extremity away from the neck by violent depression of the shoulder. The main injury is sustained by the upper roots of the plexus, which may be stretched, torn, or even avulsed from the spinal cord. There is consequent paralysis of the muscles supplied through the upper roots—chiefly the abductor and lateral rotator muscles of the shoulder and the flexors of the elbow (Erb type of paralysis). A less common type of brachial plexus injury is caused by forcible elevation of the arm and shoulder. This tends to drag on the lower roots of the plexus, with consequent motor and sensory paralysis mainly in the forearm and hand (Klumpke type of paralysis). In the most severe injuries the whole plexus is torn or avulsed and there is total paralysis of the upper limb.

Brachial plexus lesions in infants. In infants, brachial plexus injuries are usually caused during delivery (obstetrical palsy), and the risk is greatest in difficult breech deliveries. The upper arm type (Erb's palsy) is the more common. Soon after birth it is noticed that the child does not move the arm as he normally should.[1] Unopposed action of the unparalysed muscles tends to bring the arm into a position of adduction and medial rotation, and secondary contracture of the soft tissues may lead to fixed deformity in that position.

Prognosis depends upon the severity of the stretching injury. If this was mild full recovery may occur, though it may take many months ; but in a severe case there may be permanent loss of power and sensibility. The prognosis is less favourable in the rare lower arm type of lesion (Klumpke type) than in the commoner upper arm type. *Treatment.* The mother should be taught to move the limb frequently through the full range, to prevent fixed contracture. In late cases with permanent paralysis and deformity there is a place for late reconstructive operations such as corrective osteotomy, arthrodesis of the shoulder or tendon transfer operations.

Brachial plexus lesions in adults. In adults brachial plexus injuries are usually caused by forcible depression of the shoulder, especially in motor-cycle crashes. Clinical and electrical tests may indicate the approximate site of the lesion, and it is possible to determine by

---

[1] The two other main causes of failure to use the arm in infancy are birth fracture and hemiplegia.

myelography whether the roots of the plexus have been avulsed from the spinal cord.

Treatment. If the roots have been avulsed the outlook for worth-while recovery is poor, and a decision should be reached whether to attempt compensatory reconstructive operations, or in the worst cases whether to amputate a useless limb. If the roots of the plexus are not shown to be avulsed exploratory operation may be undertaken to determine the extent of the injury, and to allow repair of the nerves if it is found to be necessary and practicable. Even in a seemingly favourable case, however, the outlook for good recovery of motor and sensory function is always very doubtful.

References and bibliography, page 445.

CHAPTER THREE

Neck and Cervical Spine

THE commonest orthopaedic cause of neck disorders is degeneration of a cervical intervertebral disc. This may lead to protrusion of part of the disc contents (prolapsed cervical disc) or, more often, it may give rise to secondary osteo-arthritic changes in the intervertebral joints (cervical spondylosis). These conditions together make up a large proportion of the disabilities of the neck encountered in an orthopaedic out-patient department.

Disease of the cervical spine often interferes with the roots of the brachial plexus, causing radiating pain, muscle weakness, or sensory impairment in the upper limb. Indeed, the clinical importance of a cervical disorder often lies in its neurological effects rather than in the local lesion itself.

SPECIAL POINTS IN THE INVESTIGATION OF NECK COMPLAINTS

History

It is important to ascertain the relationship of the present symptoms to any previous neck disorder. Has there been any previous injury to the neck ? Or a sudden jerk of the head that might have jarred the cervical spine ? Is there a history of ' stiff neck '—a common feature in the early stages of prolapsed cervical disc ?

If pain in the upper limb is a prominent symptom, it is important to determine its exact distribution and its nature. Pain caused by pressure upon a nerve in the cervical region follows a clearly defined course which depends upon the particular nerve involved. It commonly extends throughout the upper arm into the forearm and hand, radiating to one or more of the digits. It is often accompanied by paraesthesiae, described as ' pins and needles ' or ' numbness.' Pain referred down the limb from a lesion of the shoulder or humerus is more diffuse, and it seldom extends below the elbow.

Exposure

The patient must be stripped to the waist. Preferably he should stand, or he may sit upon a stool.

Steps in Clinical Examination

A suggested routine for clinical examination of the neck is summarised in Table IV.

TABLE IV

ROUTINE CLINICAL EXAMINATION IN SUSPECTED
DISORDERS OF THE NECK

---

1. LOCAL EXAMINATION OF NECK, WITH NEUROLOGICAL AND
VASCULAR SURVEY OF UPPER LIMBS

Inspection	**Movements**
Bone contours	Flexion-extension
Soft-tissue contours	Lateral flexion
Colour and texture of skin	Rotation
Scars or sinuses	? Pain on movement
	? Crepitation on movement
Palpation	**Neurological state of upper limb**
Skin temperature	Muscular system
Bone contours	Sensory system
Soft-tissue contours	Sweating
Local tenderness	Reflexes

Vascular state of upper limb
    Colour
    Temperature
    Pulses

---

2. EXAMINATION OF POTENTIAL EXTRINSIC SOURCES
OF NECK SYMPTOMS

Symptoms suggestive of a neck disorder may arise from the ears or throat. Symptoms in the upper limb suggesting a neck disorder with involvement of the brachial plexus may arise from shoulder, elbow, or nerve trunks in their peripheral course.

---

3. GENERAL EXAMINATION

General survey of other parts of the body. Neck symptoms may be only one manifestation of a more widespread disease.

Movements

The movements to be examined are flexion, extension, lateral flexion to right and left, and rotation to right and left. Flexion-extension movements occur mainly at the occipito-atlantoid joint but to some extent throughout the cervical spine. Lateral flexion takes place throughout the cervical spine. Rotation occurs largely at the atlanto-axial joint, with a small range of movement at the other joints. It is important to find out whether movement causes pain and, if so, whether the pain is felt locally in the neck or whether it is referred down the upper limbs. It should be noted also whether movement is accompanied by audible or palpable crepitation.

Neurological Examination of Upper Limbs
This is an essential step in the investigation of the neck because cervical lesions so often interfere with the brachial plexus.

Muscular system. The muscles of the shoulder girdle, arm, forearm, and hand must be examined for wasting or fasciculation, a comparison being made on the two sides. The tone and power of each muscle group are then tested in turn and a comparison is made with the opposite limb.

Sensory system. Examine the patient's sensibility to touch and pin-prick. In appropriate cases test also the sensibility to deep stimuli, joint position, vibration, and heat and cold.

Sweating. Feel whether the digits are moist or dry. Sweating is dependent upon intact sudomotor nerve fibres.

Reflexes. Compare on the two sides the biceps jerk (mainly C.6), the triceps jerk (mainly C.7), and the brachioradialis jerk (mainly C.6).

From the findings elicited it should be possible to determine whether there is a neurological disturbance and, if so, whether it is of upper or lower motor neurone type, and the identity of the roots, trunks, or branches involved.

Vascular Examination of the Upper Limb
The subclavian artery is sometimes interfered with by lesions of the neck. The efficiency of the circulatory system in each upper limb must therefore be determined. Judge and compare on the two sides the colour and warmth of the forearm, hand, and fingers. Test and compare the radial pulses, first with the limb at rest, then with the shoulder depressed and the head rotated towards the side examined.

Extrinsic Causes of Neck Symptoms
Occasionally neck symptoms have their origin outside the neck itself. Thus pain may be referred to the neck from the ears or throat. These sites should be examined routinely for evidence of disease.

Symptoms in the upper limb that might suggest the possibility of a neck disorder involving the brachial plexus may, in fact, have their origin in the shoulder or elbow, or at any point along the peripheral distribution of the nerve trunk.

Radiographic Examination
Routine radiographs of the cervical spine include an antero-posterior and a lateral projection. Additional projections are often required

when it is desired to show a particular structure more clearly. For a study of the dens [odontoid process] of the axis a special antero-posterior projection is made through the open mouth. Oblique projections are essential for a proper investigation of the intervertebral foramina, and an oblique view of the lower cervical region is valuable in revealing the size and shape of a cervical rib. In cases of special difficulty stereoscopic radiography, tomography, or cineradiography may be helpful. If an intraspinal lesion is suspected, myelography is required.

CLASSIFICATION OF DISORDERS OF THE NECK AND CERVICAL SPINE

DEFORMITIES

> Infantile torticollis
> Congenital short neck
> Congenital high scapula

INFECTIONS OF BONE

> Tuberculosis of the cervical spine
> Pyogenic infection of the cervical spine

ARTHRITIS OF THE SPINAL JOINTS

> Ankylosing spondylitis
> Osteoarthritis of the cervical spine
> (cervical spondylosis)

MECHANICAL DERANGEMENTS

> Prolapsed intervertebral disc
> Cervical rib
> Cervical spondylolisthesis

TUMOURS

> Benign and malignant tumours in relation to the cervical
> spine and nerve roots

MISCELLANEOUS

> Cervical fibrositis

INFANTILE TORTICOLLIS
(' Congenital ' torticollis ; muscular torticollis)

Infantile torticollis is the commonest form of wry-neck.   The head is tilted and rotated by contracture of the sternomastoid muscle of one side.   Strictly this is not a true congenital deformity because it arises after birth.

Cause.   This is uncertain.   Probably there is interference with the blood supply of the sternomastoid muscle, caused by injury during birth.

Pathology.   In the established condition the affected muscle is replaced by contracted fibrous tissue.   In some cases contracture is known to have been preceded, in early infancy, by a tumour-like thickening of the muscle (' sternomastoid tumour '), the histology being that of muscle infarction and replacement by fibrous tissue.

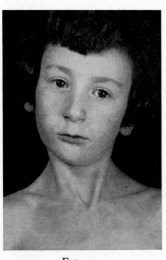

FIG. 94

Infantile torticollis.   Note the tense cord-like left sternomastoid muscle and the facial asymmetry.

Clinical features.   The child, often between 6 months and 3 years old when brought for consultation, is noticed to hold the head on one side.   *On examination*, the contracted muscle is felt as a tight cord.   The ear on the affected side is approximated to the corresponding shoulder.   In long-established cases there is retarded development of the face on the affected side, with consequent asymmetry (Fig. 94).

Diagnosis.   The condition has to be distinguished from other forms of wry-neck, including structural deformities of the cervical spine, ocular torticollis, muscle spasm from a local inflammatory lesion such as infected glands, and psychogenic (hysterical) torticollis.   The important diagnostic features are the history, the cord-like contracted muscle, and the facial asymmetry.

Treatment.   If the condition is seen at the stage of ' sternomastoid tumour,' repeated stretching of the muscle under the supervision of a physiotherapist is effective. In established cases the contracted muscle should be divided at its lower attachment.

CONGENITAL SHORT NECK
(Klippel-Feil syndrome)

This is an uncommon non-familial congenital malformation of the cervical spine characterised by short neck and limitation of head movements. The cause is unknown.

The degree of abnormality varies widely. The bony deformity consists in fusion of two or more of the cervical vertebrae. Clinically, the neck appears short or absent, and the hair-line is low. The neck may also be webbed. Movements of the head are restricted. *Radiographs* show the underlying bony abnormality.

Treatment. Operation is seldom indicated, but upper thoracoplasty is occasionally worth while simply for cosmetic improvement.

CONGENITAL HIGH SCAPULA
(Sprengel's shoulder)

Congenital high scapula is an uncommon congenital deformity characterised by an abnormally high position and relative fixity of the scapula. The cause is unknown. The anomaly represents a failure of the scapula—originally a cervical appendage—to descend during development to its normal thoracic position. The scapular muscles are ill developed and may be represented only by tough fibrous bands.

Clinically, the scapula on one or both sides is abnormally high. Its attachments seem almost rigid and it does not rotate freely during abduction of the arm. The range of shoulder abduction is consequently impaired, but the functional disability is slight.

Treatment. The condition is often best left alone, but some cases are suitable for operation. The upper part of the scapula (above its spine) is excised, the posterior scapular muscles are separated at their origins from the spinal column, the bone-and-muscle mass is displaced downwards, and the muscles are re-attached lower down to hold the scapula in its normal position.

TUBERCULOSIS OF THE CERVICAL SPINE
(Tuberculous cervical spondylitis)

Tuberculosis is far less common in the cervical spine than in the thoracic and lumbar regions. The general features of tuberculosis of bones and joints were described in Chapter II.

6

Pathology. The organisms reach the cervical spine through the blood stream from a pre-existing focus—latent or overt—elsewhere in the body. The infection begins in the front of a vertebral body, or in an intervertebral disc (Fig. 95). Destruction of bone and intervertebral disc leads to anterior collapse with consequent cervical kyphosis (Fig. 96). The degree of destruction varies

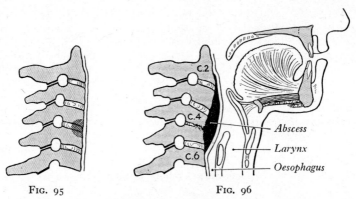

FIG. 95   FIG. 96

Tuberculosis of the cervical spine. Figure 95—The infection begins at the front margin of a vertebral body close to the intervertebral disc, or possibly in the disc itself, as indicated by the shaded area. Figure 96—The opposing surfaces of the bodies of C.4 and C.5 have been eroded and the intervening disc is destroyed. Pus has collected behind the prevertebral fascia, forming a bulging retropharyngeal abscess.

widely, depending upon the virulence of the organism and the resistance of the patient. Formation of pus leads either to a retropharyngeal abscess (behind the prevertebral fascia), which may eventually point at the posterior margin of the sternomastoid muscle, or, if the pus tracks posteriorly, to a sub-occipital abscess. The spinal cord may be damaged by direct pressure of an abscess, or by secondary thrombosis of the vessels of the cord.

Clinical features. The disease occurs mainly in children and young adults. There is pain in the neck and occiput, aggravated by movement. In addition, one or more of the following symptoms may be present : difficulty in swallowing ; abscess or sinus at the side or back of the neck ; neurological symptoms from spinal cord dysfunction, the upper limbs being affected before the lower. *On examination* the head is held rigidly, often supported by the hands. The cervical muscles stand out in spasm. One or more of the spinous processes may appear prominent, due to cervical kyphosis. There is local tenderness on firm palpation over the spinous processes. All movements of the head and neck are restricted, and cause pain if forced. An abscess may be present in the sub-occipital region, behind the sternomastoid muscle, or behind the pharynx (see below). Associated tuberculous lesions elsewhere are common. *Radiographs* always show diminution of disc space, usually some destruction of bone (Fig. 96), and sometimes an abscess shadow. *Investigations :* The erythrocyte sedimentation rate is raised in the active stage. The Mantoux test or Heaf test is positive. Pus obtained by aspiration of an abscess may yield tubercle bacilli.

Complications. *Retropharyngeal abscess :* This causes difficulty in swallowing (dysphagia). Examination through the mouth shows the posterior wall of the pharynx bulged forwards in the midline. Eventually the abscess may point behind the sterno-mastoid muscle. If neglected, it may rupture into the pharynx.

Spinal cord dysfunction. If the spinal cord is affected there will be neurological signs (sensory, motor, and visceral) at and below the level of the lesion. Unless successfully treated, dysfunction may advance to complete paralysis.

Diagnosis. Tuberculosis must be distinguished from other causes of deformity or pain in the neck, such as congenital malformations of the cervical vertebrae, deformities caused by previous injury, osteoarthritis, other infections of the spinal column, and ankylosing spondylitis. It must also be differentiated from other causes of retropharyngeal abscess and from other causes of spinal cord dysfunction. Important diagnostic features are the history (contact with tuberculosis, or tuberculous lesions elsewhere), the marked spasm of the neck muscles with restriction of all movements, abscess formation and the radiographic findings.

Treatment. The principles of treatment are the same as for other forms of skeletal tuberculosis (p. 76). *General treatment* includes rest in a country hospital and chemotherapy in the form of streptomycin, para-amino-salicylic acid (PAS), and iso-nicotinic acid hydrazide (INAH). *Local treatment* is by rest for the spine (in plaster bed or plaster case) until the disease is quiescent—often a matter of several months. Thereafter a plastic collar is worn until the lesion is shown to be well healed.

Operation is sometimes required and the following are the main indications. 1) To drain a retropharyngeal abscess that threatens to rupture or to cause asphyxia. 2) In a florid case, to remove necrotic bone and debris and then to embed a bone graft in the cavity. 3) To decompress a spinal cord damaged by pressure of abscess or granuloma. 4) In the quiescent stage, to fuse the affected region of the spine if it is judged to be unstable.

PYOGENIC INFECTION OF THE CERVICAL SPINE
(Pyogenic cervical spondylitis)

Infection of the cervical vertebrae or intervertebral discs with pyogenic organisms is uncommon. It is usually caused by the streptococcus, staphylococcus or pneumococcus, and occasionally by other bacteria, including typhoid bacilli or brucella abortus.

Pathology. The organisms reach the spinal column by the general blood stream (from a septic focus elsewhere), by lymphatic channels (from a local infection, for instance in the pharynx), or possibly by the spinal venous plexus (from a focus in the pelvis). As in tuberculous spondylitis, there is destruction of bone and intervertebral disc, with or without abscess formation. The spinal cord may be damaged by direct pressure or by thrombosis.

Clinical features. The onset is usually acute or subacute, with pyrexia. The clinical features are like those of tuberculous spondylitis (p. 153), but the course is more rapid. A suppurative process elsewhere in the body (for instance, in the pharynx or pelvis) is usually present. *Radiographs* show local osteoporosis or erosion of bone, diminution of disc space, and sometimes subligamentous new bone formation. *Investigations :* The erythrocyte sedimentation rate is raised and polymorphonuclear leucocytosis is to be expected. Appropriate agglutination tests may be positive.

Diagnosis. The condition must be distinguished from tuberculous spondylitis, which it may resemble closely. A history of pre-existing septic focus, the relatively rapid onset and course, with pyrexia and leucocytosis, and identification of the causal organism in pus, are the main diagnostic criteria.

Treatment. Appropriate antibiotic drugs (see p. 72) should be given systemically. The cervical spine must be immobilised in a plaster bed, plaster collar, or brace ; sometimes continuous head traction is required for relief of spasm. When there is an abscess it should be drained, especially if the spinal cord is threatened. Later, a plastic collar (Fig. 103, p. 164) may be required. Spontaneous fusion of the affected vertebrae usually makes operative fusion unnecessary.

ANKYLOSING SPONDYLITIS

Ankylosing spondylitis creeps up the spine from below. Only in about a third of the cases does it reach the cervical region, to cause aching pain and permanent stiffness—sometimes total rigid ankylosis—of the intervertebral joints. The general features of the disease as a whole will be described in the chapter on the spine (p. 195).

OSTEOARTHRITIS OF THE CERVICAL SPINE
(Cervical spondylosis ;   cervical spondylarthrosis)

Degenerative changes are common in the cervical spine. Beginning in the intervertebral discs, they affect the posterior intervertebral joints secondarily, causing pain and stiffness of the neck, sometimes with referred symptoms in an upper limb.

Cause. The primary degenerative changes are often initiated by injury. In other cases the condition is simply a manifestation of the widespread degenerative changes that occur with increasing age.

Pathology. Degenerative arthritis occurs most commonly in the lowest three cervical joints. The changes affect first the central intervertebral joints (between the vertebral bodies) and later the posterior intervertebral (facet) joints. In the central joints there is degenerative narrowing of the intervertebral disc, and bone reaction at the joint margins leads to the formation of osteophytes (Fig. 97). In the posterior intervertebral joints the changes are those of osteoarthritis in any diarthrodial joint—namely, wearing away of the articular cartilage and the formation of osteophytes (spurs) at the joint margins (Fig. 98).

Secondary effects. Osteophytes commonly encroach upon the intervertebral foramina, reducing the space for transmission of the cervical nerves (Fig. 98). If the restricted space in a foramen is still further reduced by traumatic oedema of the contained soft tissues, manifestations of nerve pressure are likely to occur. Exceptionally, the spinal cord itself may suffer damage from encroachment of osteophytes within the spinal canal.

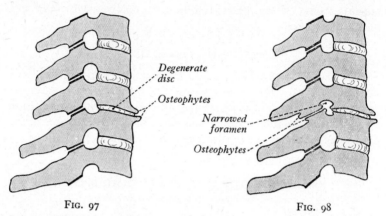

FIG. 97   FIG. 98

Osteoarthritis of the cervical spine. At first there is simply degeneration and narrowing of the intervertebral disc, with the formation of osteophytes anteriorly (Fig. 97). Later, the posterior or facet joints are affected : the articular cartilage is worn away and marginal osteophytes may encroach upon the intervertebral foramen (Fig. 98).

Clinical features. The symptoms are in the neck or in the upper limb, or both.

Neck symptoms consist chiefly of aching pain in the back of the neck or in the trapezius area, a feeling of stiffness, and ' grating ' on movement. Usually slight, they are liable to periodic exacerbations, probably from unremembered strains or repetitive movements.

In the *upper limb* there may be a vague, ill defined and ill localised ' referred ' pain spreading over the shoulder region, or there may be more serious symptoms from interference with one or more of the cervical nerves in their foramina. The main feature of nerve root irritation is radiating pain along the course of the affected nerve or nerves, often reaching the digits. There may also be paraesthesiae in the hand, in the form of tingling or 'pins and needles.' Noticeable muscle weakness is uncommon.

On examination, the neck may be slightly kyphotic. The posterior cervical muscles may be somewhat tender but they are not in spasm. Movements are not markedly diminished except during acute exacerbations or when the degenerative changes are very advanced. Audible crepitation on movement is common. In the upper limb objective findings are usually slight or absent, for

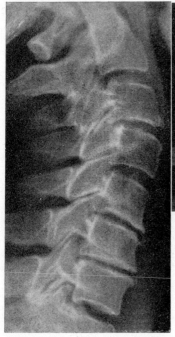
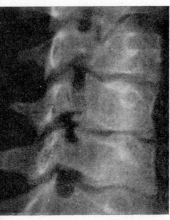

FIG. 99

Osteoarthritis of cervical spine. Note in the lateral view (left) the narrowed intervertebral space, with marginal osteophyte formation, at C.5-6 and at C.6-7. The oblique view (right) shows severe encroachment of osteophytes upon an intervertebral foramen (compare with the normal foramen below).

nerve pressure is seldom great enough to produce well defined objective neurological signs (compare prolapsed intervertebral disc). Thus demonstrable motor weakness or sensory impairment is exceptional. Depression of one or more of the tendon reflexes is, however, fairly common. *Radiographic examination :* There is narrowing of the intervertebral disc space, with formation of osteophytes at the vertebral margins, especially anteriorly (Fig. 99). Encroachment of osteophytes upon an intervertebral foramen is demonstrated best in oblique projections.

Diagnosis. Distinction has to be made 1) from other causes of neck pain, and 2) from other causes of upper limb pain (Fig. 100).

Other causes of neck pain : These include prolapsed cervical disc, tuberculous or pyogenic infection, tumours involving the vertebral column, and fibrositis.

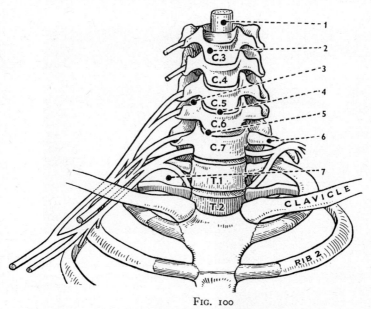

FIG. 100

Seven causes of interference with the brachial plexus or its roots. 1. Tumour of cord. 2. Tumour of spinal column. 3. Tumour of nerve root. 4. Prolapsed cervical disc. 5. Osteoarthritis. 6. Cervical rib. 7. Tumour at thoracic inlet.

Other causes of upper limb pain : These are as follows : Central lesions—Tumours involving the spinal cord or its roots ; cervical spondylolisthesis. Plexus lesions—Tumours at the thoracic inlet (Pancoast) ; cervical rib ; prolapsed intervertebral disc. Shoulder lesions with radiating pain in the upper arm. Skeletal lesions such as a tumour, infection, or Paget's disease of a bone of the upper extremity. Elbow lesions, such as ' tennis elbow ' or arthritis. Distal nerve lesions such as friction neuritis of the ulnar nerve at the elbow or compression of the median nerve in the carpal tunnel.

Osteoarthritis of the cervical spine is common in patients beyond middle life, and it is often symptomless : consequently, if osteoarthritic changes are found radiographically during the investigation of neck or upper limb pain it does not necessarily follow that the symptoms are caused by the arthritis. The diagnosis is at best presumptive, never unequivocal ; before it is justified, other causes of similar symptoms must be excluded by careful investigation (Fig. 100).

Complications. If the spinal canal is markedly narrowed by osteophytes the spinal cord may be damaged, with progressive upper motor neurone disturbance affecting all four limbs and possibly the bladder. This complication is serious but uncommon.

Treatment. There is a strong tendency for the symptoms of cervical spondylosis to subside spontaneously, though they may persist for many months and the structural changes are clearly permanent. Treatment is thus aimed towards assisting natural resolution of temporarily inflamed or oedematous soft tissues. In mild cases such measures include analgesic drugs and various forms of physiotherapy (radiant heat, short-wave diathermy, massage, traction, or exercises). Manipulation is sometimes recommended, but in the presence of extensive osteophytes it is hazardous because it may damage the spinal cord ; it should therefore be employed with extreme caution, and only by those familiar with the technique. In the more severe cases it is wise to provide rest and support for the neck by a closely-fitting collar of plaster or plastic (Fig. 103), which should be worn for one to three months according to progress.

In the exceptional cases in which the spinal cord is constricted, decompression either from in front or by laminectomy may be required, and thereafter it may be advisable to fuse the affected segments of the spinal column by a bone-grafting operation.

PROLAPSED CERVICAL DISC

Displacement of intervertebral disc material in the cervical spine is much less common than it is in the lumbar region. Even so, examples are encountered fairly frequently. The condition is characterised by pain and stiffness in the neck, often with neurological manifestations in the upper limb and sometimes with signs of spinal cord compression.

6*

Cause. Injury is a predisposing factor, though a history of injury cannot be obtained in every case. Probably an intrinsic change in the substance of the disc makes it prone to rupture and displacement.

Pathology. The disc between C.5-6 and that between C.6-7 are those most frequently affected. Part of the gelatinous nucleus pulposus protrudes through a rent in the annulus fibrosus at its weakest part, which is postero-lateral ; or part of the annulus

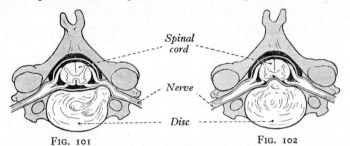

FIG. 101   FIG. 102

Prolapsed cervical disc. Figure 101 shows a lateral prolapse, with compression of the issuing nerve. Figure 102 shows the much less common central prolapse, with impingement upon the spinal cord.

itself may be displaced. If slight, the protrusion bulges the pain-sensitive posterior longitudinal ligament, causing local pain in the neck. If large, the protrusion herniates through the posterior ligament and may impinge upon the nerve leaving the spinal canal at that level (lateral prolapse) (Fig. 101), or occasionally upon the spinal cord itself (central prolapse) (Fig. 102). Healing is probably by shrinkage and fibrosis of the extruded material rather than by its reposition within the disc. *Secondary effects :* Prolapse of a disc accelerates its degeneration and predisposes to the development of osteoarthritis in later years.

Clinical features. *Central protrusions :* These lead to manifestations of spinal cord compression and may be confused with spinal cord tumours or other central neurological disorders. They fall within the province of the neurosurgeon rather than the orthopaedic surgeon. *Lateral protrusions :* The characteristic clinical picture is as follows. The patient sustains an injury to the neck—often a jarring or twisting strain—which may seem slight at the time and may cause no immediate effects. Hours or days later there is a rapid development of acute ' stiff neck, with severe pain made worse by coughing or similar strains. Hours or days later still, the pain begins to radiate over the shoulder and throughout the length of the upper limb ; it is felt strictly in the course of a cervical nerve. Paraesthesiae are felt in the digits. *On examination*, there is limitation of certain neck movements by pain, but movement in at least one direction (often lateral flexion away from the affected side) is free. In the upper limb there is a full range of joint movements. There are slight muscle wasting and slight sensory impairment in the distribution of a cervical nerve. The corresponding tendon reflex (biceps jerk in C.5-6 lesions ; triceps jerk in C.6-7 lesions) is depressed or absent.

Variations. The characteristic features described are not always present. Variations are common. Thus a history of injury is not always obtainable. The symptoms may be confined to the neck, the upper limb being spared ; or they may be confined entirely to the upper limb. Motor changes (wasting and weakness) may be marked, sometimes amounting to almost complete paralysis of a muscle or a group of muscles ; or, on the other hand, they may be absent. Similarly, wide variations in the degree of sensory impairment are noted.

Radiographs characteristically show a normal appearance in the first attack, but narrowing of one of the disc spaces (usually C.5-6 or C.6-7) is often demonstrable. Such narrowing denotes previous disc degeneration ; it cannot be explained simply by extrusion of disc substance because the extruded matter forms only a small proportion of the total volume of the disc.

Diagnosis.[1] Prolapsed cervical disc has to be differentiated 1) from other causes of neck pain, and 2) from other causes of upper limb pain (Fig. 100). The main conditions that may be confused with it are the same as those listed in the differential diagnosis of cervical osteoarthritis (p. 160). Diagnosis is presumptive and never unequivocal (unless confirmed at operation). A confident diagnosis is justified only when a suggestive history is associated with the signs of a lesion of a single cervical nerve, and provided always that other possible causes have been excluded by careful investigation. Diagnostic myelography is seldom justified unless

---

[1] Lateral protrusions only are considered here. Central protrusions with spinal cord compression fall within the province of the neurosurgeon.

a spinal tumour is seriously suspected, or unless there are signs of compression of the spinal cord.

Relationship between prolapsed disc and osteoarthritis.   The clinical features of the two conditions are similar.   Distinction is difficult if the radiographs show arthritic changes, because the arthritis may be only incidental and itself symptomless.   Nerve pressure is probably greater in prolapsed disc than in osteoarthritis ; consequently the symptoms tend to be more clearly defined and the objective signs more marked.   Fortunately differentiation is not important in practice, because the treatment of both conditions is usually similar.

Course.[1]   There is a strong tendency to spontaneous recovery, but symptoms often persist with decreasing severity for as long as six months or more.

Treatment.[1]   This depends upon the nature and severity of the individual case.   When the symptoms are slight no treatment other than perhaps a mild analgesic drug is required.   In the more severe cases treatment is advisable, especially in the early acute stage.   If the neck is ' stiff ' and if movements aggravate the neck and limb pain, rest for six weeks in a supportive collar made from plaster-of-Paris or from plastic (Fig. 103) is the most satisfactory method.   Continuous head traction in recumbency is a useful alternative.   Apart from these measures, reliance must be placed upon palliative treatment such as physiotherapy in the form of intermittent manual traction, short-wave diathermy, radiant heat, or massage.   Operative removal of lateral disc protrusions is potentially dangerous and is seldom justified.

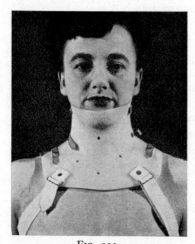

Fig. 103

Plastic collar for immobilising the cervical spine in severe cases of prolapsed disc or osteoarthritis.

------

[1] Lateral protrusions only are considered here.   Central protrusions with spinal cord compression fall within the province of the neurosurgeon.

CERVICAL RIB

A cervical rib is a congenital over-development, bony or fibrous, of the costal process of the seventh cervical vertebra. It often exists without causing symptoms, but it may cause neurological or vascular disturbance in the upper limb.

Cause. The cause of the congenital error is unknown. The tendency to dropping of the shoulder girdle that occurs in adult life is held responsible for the onset of symptoms.

Pathology. The over-developed costal process may be unilateral or bilateral. It may be of any size from a small bony protrusion, often with a fibrous extension, to a complete supernumerary rib. The subclavian artery and the lowest trunk of the brachial plexus arch over the rib. In a proportion of cases the nerve trunk suffers damage at the site of pressure against the rib ; this accounts for the neurological manifestations. The vascular changes are probably similarly accounted for by local damage to the subclavian artery, from which emboli may be repeatedly discharged into the peripheral vessels of the upper limb.

Clinical features. Cervical rib is often symptomless. When symptoms occur, they usually begin during early adult life. They may be neurological, vascular, or combined.

Neurological manifestations. The sensory symptoms are pain and paraesthesiae in the forearm and hand, most marked towards the medial (ulnar) side, and often relieved temporarily by changing the position of the arm. The motor symptoms include increasing weakness of the hand, with difficulty in carrying out the finer movements. *On examination*, there is usually an area of sensory impairment—sometimes complete anaesthesia—in the forearm or hand. The affected area does not correspond in distribution to any of the peripheral nerves, but may be related to the lowest trunk of the brachial plexus. There may be wasting of the muscles of the thenar eminence or of the interosseous and hypothenar muscles.

Vascular manifestations. The changes that have been observed range from dusky cyanosis of the forearm and hand to gangrene of the fingers. The radial pulse may be weak or absent.

Radiographs show the abnormal rib : if small, it is seen best in oblique projections (Fig. 104).

Diagnosis. Radiographic demonstration of a cervical rib does not prove that it is the cause of symptoms. The condition has to be distinguished 1) from other causes of pain and paraesthesiae in the forearm and hand, 2) from other causes of muscle wasting in the hand, and 3) from other causes of peripheral vascular changes in the upper limb.

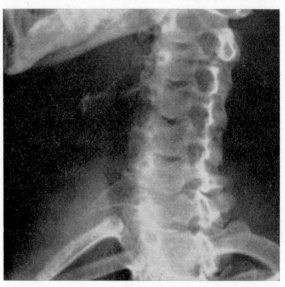

FIG. 104

Cervical rib. Typical appearance of a small supernumerary rib. This one caused severe neurological symptoms and signs. A cervical rib is shown best by an oblique radiograph such as this.

Other causes of pain in the forearm and hand (Fig. 100). The important alternative causes are as follows : *Central lesions*— Tumours involving the spinal cord or its roots ; cervical spondylolisthesis. *Plexus lesions*—Tumours at the thoracic inlet (Pancoast) ; prolapsed cervical disc ; cervical osteoarthritis. *Distal nerve lesions*—Friction neuritis of the ulnar nerve at the elbow ; pressure upon the median nerve in the carpal tunnel. *Other causes of muscle wasting in the hand.* These include the following : *Central lesions*—Syringomyelia ; tumour of spinal cord ; poliomyelitis ; progressive muscular atrophy (motor neurone disease) ; cervical spondylolisthesis. *Plexus lesions*—Tumours at the thoracic inlet (Pancoast) ; prolapsed cervical disc (especially at C.7-T.1). *Distal nerve lesions*—Friction neuritis of the ulnar nerve at the elbow ; pressure upon the median nerve in the carpal tunnel ; toxic neuritis. *Muscle lesions*—Muscular dystrophy.

Other causes of upper limb peripheral vascular lesions. These include peripheral arterial disease and Raynaud's disease.

The diagnosis of symptomatic cervical rib depends upon the detection of the characteristic neurological signs or vascular disturbance in association with a demonstrable supernumerary rib. Prolapsed intervertebral disc at C.7-T.1 gives a similar clinical picture neurologically, and indeed it may often be the true cause of symptoms ascribed to a cervical rib ; but in cases of prolapsed disc there is a strong tendency to spontaneous recovery.

Treatment. This depends upon the severity of the subjective and objective manifestations. In mild cases physiotherapy in the form of ' shrugging ' exercises, to improve the tone of the elevator muscles of the shoulder girdle, is adequate. But if the neurological or vascular signs are well marked, and especially if they are increasing, operation is advisable. First the scalenus anterior muscle is divided. If this does not demonstrably release the lowest nerve trunk from constricting pressure the scalenus medius should be divided and the abnormal rib removed.

Occlusion of the subclavian artery may be amenable to surgery if the diagnosis is made before irreversible changes have occurred.

SCALENUS SYNDROME (First rib syndrome)

Occasionally the neurological manifestations characteristic of cervical rib occur in the absence of a demonstrable skeletal abnormality. They have been ascribed to trapping of nerves between the first rib and the clavicle (costo-clavicular compression), and to stretching of the lowest trunk of the brachial plexus over the normal first rib. In fact, however, they are usually due to the presence of a tough fibrous band in the scalenus medius muscle, which may cause kinking of the lowest trunk of the brachial plexus, demonstrable at operation. The symptoms are easily confused with those from a prolapsed intervertebral disc between C.7 and

T.1. Treatment should therefore be conservative at first, as for prolapsed disc. Gradual improvement would support that diagnosis. But if the symptoms persist with undiminished intensity for a long time a true scalenus syndrome is probably the cause. In that event it may be justifiable to explore the plexus, divide the scalenus anterior and remove the causative band in the scalenus medius.

CERVICAL SPONDYLOLISTHESIS
(Spontaneous subluxation of the cervical spine)

In cervical spondylolisthesis there is spontaneous displacement, usually forwards, of one cervical vertebra upon the next below it.

Causes and pathology. There are three types, caused by 1) congenital failure of fusion of the dens [odontoid process] with the axis, 2) inflammatory softening of the transverse ligament of the atlas, and 3) instability from previous injury.

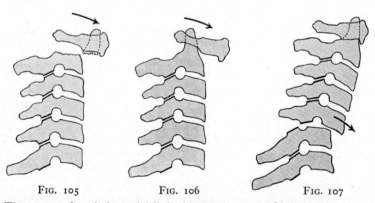

FIG. 105   FIG. 106   FIG. 107

Three types of cervical spondylolisthesis or spontaneous subluxation. Figure 105 —Displacement of atlas with the dens permitted by congenital or post-traumatic non-fusion of the dens with the axis. Figure 106—Displacement of atlas on axis, from softening of the transverse ligament of the atlas. Figure 107— Subluxation of the fifth on the sixth cervical vertebra due to instability of the intervertebral joint after previous injury.

Congenital non-fusion of dens. Occasionally the dens fails to fuse with the body of the axis by bone, being attached only by fibrous tissue. Under the constant stress of superimposed weight the fibrous bond slowly stretches, allowing the dens, and with it the atlas and skull, to slide gradually forwards upon the axis (Fig. 105). A similar condition may be caused by fracture of the dens.

Inflammatory softening of the transverse ligament of the atlas. In this type the underlying cause is an inflammatory lesion in the upper part of the neck, such as rheumatoid arthritis or an infection of the throat or glands. There is rarefaction of the atlas, with softening of the transverse ligament. In consequence the atlas is able to slide forwards upon the axis (Fig. 106).

Post-traumatic instability. A traumatic fracture-dislocation or subluxation at any level in the cervical spine may cause permanent instability, with a liability to slow redisplacement months or years after the initial injury (Fig. 107).

In all types the upper segment is displaced forwards in relation to the lower. The spinal canal becomes progressively more flexed and narrowed, and there is always a grave risk of compression of the spinal cord.

Clinical features. In the inflammatory type the patient is often a child with an acute infective lesion in the ear, throat, or neck, or an adult with rheumatoid arthritis. There is complaint of ' stiff neck.' The head is held rigidly, the cervical muscles being in spasm. In subluxation from congenital or post-traumatic instability there are discomfort and stiffness in the neck, and flexion deformity is apparent.

Complications. In all types the complication to be feared is compression of the spinal cord. The first symptoms appear in the upper limbs and consist of root pain, paraesthesiae, motor weakness, or sensory impairment. Eventually, increasing cord compression may lead to spastic paralysis below the level of the lesion, and to bladder and bowel dysfunction.

Treatment. This depends upon the underlying cause and upon whether or not neurological disturbance is present.

Inflammatory type: The displacement is reduced by head traction, which is continued for two weeks. Thereafter the neck is immobilised in extension in a plaster jacket for two months. Atlanto-axial fusion may be required.

Congenital or post-traumatic instability: If subluxation is not complicated by neurological disturbance, treatment may be expectant (observation only), by a plastic collar to give support (Fig. 103), or by local fusion of the spine, according to the severity of the displacement and of the local symptoms. If neurological disturbance is present, treatment is by preliminary skull traction to reduce the displacement, followed by operative fusion of the affected segments of the spine.

TUMOURS IN RELATION TO THE CERVICAL SPINE AND NERVE ROOTS

Classification and pathology. These tumours are best classified according to their site and nature. *Tumours of the spinal cord or meninges :* These include meningioma, intradural neurofibroma, and, more rarely, glioma. *Tumours of nerves :* The important one is neurofibroma, which may be single or multiple. If it arises from a nerve in the intervertebral foramen it may grow inwards to compress the spinal cord and outwards towards the surface (' dumb-bell ' tumour). *Tumours of the bony spinal column :* Benign tumours of the spinal column are rare. Malignant tumours may be primary (sarcoma, multiple myeloma) or metastatic (carcinoma, sarcoma). *Tumours at the thoracic inlet :* Pancoast's tumour at the thoracic inlet (usually an apical lung carcinoma) invades the base of the neck and is appropriately included here. Metastatic tumours in this area are usually lymph gland metastases.

Clinical features. The effects of these tumours vary according to their site. Broadly, the effects may be placed in three groups : 1) spinal cord compression, 2) local destruction and collapse of cervical vertebrae, and 3) interference with the brachial plexus. *Spinal cord compression.* Interference with the function of the spinal cord may be caused by tumours of the cord itself or of its meninges, by tumours of nerves (neurofibroma), or by tumours of the bony spinal column. The clinical manifestations depend upon the exact location of the tumour. Typically, root pains at the level of the lesion are followed by lower motor neurone changes at the same level and by progressive upper motor neurone paralysis and visceral dysfunction below the lesion.

Destruction and collapse of cervical vertebrae. The commonest cause is a metastatic carcinoma (Fig. 108). The clinical features are local pain and, usually, flexion deformity. The spinal cord or the issuing cervical nerves may be involved, with corresponding signs of spinal cord compression or peripheral nerve defect.

Interference with the brachial plexus. Nerves forming the plexus may be involved by tumours of the nerves themselves (neurofibroma), by bone tumours, or by tumours at the thoracic inlet. The predominant features are severe pain along the course of the nerve or nerves affected (neck or upper limb) and increasing motor and sensory impairment in the distribution of the nerves.

Radiographic features. Plain radiographs will usually help in discovering a tumour arising in the bones of the spinal column or eroding the bones from outside (Fig. 108). They may also reveal a tumour at the thoracic inlet. Myelography is helpful in the diagnosis of intraspinal tumours. Radiographs of the chest may reveal an apical lung tumour or pulmonary metastases. Radiographs of other bones are required if a widespread skeletal tumour such as multiple myeloma is suspected.

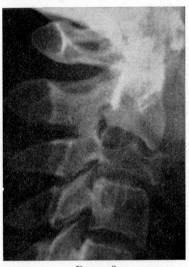

FIG. 108

Partial destruction of the body of the third cervical vertebra by a metastasis from a hypernephroma.

Treatment. This depends upon the nature and site of the tumour. In general, the choice lies between excision, for those that are amenable to it, and palliative radiotherapy for malignant tumours that cannot be removed. Hormone therapy (stilboestrol or testosterone) is appropriate for certain prostatic or breast metastases.

CERVICAL FIBROSITIS
(Muscular rheumatism)

The existence of fibrositis has been questioned, and it is admitted that it cannot be supported on pathological grounds. Nevertheless the term ' cervical fibrositis ' is a useful label for a fairly clear-cut clinical condition characterised by pain and tenderness in the muscles at the base of the neck, but without other objective signs. The cause is unknown.

Pathology. There are no demonstrable pathological changes. So-called fibrositic nodules cannot be identified histologically.

Clinical features. There is pain at the base of the neck posteriorly, with radiation towards the back of the shoulder on one or both sides. The pain is inconstant and varies in severity, often with climatic changes. There may be complaint of similar pain in other muscle groups. *On examination,* the only sign is local tenderness on firm pressure over the affected muscles or on squeezing them between the fingers. The trapezius and levator scapulae are most commonly affected. Radiography and other investigations show normal findings.

Diagnosis. Other causes of neck pain must be excluded by a careful history, clinical examination, and radiography.

Treatment. Often reassurance alone is required. When discomfort is marked, physiotherapy in the form of local heat and deep massage hastens spontaneous relief.

References and bibliography, page 445.

CHAPTER FOUR

Trunk and Spine

PAIN in the back is the commonest symptom encountered in orthopaedic practice. Indeed, if accident cases are excluded, it accounts for nearly a third of all orthopaedic out-patient attendances.

When this huge mass of material is sifted and categorised it is found that the cases fall into two broad groups. In the first group clear-cut physical signs, with or without distinctive radiographic changes or other abnormal findings, allow a precise determination of the nature of the lesion and of its site. The diagnosis is positive, and rational treatment can be applied. In the second group, almost as large as the first, there are no abnormal findings on clinical and radiographic examination. Diagnosis is largely a matter of conjecture, and treatment is empirical. For want of more accurate knowledge these rather vague and unsatisfactory cases are generally classed as ' chronic ligamentous strain ' or ' postural back pain.'

Lumbar back pain is often accompanied by radiating pain in the buttock, thigh or leg, usually on one side but occasionally on both. This pain is generally referred to as sciatica, though the term should strictly be reserved for pain in the distribution of the sciatic nerve. It should be noted that sciatica is often a much more disturbing symptom of back disorders than the back pain itself, which indeed may be slight or transient.

SPECIAL POINTS IN THE INVESTIGATION OF BACK AND SCIATIC SYMPTOMS

History

Special attention should be paid to the mode of onset of the symptoms, whether they are periodic or constant, whether they are getting worse or better, and what relieves them or aggravates them. The precise location of the back pain and its character should be determined. The patient should be asked to what he attributes his

173

symptoms : a history of a jarring strain, a fall, or an unaccustomed lifting job may be pertinent.

Significance of sciatica. If pain radiates into the lower limb its character and exact distribution must be ascertained. Two distinct

TABLE V

ROUTINE CLINICAL EXAMINATION IN SUSPECTED DISORDERS OF THE BACK

---

1. LOCAL EXAMINATION OF THE BACK, WITH NEUROLOGICAL SURVEY OF THE LOWER LIMBS

(*Patient standing*)

Inspection

Bone contours and alignment
Soft-tissue contours
Colour and texture of skin
Scars or sinuses

Palpation

Skin temperature
Bone contours
Soft-tissue contours
Local tenderness

Movements

Spinal joints
Flexion
Extension
Lateral flexion
Rotation
? Pain on movement
? Muscle spasm

Costo-vertebral joints
Range indicated by chest expansion

Sacro-iliac joints
(Impracticable to assess range)
? Pain on movement imparted by lateral compression of pelvis

(*Patient recumbent*)

Palpation of iliac fossae

Examine specifically for abscess

Neurological state of lower limbs

Straight leg raising test
Muscular system
Sensory system
Reflexes

---

2. EXAMINATION OF POTENTIAL EXTRINSIC SOURCES OF BACK PAIN AND SCIATICA

This is important if a satisfactory explanation for the symptoms is not found on local examination. The investigation should include : 1) the abdomen ; 2) the pelvis, including rectal examination ; 3) the lower limbs ; and 4) the peripheral vascular system.

---

3. GENERAL EXAMINATION

General survey of other parts of the body. The local symptoms may be only one manifestation of a widespread disease.

---

types of sciatica can be recognised. If the pain is severe and radiates in a well defined course, and especially if it is accompanied by motor, sensory, or reflex impairment, it suggests mechanical interference with nerve fibres of the lumbar or sacral plexus. On the other hand, if it takes the form of a vague diffuse ache, ill defined in its distribution, it is more likely to be a ' referred ' pain originating in a disordered joint or ligament.

Exposure

The patient should be stripped completely, except for short underpants or a special pelvic slip and, in women, a brassiere.

Steps in Routine Examination

A suggested plan for the routine clinical examination of the back is summarised in Table V.

Movements of the Spinal Column and Related Joints

The spinal column. The joints of the spinal column must necessarily be considered as a group, for it is impracticable to study the movement of each joint independently. The movements to be examined are flexion, extension, lateral flexion to right and left, and rotation to right and left. It should be noted particularly whether the spinal muscles go into protective spasm when movement is attempted. *Flexion:* Instruct the patient to stretch his fingers towards his toes, keeping the knees straight. It is important to judge what proportion of the movement occurs at the spine and how much is contributed by hip flexion (Figs. 109 and 110). Some patients can almost reach

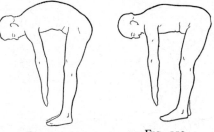

FIG. 109   FIG. 110

Figure 109—Normal flexion of lumbar spine. Figure 110—Apparent or false flexion due entirely to movement at the hips, the hamstrings being unusually lax. In estimating trunk flexion it is important to judge how much of the movement occurs at the spinal joints and how much at the hips.

their toes, despite a stiff back, simply by flexing unusually far at the hips. (Normally the hamstrings limit hip flexion to about 90 degrees when the knees are straight.) The range may be expressed as a percentage of the normal, or as the distance by which the fingers fail to reach the floor. *Extension :* Instruct the patient to arch the spine backwards, looking up at the ceiling. Judge the range and express approximately as a percentage of the normal. *Lateral flexion :* Instruct the patient to slide each hand in turn down the lateral side of the corresponding thigh. Observe the range. *Rotation :* With the feet fixed, the patient rotates the shoulders towards each side in turn. Note the range of spinal rotation as distinct from that which occurs at the knees and hips.

Related joints. *The costo-vertebral joints :* The mobility of the costo-vertebral joints is judged from the range of chest expansion. The normal difference in chest girth at full inspiration and full expiration is about 7 or 8 centimetres. A marked reduction of chest expansion is of particular significance when ankylosing spondylitis is suspected. *The sacro-iliac joints :* It is not practicable to measure the range of sacro-iliac movement. But the joints should be moved passively to determine whether pain is produced, as it will be in arthritic conditions of the joints. A simple method is to grip each iliac crest and compress the pelvis strongly from side to side.

Palpation of the Iliac Fossae and Groins

Palpation of the iliac fossae and groins is an essential step in the examination of the back. Its specific purpose is to determine whether

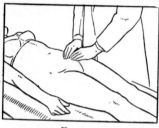

Fig. 111

Palpating the iliac fossae for abscess. This is an essential step in the routine examination of the spine.

or not there is a soft-tissue thickening or abscess. It should be remembered that the ' psoas ' abscess originating from a tuberculous lesion of the lumbar spine first becomes palpable deep in the iliac fossa. Such an abscess is felt most easily by pressing the flat palmar surface of the hand and fingers against the flat inner aspect of the iliac bone. To do this the surgeon must stand at the side of the couch corresponding to the side being examined—that is, he must stand on the right of the patient to examine the right iliac fossa and on the left to examine the left iliac fossa (Fig. 111).

Neurological Examination of the Lower Limbs

Disorders of the back are so frequently accompanied by radiating pain, paraesthesiae, or other manifestations in the lower limb that a neurological survey should be carried out as a routine. **Straight leg raising test.** Holding the knee straight, lift each lower limb in turn to determine the range of pain-free movement (normal = 90 degrees ; often more in women) (Fig. 112). When associated with clearly defined sciatica (and in the absence of gross disease of the hip), marked impairment of straight leg raising

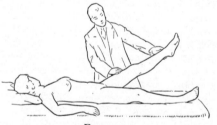

Fig. 112

The straight leg raising test, an important part of the neurological examination of the lower limbs.

by pain suggests mechanical interference with one or more of the roots of the sciatic nerve. The pain is easily explained. Even a normal sciatic nerve is tautened by straight leg raising, though not to the point of causing pain by dragging on the meningeal sheath that encloses the nerve root. If a nerve is already stretched or anchored, as by a protruded piece of an intervertebral disc or a tumour, the further tautening entailed in lifting the limb is sufficient to cause pain.

Muscular system. Examine the muscles for wasting, hypertrophy, and fasciculation. Note the tone and test the power of each muscle group, comparing it with its counterpart in the opposite limb. Circumferential measurement is a reliable method of comparing the bulk of the calf muscles, the girth being measured at the widest part or ' equator ' (Fig. 113). Circumferential measurement of the thighs, on

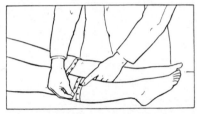

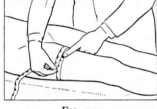

FIG. 113 FIG. 114

Figure 113—Girth measurement at the widest part is a reliable method of comparing the bulk of the calf muscles on the two sides. Figure 114—Measurement is unreliable in comparing the bulk of the thigh muscles because of the conical shape of the thigh and the difficulty of taking the measurement at an exactly comparable level on each side.

the other hand, tends to be inaccurate, and may be misleading, on account of the conical shape of the thigh (Fig. 114). Often a more accurate assessment of the relative volume of the two thighs is obtained from inspection and palpation. If the thighs are measured the girth should be taken on each side at an equal distance above the knee— 12 or 15 centimetres above the upper margin of the patella is usually a convenient level.

Sensory system. Examine the patient's sensibility to touch and pin-prick. When indicated, test also the sensibility to deep stimuli, joint position, vibration, and heat and cold.

Reflexes. Compare on the two sides the knee jerk (mainly L.4) and the ankle jerk (mainly S.1). It is important to note not only the presence or absence of the response, but also any difference of intensity (Figs. 115 and 116). Test the plantar reflex.

Radiographic Examination

If the complaint is clearly localised to the thoracic spine, antero-posterior and lateral radiographs of that area alone will usually suffice. If the lumbar spine is the part complained of, radiographs should include not only antero-posterior and lateral views of the lumbar spine but also at least one view of the sacro-iliac joints, pelvis, and hip joints.

In cases of doubt additional projections may be required. Oblique projections—from half right and half left—are essential for the proper study of the sacro-iliac joints and the posterior intervertebral (facet) joints of the lumbar region. For doubtful lesions of the vertebral bodies tomographs are often helpful. If a spinal tumour is suspected, myelography is required.

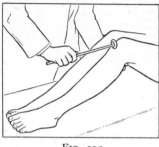
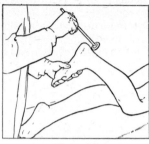

FIG. 115   FIG. 116

Figure 115—The patellar reflex is dependent mainly on L.4 nerve. Figure 116—In testing the calcaneal reflex (mainly S.1 nerve), slight inequalities between the two sides can best be detected if the patient lies prone, with the knee flexed 45 degrees and the ankle at 90 degrees.

Extrinsic Sources of Back Pain and Sciatica

The back offers many pitfalls in diagnosis. Sometimes there are no local symptoms to indicate that the spine is the seat of the disorder, pain being referred entirely to the buttock or to the lower limb. Thus patients often complain only of pain 'in the hip' or 'in the leg' when the true source of the trouble is the lumbar spine. Conversely, the symptoms may suggest a spinal lesion when in fact they arise from an affection of the abdomen, pelvis, or lower limb, or from occlusion of a major artery. Finally, it should always be remembered that back symptoms may be no more than a local manifestation of a generalised skeletal disease.

Thus the investigation of back or sciatic symptoms must extend further than a study of the spine itself; it must include an examination of the abdomen, pelvis, and lower limbs, and a general survey of the rest of the body.

CLASSIFICATION OF DISORDERS OF THE TRUNK AND SPINE

CONGENITAL ABNORMALITIES
    Lumbar and sacral variations
    Hemivertebra
    Spina bifida

DEFORMITIES
Scoliosis
Kyphosis
Lordosis

INFECTIONS OF BONE
Tuberculosis of the thoracic or lumbar spine
Pyogenic infection of the thoracic or lumbar spine

ARTHRITIS OF THE SPINAL JOINTS
Rheumatoid arthritis
Osteoarthritis
Ankylosing spondylitis

OSTEOCHONDRITIS
Scheuermann's vertebral osteochondritis
Calvé's vertebral osteochondritis

MECHANICAL DERANGEMENTS
Prolapsed lumbar intervertebral disc
Acute lumbago
Spondylolysis
Spondylolisthesis

TUMOURS
Tumours in relation to the sipnal column, spinal cord, or nerve
  roots
Other tumours of the trunk

CHRONIC STRAINS
Chronic lower lumbar ligamentous strain
Coccydynia

MISCELLANEOUS
Fibrositis
Senile osteoporosis

DISORDERS OF THE SACRO-ILIAC JOINTS
Tuberculosis of a sacro-iliac joint
Ankylosing spondylitis
Other forms of arthritis
Sacro-iliac ligamentous strain

LUMBAR AND SACRAL VARIATIONS

Minor variations of the bony anatomy are common, especially in the lumbar and sacral regions. They are of little practical importance. They include : deficient or rudimentary lowest ribs ; incomplete or complete incorporation of the fifth lumbar vertebral body in the sacrum (sacralisation of the fifth lumbar vertebra) ; persistence of the first sacral segment as a separate vertebra (lumbarisation of first sacral vertebra) ; and over-development of the fifth lumbar transverse process on one or both sides with, in marked cases, a false joint between the hypertrophied process and the ilium (Fig. 117). In the last-mentioned condition the false joint is sometimes a source of pain.

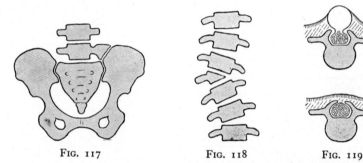

FIG. 117   FIG. 118   FIG. 119

Three congenital anomalies of the spine. Figure 117—Hypertrophied transverse process forming false joint with ilium. Figure 118—Hemivertebra, an occasional cause of scoliosis. Figure 119—Two examples of spina bifida. In both, the neural arch is deficient posteriorly. In the upper drawing the overlying soft tissues are also deficient and the spinal theca bulges backwards to form a meningocele. The lower drawing shows the much commoner and less severe defect, with the skin and soft tissues intact—spina bifida occulta.

HEMIVERTEBRA

In this anomaly a vertebra is formed in one lateral half only. The defect may occur at any level. The body of the half-vertebra is wedge-shaped, and the spine is angled laterally at the site of the defect (Fig. 118). This anomaly is a rare cause of scoliosis.

SPINA BIFIDA
(Spinal dysraphism)

The basic fault in spina bifida is a failure of the embryonic neural plate to fold over to form a closed neural tube, or of meso-dermal tissue fully to invest the neural tube as it does in the normal embryo to form the vertebral arch with its spinous process, and the surrounding muscles and ligaments.

The defect varies in degree from the very mild to the very severe. In the mildest form there is no more than a dimple in the skin or a split spinous process (spina bifida occulta). In more severe examples there is a wide defect in the vertebral arch, with cystic herniation of the dura to form a bulge under the skin (meningocele) (Fig. 119); or, worse still, nerve tissue also lies within the backward-bulging sac (myelo-meningocele). In the worst form of the anomaly there is total failure of closure of skin, vertebrae and dura, and nerve tissue is exposed on the surface of the body.

The main significance of spina bifida relates to the neurological deficit, and the condition was described more fully in the section on neurological disorders (p. 141).

SCOLIOSIS

The term scoliosis denotes lateral curvature of the spine. The deformity may be ' structural,' implying a permanent change in the bones or soft tissues, or it may be no more than a temporary disturbance produced by reflex or postural activity of the spinal muscles. Four types can be recognised : 1) primary or idiopathic structural scoliosis, a well defined group of unknown cause arising in children ; 2) secondary structural scoliosis, a miscellaneous group in which the curvature is secondary to a demonstrable underlying disorder ; 3) sciatic scoliosis, a temporary deformity ; and 4) compensatory scoliosis.

IDIOPATHIC STRUCTURAL SCOLIOSIS

Idiopathic scoliosis is the most important type of structural scoliosis. It begins in childhood or adolescence and tends to increase progressively until the cessation of skeletal growth. It sometimes leads to severe and ugly deformity, especially when the thoracic region is the part affected. The cause is unknown.

Pathology. Any part of the thoraco-lumbar spine may be affected. There is a primary curve, with secondary compensatory curves. The pattern of curve and its natural evolution are fairly constant for each site, and the following types are recognised : lumbar scoliosis, thoraco-lumbar scoliosis, thoracic scoliosis (Fig. 120). The lateral curvature is constantly accompanied by rotation of the vertebrae on a vertical axis, the body of the vertebra rotating towards the convexity of the curve and the spinous process away from the convexity. By thrusting the ribs backwards on the convex side this rotation increases the ugliness of the deformity (Figs. 120 and 121).

Clinical features. The onset may be at any time from infancy to adolescence—often between the ages of 10 and 12 years.

In children deformity is usually the only symptom. Pain is occasionally a feature in adults with long-standing deformity.

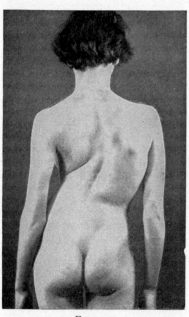

Fig. 120

Idiopathic scoliosis in an adolescent girl. The main curve is in the thoracic region. There is marked rotation of the vertebrae, causing posterior prominence of the ribs on the side of the convexity. In lumbar scoliosis the deformity is much less noticeable.

Course and prognosis. The outlook depends upon the age at onset and upon the site of the primary curve. The ultimate visible deformity tends to be worst in thoracic scoliosis and least in lumbar scoliosis. The curvature tends to increase until the end of the period of spinal growth, but not thereafter. In general, therefore, the earlier the onset the worse the prognosis.

Treatment. The first essential is to assess the prognosis from a consideration of the age at onset and the site of the curve. When the prognosis is good (for instance, in most cases of lumbar scoliosis) expectant treatment, with review every six months, is all that is required. When the prognosis is poor (as in thoracic scoliosis arising early) active treatment is advised. The method that has hitherto been most widely accepted is to correct the deformity so far as possible by a hinged plaster jacket controlled by turnbuckles, and subsequently to fuse the whole length of the primary curve by bone grafting to maintain the correction.

This method can certainly give correction that is well worth while, but it often leaves much to be desired, a considerable deformity often remaining. Because of this, much surgical endeavour has been spent in attempts to find a more effective operation. One method aims to correct the primary inequality of vertebral growth on the two sides. The epiphysial growth cartilages of several vertebral bodies are extirpated on the convex side of the curve, in the hope that growth will be arrested there while it continues on the concave side. This operation is best under-taken well before the age at which growth ceases. In another type of operation telescopic metal rods (Harrington's rods) are wedged between vertebrae on the concave side and then forcibly elongated to open the curve. The results of both these operations are encouraging, but it is too early yet to define their place in the treatment of scoliosis.

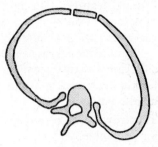

FIG. 121

With rotation of the vertebrae the ribs are thrust backwards on the convex side, increasing the ugliness of the deformity. This rotation is a constant feature of structural scoliosis.

In young children in whom spinal fusion is to be deferred until a later age, further increase of the curvature may sometimes be pre-vented by a special distraction appliance (the Milwaukee brace) which rests upon the pelvis below and is extended to support the chin and occiput above. The brace is worn continuously, night and day. Though rather uncomfortable, it is the only type of external appliance that is effective in controlling a scoliotic curve.

It must be emphasised that it is impossible to prevent the increase of a progressive deformity by exercises or by ordinary spinal jackets ; and that it is impracticable to correct long-standing deformity in adults by any method.

SECONDARY STRUCTURAL SCOLIOSIS

In this group the spinal curvature is secondary to a demonstrable underlying abnormality.

Causes. The three commonest underlying causes are congenital

References and bibliography, page 445.

abnormalities (especially hemivertebra), poliomyelitis with residual weakness of the spinal muscles, and neurofibromatosis.

Pathology. In *congenital hemivertebra* there is a sharp angulation at the site of the anomaly, with compensatory curves above and below (Fig. 118). Scoliosis following *poliomyelitis* is explained by unequal pull of the muscles on the two sides. The mechanism of scoliosis complicating *neurofibromatosis* is not clear ; in this type the deformity may be very severe.

Clinical features. In most cases the visible deformity is the only symptom. The age of onset, site, nature, and severity of the curve vary with the underlying cause.

In exceptional cases of severe long-standing scoliosis the sharp angulation of the spinal cord over the apex of the deformity may lead to interference with its function, with consequent neurological manifestations.

Treatment. In most cases treatment is along the lines suggested for idiopathic scoliosis.

SCIATIC SCOLIOSIS

Sciatic scoliosis is a temporary deformity produced by the protective action of muscles in certain painful conditions of the spine.

Cause. In many cases the underlying cause is a prolapsed intervertebral disc impinging upon a lumbar or sacral nerve. But the deformity may also be observed in some cases of acute lumbago (p. 207) and is then possibly caused by strain of one of the posterior intervertebral (facet) joints.

Pathology. The curve is in the lumbar region. The abnormal posture is assumed involuntarily in an attempt to reduce as far as possible the painful pressure upon the nerve.

Clinical features. The predominant feature is severe back pain or sciatica, aggravated by movements of the spine (see prolapsed intervertebral disc, p. 202). The onset is usually sudden. The scoliosis is poorly compensated ; so the trunk may be tilted over markedly to one side (Fig. 138, p. 204). The curvature is not associated with rotation of the vertebrae.

Treatment. The treatment is that of the underlying condition.

COMPENSATORY SCOLIOSIS

Lumbar scoliosis is seen as a compensatory device when the pelvis is tilted laterally—as, for instance, when the lower limbs are unequal in length, or when there is a fixed abduction or adduction deformity at one hip joint. In such a case it is only by curving the lumbar spine through an angle equal to the pelvic tilt that the trunk can be held vertical. Usually there is no intrinsic abnormality of the spine itself, and the scoliosis disappears automatically when the pelvic tilt is corrected. In cases of many years' duration, however, the lumbar scoliosis may become fixed by adaptive shortening of the tissues on the concave side.

KYPHOSIS

Kyphosis is the general term used to define excessive posterior curvature of the spinal column. The deformity may take the form of a long rounded curve (' round back '), or there may be a localised sharp posterior angulation (' hump back ').

In the thoracic region there is normally a considerable posterior curvature : thoracic kyphosis exists only if this curve is excessive. In the cervical and lumbar regions there is normally an anterior curvature : any reversal of this constitutes cervical or lumbar kyphosis.

Causes. Kyphosis is a manifestation of an underlying disorder of the spine. The causes are numerous. The following are the most important : 1) tuberculosis of the spinal column (Fig. 123) ; 2) unreduced vertebral compression fracture ; 3) Scheuermann's osteochondritis ; 4) ankylosing spondylitis ; 5) senile osteoporosis ; and 6) tumour of the spinal column (especially metastatic carcinoma).

Treatment. The treatment is that of the underlying condition.

LORDOSIS

Lordosis is the opposite deformity to kyphosis. The term denotes excessive anterior curvature of the spinal column. In practice, lordosis is seen only in the lumbar region, where a slight anterior curve is normal. Strictly, the term lordosis should be used only when this normal curve is exaggerated.

7

Causes. Spinal disorders tend to cause kyphosis or scoliosis rather than lordosis. In many cases lordosis is simply a postural deformity, predisposed to by lax muscles and heavy abdomen. Sometimes it is compensatory, balancing a kyphotic deformity above or below, or a fixed flexion deformity of a hip.

TUBERCULOSIS OF THE THORACIC OR LUMBAR SPINE
(Tuberculous spondylitis ; Pott's disease)

Tuberculosis of thoracic or lumbar vertebral bodies is one of the commonest forms of skeletal tuberculosis.

Pathology. The infection begins at the anterior margin of a vertebral body, near the intervertebral disc (Fig. 122). The disc itself is usually involved at an early stage. The extent of the

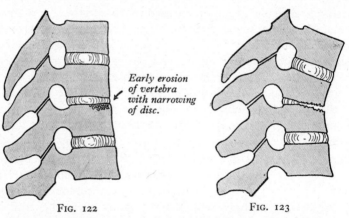

Early erosion of vertebra with narrowing of disc.

FIG. 122   FIG. 123

Tuberculosis of the spine. The infection begins anteriorly near an intervertebral disc, which is soon destroyed (Fig. 122). It may spread to adjacent vertebrae, which collapse in front, with consequent angular kyphosis (Fig. 123).

destruction varies widely from case to case. Commonly there is complete destruction of one intervertebral disc with partial destruction of the two adjacent vertebrae, most marked anteriorly (Fig. 123). But the changes may extend over several spinal segments ; or, on the other hand, they may be confined to a single intervertebral disc, without evident bone involvement (Fig. 124). Anterior collapse of the affected vertebrae leads to an angular kyphosis. Abscess formation is usual. In the thoracic region pus collects around the spinal column, forming a fusiform para-spinal abscess (Fig. 126) ; or it may track towards the surface between ribs. From the lower thoracic or lumbar region pus tracks downwards behind the fascial sheath of the psoas muscle and generally bursts into the compartment behind the iliacus fascia to

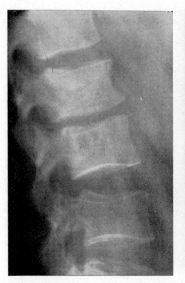 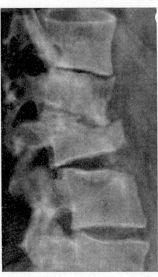

FIG. 124   FIG. 125

Figure 124—Early tuberculous lesion causing a narrowed lumbar disc space in a young adult. Narrowing of a disc space without osteophytic spurring of the vertebral margins always suggests infection. Figure 125—Severe tuberculous erosion of two lumbar vertebrae, with anterior collapse. The vertebra below also shows erosion at its upper anterior corner. One intervertebral disc is destroyed and the one above is much narrowed.

form a palpable abscess in the iliac fossa (psoas abscess). An abscess occasionally points posteriorly, or in the thigh.
Secondary effects : An abscess or mass of granulation tissue encroaching upon the spinal canal may interfere with the spinal cord or with a spinal nerve. In cases of long-standing severe kyphosis the spinal cord is occasionally damaged by the bony ridge at the site of deformity.

Clinical features. The disease is commonest in young adults. One or more of the following symptoms may be present : 1) pain in the back ; 2) stiffness of the back ; 3) visible deformity of the back ; 4) localised swelling (abscess) ; 5) weakness of legs or visceral dysfunction (involvement of spinal cord). *On examination,*

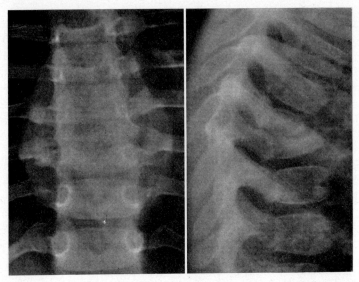

FIG. 126

Tuberculosis of the thoracic spine in a child. Note in the antero-posterior view the typical fusiform appearance of a paraspinal abscess, an almost constant feature of thoracic spinal tuberculosis. In the lateral view two vertebral bodies are seen partly collapsed into a wedge-shaped mass ; the disc between them has been destroyed.

the patient often looks ill. There may be visible or palpable angular kyphosis. There is local tenderness on firm palpation or percussion over the affected vertebrae. All spinal movements are restricted and when they are attempted the spinal muscles go into protective spasm. An abscess may be detected over the thoracic wall or in the flank, iliac fossa, or upper thigh. Signs of spinal cord compression (' Pott's paraplegia ') or of a nerve root lesion may be present. Tuberculous lesions are often manifest elsewhere. *Radiographic examination :* The earliest signs are narrowing of an intervertebral space (Fig. 124) and local vertebral osteoporosis. Later, there is usually destruction of bone at the anterior margin of one or more of the vertebral bodies, leading to anterior collapse and wedge-shaped deformity of the affected vertebrae (Figs. 125 and 126). An abscess shadow is nearly always visible : in the thoracic region it is seen as a fusiform paraspinal shadow (Fig. 126) ; in the lumbar region it is indicated by lateral bulging of the psoas outline, usually on one side. In the healing stage the bone outline in the area of destruction becomes sharper, and normal density is regained. Abscesses may become calcified. *Investigations :* The erythrocyte sedimentation rate is raised in the active stage. The Mantoux test is positive. Tubercle bacilli can sometimes be isolated from aspirated pus.

Diagnosis. The condition has to be distinguished : 1) from other causes of back pain with localised bony destruction or kyphosis (non-specific pyogenic spondylitis ; ankylosing spondylitis ; spinal tumours ; osteochondritis ; old compression fracture), and 2) from other causes of dysfunction of the spinal cord or cauda equina (prolapsed intervertebral disc ; spinal tumour).

Important diagnostic features are : a history of contact with tuberculosis, or of previous tuberculous infection ; restriction of *all* spinal movements by protective muscle spasm ; abscess formation ; the characteristic radiographic changes (including destruction of an intervertebral disc, which is not usual in cases of tumour and not marked in osteochondritis) ; and the raised erythrocyte sedimentation rate.

Complications. These include : 1) chronic discharging sinus ; 2) interference with the spinal cord, causing weakness or paralysis in the lower limbs with or without sensory impairment or disturbance of bladder and bowel function (' Pott's paraplegia ') ; and 3) tuberculous infection of other organs, such as meninges, kidneys, or lungs.

Prognosis. In most cases the ultimate outlook is good. In a few there is severe permanent kyphosis. There is a small risk of death from spread of the infection to other organs, or from the effects of paraplegia. The prognosis is worse in certain Asian and African countries where the disease tends to be florid, than in Britain, North America, and the Antipodes where it is usually mild.

Treatment. The treatment of spinal tuberculosis has undergone important changes in the last few years. Whereas previously treatment was almost entirely conservative, by constitutional measures designed to build up the patient's resistance, there is now a tendency to advise operation in a large proportion of cases and at a relatively early stage.

Constitutional treatment is still important because tuberculosis is always to some extent a generalised disease with widespread constitutional effects. But with the aid of modern antibiotics and other drugs, and with better all-round conditions, the period of treatment can often be reduced from a matter of years to a matter of months. Constitutional treatment entails rest in a healthy fresh-air environment, good diet, and chemotherapy in the form of streptomycin, para-amino-salicylic acid, and isonicotinic acid hydrazide given together in a six-months' course if well tolerated.

Local treatment is at first by rest for the spine, either on a plaster bed or frame or by recumbency alone. In most cases one or more of the following surgical procedures will be carried out at the appropriate time.

Drainage of abscess. 1) An abscess that is superficial should be either aspirated or drained by simple incision (followed by immediate suture of the skin). 2) A paraspinal abscess in the thoracic region may be drained from the back by removing the head and neck of a rib and the adjacent transverse process (costo-transversectomy). 3) Alternatively—and preferably if there is much necrosis of the vertebral bodies—the focus may be exposed by a direct approach (trans-thoracic or lateral lumbar, depending upon the site of the lesion) to allow thorough emptying of the abscess cavity and removal of all dead bone and fibrinous débris.

Relief of paraplegia. If paraplegia from compression of the spinal cord does not show rapid improvement after one month's treatment by rest and chemotherapy the spinal canal should be decompressed by operation. Occasionally this may be achieved by costo-transversectomy alone, particularly if a paraspinal abscess is the chief factor responsible for the compression. More reliably, it may be done by removing on one side the pedicles of three or four vertebrae in order to expose the spinal theca and thus permit the removal of fragments of bone or disc, or of other débris, under direct vision (antero-lateral decompression).

Spinal fusion. In the quiescent stage of the disease the affected region of the spine may be fused by bone grafting if it is judged to be unstable. Bone grafts may be fitted posteriorly or they may be let into the spinal column from in front after thorough removal of all dead bone and débris.

Assessment of cure. Signs of quiescence are : good general health, diminishing blood sedimentation rate, and arrest of the destructive process with hardening of the bony outlines as seen radiographically. When the disease is quiescent the patient is allowed up with the protection of a plaster jacket or spinal brace, which is worn for about a year.

COMMENT

Operation is being undertaken increasingly for drainage of a paraspinal abscess, which it is believed may retard healing and favour spread of the disease up and down the spinal column. Many now go further and advise the thorough removal of débris and necrotic bone through a direct approach as a routine method of treatment. On the other hand many surgeons now consider that spinal fusion is seldom necessary for tuberculosis. When it is done now it is often by the anterior route rather than the posterior, and is combined with curettage of the diseased area.

It is important to appreciate that spinal tuberculosis tends to be a much more florid disease in certain countries of the East than it is in Britain and the West, and therefore that whereas radical surgery may be the method of choice in the former countries it will often be needlessly drastic in those where the disease is relatively mild.

PYOGENIC INFECTION OF THE THORACIC OR LUMBAR SPINE
(Pyogenic spondylitis ; osteomyelitis of the spine)

Pyogenic infection of the spine is rather uncommon. It has often been confused with tuberculous spondylitis, which it resembles clinically and radiographically.

Cause. It is caused by infection with the streptococcus, staphylococcus, pneumococcus, or occasionally with other bacteria such as the typhoid bacillus or brucella abortus.

Pathology. Organisms usually reach the spinal column through the general blood stream, from a septic focus elsewhere. Other possible routes are through the spinal venous plexus from a focus in the pelvis, or through lymphatic channels from a neighbouring focus. As in tuberculous spondylitis, there is destruction of bone and intervertebral disc, with or without abscess formation. The spinal cord may be damaged by pressure, or by thrombosis of its vessels.

Clinical features. The clinical picture is inconstant : there are remarkable variations in the severity of the symptoms from case to case. The onset is often acute or subacute, and may be accompanied by pyrexia. In many respects the features are like those of tuberculous spondylitis (p. 186), the predominant findings being local pain and restriction of all movements by muscle spasm. A suppurative process elsewhere in the body is usually present or has recently subsided. *Radiographs* show local rarefaction or erosion of bone, diminution of disc space, and sometimes sub-ligamentous new bone formation. After healing, spontaneous bony fusion of affected vertebrae is often observed. *Investigations :* The erythrocyte sedimentation rate is raised. Polymorphonuclear leucocytosis is to be expected. Serological studies can occasionally incriminate a particular organism, such as one of the Salmonella group.

Diagnosis. Pyogenic infection has to be distinguished mainly from tuberculous spondylitis, which it may resemble closely. The relatively acute onset, history of pre-existing infection or septic focus, pyrexia, leucocytosis, and identification of the causal organism in pus, are the main diagnostic criteria.

Prognosis. If the infection is overcome, complete healing of the spinal lesion—often with bony fusion of affected vertebrae— is usual.

Treatment. Appropriate chemotherapy is given. The spine is rested, at first in bed, and later in a plaster jacket or by a suitable brace, until healing occurs. Abscesses may require drainage, especially if the spinal cord is threatened.

RHEUMATOID ARTHRITIS OF THE SPINAL JOINTS

(General description of rheumatoid arthritis, p. 46.)

The term ' rheumatoid spine ' is sometimes used loosely to denote ankylosing spondylitis. Such terminology is inaccurate and leads to confusion. In point of fact, rheumatoid arthritis of the spinal joints is quite distinct from ankylosing spondylitis.

Pathology. The joint changes are like those of rheumatoid arthritis elsewhere. Unlike ankylosing spondylitis, which always begins in the sacro-iliac joints and creeps upwards, rheumatoid changes in the spinal joints may begin in the cervical region.

Clinical features. The changes in the spinal joints usually form only part of a widespread rheumatoid polyarthritis. The spinal manifestations consist in aching pain of a rather diffuse type, with impairment of spinal movements. The symptoms develop insidiously, without preceding injury. Examination of the limbs will usually reveal typical rheumatoid changes in several joints. *Radiographs* are not distinctive, but in cases of considerable duration there is rarefaction of the vertebrae with thinning of the intervertebral disc spaces. These changes do not progress to bony ankylosis like the changes of ankylosing spondylitis.

Treatment. This is along the lines recommended for rheumatoid arthritis of other joints (p. 49).

OSTEOARTHRITIS OF THE THORACIC AND LUMBAR SPINE
(Spondylosis ; spondylarthrosis)

Osteoarthritis of the thoracic or lumbar intervertebral joints is found very commonly in those used to heavy work, but it is not necessarily accompanied by symptoms.

Cause. Predisposing factors are : 1) previous injury to the spinal joints ; 2) previous disease involving the joints (for example, Scheuermann's osteochondritis) ; and 3) intervertebral disc lesions. In other cases the degenerative changes are simply a manifestation of increasing age.

Pathology. The changes affect the central intervertebral (body-to-body) joints and the posterior intervertebral (facet) joints. One or several segments may be affected. In the central joints, which are affected first, there is degeneration with consequent narrowing of the intervertebral disc, and hypertrophy of bone at the joint margins leads to the formation of osteophytes (Fig. 127). In the posterior intervertebral joints the changes are those of osteoarthritis in any diarthrodial joint—namely, attrition of the articular cartilage and osteophyte formation (spurring) at the joint margins. These changes in the facet joints are probably the more important from a clinical point of view.

7*

Secondary effects : Rarely, osteophytes encroach upon an inter-vertebral foramen sufficiently to interfere with the function of the issuing nerve. Thinning of the articular cartilage of the posterior intervertebral (facet) joints reduces the stability of the affected segment and predisposes to one type of spondylolisthesis (p. 209).

Clinical features. Spinal osteoarthritis can exist in quite marked degree without causing symptoms. But there is often a complaint of aching pain in the affected area, worse on activity. In the lumbar region there is a tendency to acute exacerbations of pain, usually arising suddenly and lasting a few weeks (acute lumbago). These are possibly explained by strain or momentary subluxation of an unstable degenerate joint. Interference with a nerve in a narrowed intervertebral foramen leads to radiating pain in the distribution of the affected nerve (girdle pain or sciatica according to the level affected). *On examination* in the quiet phase, the objective findings are slight. Spinal movements may be moderately restricted, especially flexion ; but there is no muscle spasm. If there is interference with a lumbar nerve root straight leg raising on the affected side is likely to be restricted. Apart from this, objective neurological signs are exceptional. During an acute exacerbation of pain there may be marked impairment of spinal movements, with muscle spasm (see *acute lumbago*, p. 207). *Radiographic examination :* The changes are most obvious in the central (body-to-body) intervertebral joints, which show narrowing of the intervertebral space and osteophyte formation (spur-ring) at the joint margins (Figs. 127 and 132). Later the posterior interverte-bral (facet) joints also show changes : there is narrowing of the joint space with sharpening of the margins of the facets. These changes are seen clearly only in oblique projections.

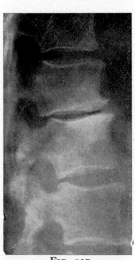

FIG. 127

Osteoarthritis of the lumbar spine. Marked narrowing of an intervertebral disc, with anterior osteophytes. Note also the slight pos-terior subluxation. (See also Figure 132.)

Diagnosis. Osteoarthritis has to be distinguished from other causes of back pain and from other causes of radiating nerve pain (girdle pain or sciatica) (Fig. 139, p. 205). It should be remembered that the demonstration of osteoarthritic changes in the radiographs does not necessarily mean that the arthritis is the cause of the patient's symptoms, for spinal osteoarthritis is often painless. The diagnosis is always presumptive rather than proved, and it is justified only when other possible causes have been excluded by careful consideration of the history, clinical examination and radiographs.

Treatment. This depends upon the severity of the disability. In mild cases treatment is unnecessary.

Thoracic spine. In osteoarthritis of the thoracic spine the symptoms are seldom severe, and if treatment is required a course of active spinal exercises to strengthen the muscles is usually sufficient.

Lumbar spine. In lumbar osteoarthritis with moderate disability a well fitted surgical corset will usually afford adequate relief. Heavy lifting and similar strains to the back should be strictly avoided. Occasionally, if the pain from a localised lesion is bad enough to cause serious hardship, operative fusion of the affected segments of the spine may be required.

Spinal fusion. Fusion, or arthrodesis, of spinal segments is effected by bridging the vertebrae with bone grafts, usually obtained from the ilium but sometimes from the tibia or fibula. In *posterior fusion* the grafts are fitted between or alongside the spinous processes, superficial to the laminae. In *anterior fusion* blocks of bone are inlayed in deep slots cut in the vertebral bodies after excision of most of the intervertebral disc from the front. In *lateral fusion* bone grafts are wedged between the transverse processes or, in the case of the lumbo-sacral joint, between transverse processes above and the lateral masses of the sacrum below. Each method has its special applications, but the choice also depends largely on the surgeon's individual preference.

ANKYLOSING SPONDYLITIS

In ankylosing spondylitis there is chronic inflammation, progressing slowly to bony ankylosis, of the joints of the spinal column and occasionally of the major limb joints.

Cause. This is unknown. The condition is distinct from rheumatoid arthritis, although it is sometimes loosely termed ' rheumatoid spine.' There is evidence of an inheritable predisposition to the disease.

Pathology. The disease always begins in the sacro-iliac joints, whence it usually extends upwards to involve the lumbar, thoracic, and often the cervical spine. Occasionally the hips or shoulders are also affected. The articular cartilage, synovium, and ligaments show chronic inflammatory changes and eventually they become ossified. After several years the inflammatory process ' burns itself out.'

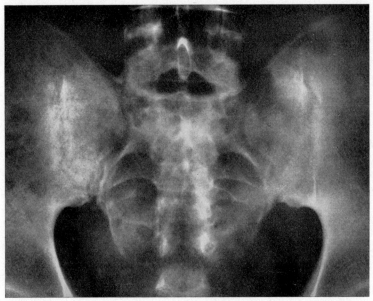

FIG. 128

Ankylosing spondylitis. Characteristic fuzziness with loss of sharp outline of both the sacro-iliac joints. Later, these joints undergo spontaneous bony fusion, and similar changes may creep upwards, sometimes affecting the whole of the spinal column.

Clinical features. With few exceptions the disease is confined to men, and it nearly always begins between the ages of 18 and 30. The early symptoms are pain in the lower back and increasing stiffness. Later, the pain migrates upwards. Diffuse radiating pain down one or both lower limbs is also common. *On examination* the predominant finding is marked limitation of all movements in the affected area of the spine (' poker back '). When the thoracic region is involved chest expansion is markedly reduced, from ankylosis of the costo-vertebral joints. In a few cases the

hips or shoulders are affected, with pain and limitation of movement. *Radiographic examination :* In the early stages there is
fuzziness of both the sacro-iliac joints, so that the joint outline is

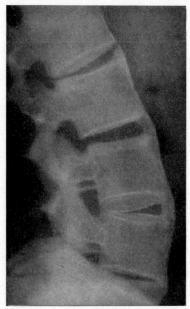 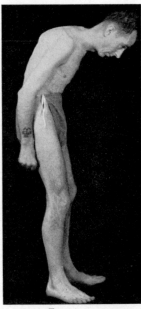

FIG. 129   FIG. 130

Figure 129—Ossification of the anterior longitudinal ligament in
ankylosing spondylitis. In severe cases the spinal column may become
rigid throughout its length. Figure 130—Rigid flexion deformity of spine
complicating old ankylosing spondylitis. This complication should
never be allowed to occur. It can be prevented simply by ensuring that
the patient sleeps on his back upon a flat hard mattress, with only a
single thin pillow for the head.

no longer clearly defined (Fig. 128). Later, the sacro-iliac joints
are completely obliterated and, if the disease progresses, the
intervertebral joints in the lumbar, thoracic, and sometimes even
the cervical region undergo bony ankylosis (Fig. 129). *Investigations :* The erythrocyte sedimentation rate is raised while the
disease is active.

Diagnosis. Ankylosing spondylitis has to be distinguished from
other causes of back pain and sciatica (Fig. 139). The marked
limitation of spinal movement, reduced chest expansion, typical

radiographic features, and raised erythrocyte sedimentation rate are diagnostic.

Course and complications. The disease usually ceases to progress after ten or fifteen years, leaving permanent stiffness, the extent of which varies widely from case to case. Some patients become bedridden. Complications include fixed flexion deformity of the spine (Fig. 130), intercurrent respiratory infections, and iridocyclitis, which in severe cases may lead to blindness.

Treatment. Radiotherapy has in the past been widely advocated as the mainstay of treatment. It is certainly often effective in relieving pain, and many believe that it arrests or at least retards the progress of the disease. Its great disadvantage is that it entails a risk of leukaemia—though probably a very slight one if the dosage is carefully judged. A further objection in women is that the ovaries may be damaged by irradiation of the base of the spine. The future of this method must depend upon a further long-term assessment of its efficacy and of the magnitude of the risk involved. As an alternative phenylbutazone may be found effective in relieving pain. Other mild anti-inflammatory drugs may also be tried, but corticosteroids should have no place in treatment except for ophthalmic complications. Apart from these measures, treatment should be directed towards preserving function. Activity rather than rest should be enjoined. Special exercises should be practised to make the most of such movement as remains. The patient should adopt the habit of sleeping flat upon his back on a firm mattress, with only a single pillow, to prevent increasing flexion deformity of the spine. If severe flexion deformity occurs through neglect of this precaution (Fig. 130) it may be corrected by wedge osteotomy of the spine in the lumbar region.

SCHEUERMANN'S VERTEBRAL OSTEOCHONDRITIS
(Adolescent vertebral osteochondritis ; adolescent kyphosis)

The term osteochondritis has retained a place in the nomenclature of this disease mainly through long usage. Scheuermann's disease was formerly thought to be homologous with other examples of osteochondritis juvenilis (p. 97), but it is now recognised that it behaves differently from typical osteochondritis, and is probably unrelated to it. The cause and precise nature of the affection require further elucidation.

Pathology. The vertebral bodies ossify from three centres—a primary centre for the middle of the body, and secondary centres for the upper and lower surfaces. These secondary centres, known as the ring epiphyses, appear at about the time of puberty in the cartilaginous end-plates that separate the vertebral bodies from the adjacent intervertebral discs. In Scheuermann's disease

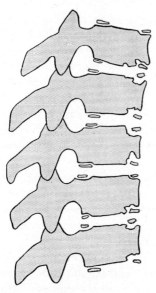
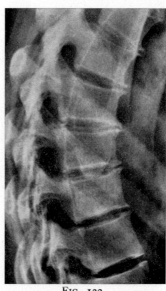

FIG. 131   FIG. 132

Figure 131—Scheuermann's vertebral osteochondritis in the active stage (diagrammatic). The upper and lower margins of the vertebral bodies are irregularly indented in front, and the corresponding parts of the ring epiphyses appear isolated from the main mass of the vertebral body. It is believed that these changes may be caused by bursting of the disc contents through the cartilage plates. Figure 132—The late effect of Scheuermann's disease. Slight wedging of several thoracic vertebral bodies with consequent rounded kyphosis and secondary osteoarthritis.

there is a disturbance of the normal development of the cartilage plates and ring epiphyses, possibly because they are damaged by bursting of the disc contents through the cartilage into the subjacent vertebral body (Fig. 131). The changes occur predominantly near the anterior margins of the vertebrae, where the greatest weight-thrust is borne. In consequence the disc is somewhat narrowed anteriorly, and through deficient growth of the affected part of the ring epiphysis the vertebral body becomes slightly wedge-shaped. The deformity predisposes to the later development of osteoarthritis (Fig. 132).

Characteristically Scheuermann's disease affects several vertebrae in the thoracic region. Occasionally similar changes are confined to a single vertebra, and this localised form of the disease is probably as common in the lumbar as in the thoracic region.

Clinical features. The patient is usually 13 to 16 years old. In the active stage there is pain in the thoracic spine, with ' round ' back. After some months the pain subsides, leaving a slight rounded kyphosis. In later life there may be renewed pain from the development of osteoarthritis. *On examination*, there is a slight or moderate rounded kyphosis in the thoracic region. In the active stage there is tenderness on firm palpation over the affected vertebrae. *Radiographic examination :* In the active stage of the disease the affected vertebral bodies show deep notched defects at their anterior corners, and the corresponding parts of the ring epiphyses may be irregular in shape and size (Fig. 131). The disc spaces are slightly narrowed but never totally destroyed. After healing, there is slight antero-posterior wedging of the affected vertebral bodies. Years later, osteoarthritic spurring of the anterior vertebral margins is observed (Fig. 132).

Diagnosis. In its characteristic form the affection is easily diagnosed from the history, clinical appearance, and radiographs. If localised to a single vertebra it may easily be confused with tuberculous spondylitis. Radiologically, the chief points of distinction are that in osteochondritis the margins of the notched defect in the vertebral body tend to be sclerotic rather than rarefied, and a paraspinal abscess shadow (almost a constant feature of thoracic spinal tuberculosis) is never seen. Furthermore, the erythrocyte sedimentation rate is not raised in osteochondritis.

Course and prognosis. The affection is self-limiting, the active stage lasting about two years. If the epiphyses become deformed, permanent wedging of the affected vertebrae, with consequent slight or moderate kyphosis, remains. Osteoarthritis often supervenes in later life but it is of little clinical significance.

Treatment. Theoretically it might seem wise to try to prevent deformity by protecting the spine from pressure stresses until the epiphysial plates are fully developed, but this would necessitate the child's lying recumbent in a plaster bed for many months. Such prolonged immobilisation is seldom desirable, and it is usual to adopt a compromise. If the initial symptoms are severe the child should rest in a plaster bed for two to three months. This allows the pain to subside. Thereafter a spinal brace is worn for a further six months, and active exercises to strengthen the posterior spinal muscles are encouraged.

In the milder cases—the great majority—rest in a plaster bed is unnecessary, and a spinal brace with exercises, or even exercises alone, will suffice.

CALVÉ'S VERTEBRAL OSTEOCHONDRITIS
(Vertebra plana)

Whereas in Scheuermann's disease it is the vertebral ring epiphyses that are affected, Calvé's disease affects the central bony nucleus of a vertebral body. It is much less common than Scheuermann's disease, and it is confined to a single vertebra.

Pathology. Mainly from its radiological features and from its benign course, Calvé's disease has been regarded as homologous with osteochondritis of other developing bony nuclei (p. 97), and it is possible that this is indeed the true explanation in some cases. Histological studies have shown, however, that in at least some instances the characteristic vertebral collapse has been caused by an eosinophilic granuloma (p. 123), and it is possible that this will be found to be the usual pathology.

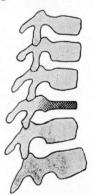

FIG. 133

Calvé's disease of vertebral body. The bony nucleus has shrunk into a thin dense wafer. The adjacent intervertebral discs are intact.

In a typical case the bony nucleus of one of the vertebral bodies, usually in the thoracic region, becomes soft and is condensed into a thin wafer. Later, the bone may re-develop surprisingly well, but it is doubtful if it is ever restored quite to its full depth. The intervertebral discs above and below are usually unaffected.

Clinical features. The affection occurs in children of from 2 to 10 years of age. The complaint is of pain, usually in the thoracic region of the spine. *On examination*, there may be slight localised kyphosis. Percussion of the spinal column reveals deep tenderness in the affected region. Movements of the spine as a whole are impaired but little, if at all. *Radiographs* show the characteristic extreme flattening of the affected vertebral body, which appears greatly increased in density (Fig. 133) : it has been likened to a coin seen end on. The intervertebral disc spaces above and below are of normal depth ; or they may even appear to be increased in depth, for the cartilage of the vertebral body shrinks less than its bony nucleus.

Diagnosis. The radiographic appearance is distinctive. It serves to differentiate the condition from tuberculous disease, which always destroys the intervertebral disc.

Treatment. Calvé's disease is non-progressive, and in practice treatment is required only for as long as the symptoms last. While the pain persists the child should be kept recumbent in bed, but in most cases he may safely resume an active life without external support within two or three months.

PROLAPSED LUMBAR INTERVERTEBRAL DISC

Herniation of part of a lumbar intervertebral disc is a common cause of combined back pain and sciatica.

Cause. Prolapse of a disc is often precipitated by injury, but it is believed that spontaneous age-degeneration of the disc is an important predisposing factor.

Pathology. The discs between L.5 and S.1 and between L.4 and L.5 are those most often affected. Part of the gelatinous nucleus pulposus protrudes through a rent in the annulus fibrosus at its weakest part, which is postero-lateral (Figs. 134-137) ; or sometimes the torn annulus itself protrudes backwards. If it is small, the protrusion bulges the pain-sensitive posterior longitudinal ligament, causing pain in the back. If it is large, the protrusion herniates through the posterior ligament and may impinge upon an issuing nerve to cause sciatic pain. The nerve affected is that which leaves the spinal canal at the interspace next below the site of the disc lesion. Thus the first sacral nerve is impinged upon by a prolapse between L.5 and S.1, the fifth lumbar nerve by a prolapse between L.4 and L.5, and so on.

Natural healing is probably by shrinkage and fibrosis of the extruded disc material rather than by its spontaneous reposition within the disc. *Secondary effects :* Progressive degeneration of the disc leads, after months or years, to osteoarthritis, with

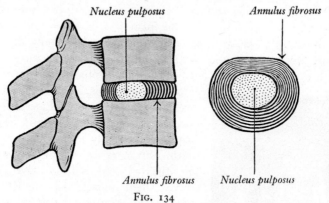

Nucleus pulposus   *Annulus fibrosus*

Annulus fibrosus   *Nucleus pulposus*

FIG. 134

A normal intervertebral disc seen in sagittal section (left) and in horizontal section (right).

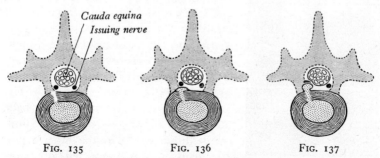

Cauda equina
Issuing nerve

FIG. 135   FIG. 136   FIG. 137

Stages in prolapse of an intervertebral disc. Figure 135—The annulus fibrosus is torn but there has been no extrusion of the nucleus pulposus. Figure 136— Extrusion of nuclear material through the rent. The posterior longitudinal ligament is stretched but the protrusion has not reached the nerve. Figure 137—The protrusion is larger and the nerve is stretched over it. Sometimes a fragment of the torn annulus itself protrudes backwards.

ultimate involvement of the posterior intervertebral (facet) joints as well as the central (body-to-body) joints.

Clinical features. In a typical case the clinical picture is clearly defined. The patient is aged between 18 and 60. A few hours or days after jarring or straining the back he is seized, while twisting, stooping or coughing, with agonising pain in the lumbar region. He is unable to move. The acute pain gradually lessens in severity, but after a few days a radiating pain is felt in one or other buttock and down the back or side of the thigh to the calf and foot. Tingling or numbness is felt in the calf or foot. The pain is aggravated by coughing or sneezing. *On examination* the patient with a fully developed acute attack stands either with a lumbar scoliosis (sciatic scoliosis) (Fig. 138) or with the normal anterior lumbar curve obliterated.

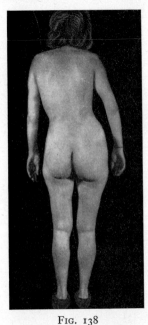

FIG. 138

Sciatic scoliosis. A temporary tilt to one or other side is a common feature of severe prolapsed lumbar disc. The posture is adopted involuntarily to relieve the pressure upon the nerve at the site of the prolapse.

Forward flexion is greatly restricted, as also may be extension. Lateral flexion, on the other hand, is usually free and painless—certainly to one side if not to both. Straight leg raising is restricted on the affected side. Careful tests reveal slight muscle wasting or weakness in the distribution of the affected nerve, and the corresponding tendon jerk (knee jerk in L.3-L.4 lesions; ankle jerk in L.5-S.1 lesions) is impaired or absent.

Variations. Atypical cases are common. Thus a definite history of injury or strain is often lacking. The pain may begin gradually rather than suddenly. The symptoms may be confined to the back and never radiate to the lower limb (acute lumbago). On the other hand, the pain is sometimes felt predominantly in the limb and is scarcely perceptible in the back. The severity of the pain varies greatly from case to case, and its exact distribution depends upon the level of the disc prolapse; for instance, in the relatively uncommon cases of high lumbar or mid-lumbar prolapse the pain radiates towards the groin and the front of the thigh rather than to the back of the thigh and leg.

Radiographic examination. In a case of acute prolapsed disc radiographs do not show any abnormality, and the purpose of radiography is mainly to exclude other causes of back pain and sciatica. It is only when a disc has been deranged for many months or years that appreciable narrowing of the disc space and spurring of the joint margins (denoting secondary osteoarthritis) are observed.

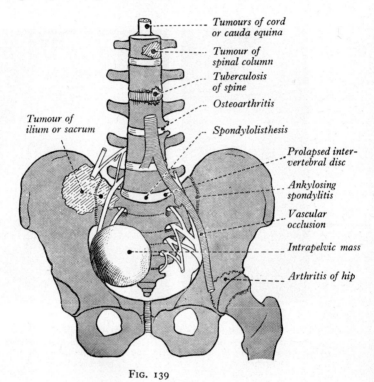

Tumours of cord or cauda equina

Tumour of spinal column

Tuberculosis of spine

Osteoarthritis

Tumour of ilium or sacrum

Spondylolisthesis

Prolapsed intervertebral disc

Ankylosing spondylitis

Vascular occlusion

Intrapelvic mass

Arthritis of hip

FIG. 139

Eleven causes of pain in the back or lower limb. All must be considered in differential diagnosis.

Investigations. Lumbar puncture reveals either normal cerebrospinal fluid or, commonly, a slight increase of protein content.

Correlation of pathology with clinical features. The initial injury or strain marks the time when the annulus fibrosus is torn or damaged. The nucleus pulposus is very gelatinous and an interval elapses before it becomes extruded. Bulging of the extruded material beneath the posterior longitudinal ligament corresponds to the stage of acute back pain. Herniation through the ligament with impingement against the adjacent nerve is responsible for the radiating limb pain.

Diagnosis. Prolapsed intervertebral disc must be differentiated from other causes of pain in the back or leg (Fig. 139). The

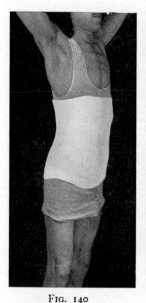 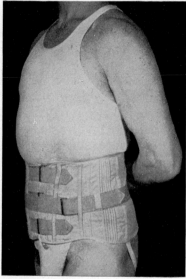

FIG. 140

Plaster jacket used in the conservative treatment of prolapsed lumbar intervertebral disc.

FIG. 141

Steel-reinforced surgical corset used for mild cases of prolapsed intervertebral disc and for certain types of chronic low back pain.

conditions with which it is most likely to be confused are : tuberculosis of the spine or sacro-iliac joints ; intraspinal tumour ; tumour of the spine or pelvis ; spondylolisthesis ; ankylosing spondylitis ; osteoarthritis of the spine ; arthritis of the hip ; and occlusion of the aorta or of the iliac or femoral artery, with consequent ischaemic pain in the proximal limb muscles on exercise. Diagnosis rests upon the recognition of the characteristic features of disc prolapse and upon the exclusion of other possible causes of the symptoms by careful consideration of the history, clinical examination (including rectal examination), and radiographs. A dramatically sudden onset is always suggestive of a mechanical derangement and especially of a prolapsed disc, whereas pain that increases relentlessly without intermission suggests a progressive lesion, inflammatory or neoplastic. In doubtful cases lumbar puncture and myelography, and sometimes discography, are required.

Treatment. *Non-operative treatment* is successful in relieving the symptoms in a high proportion of cases—probably at least nine out of ten. The principle is to provide rest for the lumbar spine. This is preferably secured by a plaster jacket (Fig. 140), which allows the patient to be up and about ; but rest in bed is a commonly used alternative, and it is often combined with continuous or intermittent traction on the legs or pelvis. In either case rest for the spine must be continued for six to twelve weeks according to progress. Thereafter a surgical corset (Fig. 141) should be worn for several months if minor symptoms persist.

Operative treatment : Excision of the displaced disc material is indicated in the following circumstances : 1) when the sciatic pain is so excruciating from the beginning that it prevents sleep and leads to deterioration of the general health ; 2) when severe neurological disturbance suggests massive prolapse with compression of the cauda equina ; 3) when severe sciatic pain is unrelieved by efficient conservative treatment for twelve weeks.

At operation the disc is exposed from behind by retraction of the posterior spinal muscles away from the midline, excision of the ligamentum flavum and perhaps part of a lamina at the appropriate level, and gentle retraction of the theca. The protruded part of the disc forms an obvious rounded bulge, over which the emerging spinal nerve may be seen tightly stretched. The extruded material is removed, together with as much of the remaining nuclear tissue as can be pulled out from between the vertebral bodies.

ACUTE LUMBAGO

Lumbago is a symptom rather than a disease. In a typical attack of acute lumbago the patient is suddenly seized with agonising pain in the lumbar region of the spine, usually while stooping, lifting, turning, or coughing. The pain is often so severe that any movement is difficult and the patient is ' stuck.' With rest, the pain gradually subsides, but in some cases the acute back pain is succeeded by sciatica, suggesting irritation of a lumbar or sacral nerve.

It seems fairly certain that there is more than one cause for symptoms of this type. Probably in many cases the underlying lesion is a prolapsed disc that has not yet been retropulsed far enough to interfere with a nerve root. It is in these cases that sciatica may develop later, as the size of the prolapse increases. But other examples of acute lumbago are more convincingly ascribed to some other mechanical disorder of the spine, such as sudden nipping of the synovial membrane in one of the facet oints, or momentary subluxation with consequent ligamentous strain, especially at an intervertebral joint that is unstable on account of disc degeneration or osteoarthritis. In such a case acute attacks of pain may recur at intervals of months or years.

Treatment should usually be to provide rest for the spine, either by recumbency or by a plaster jacket or surgical corset, as for a prolapsed intervertebral disc.

SPONDYLOLYSIS

In spondylolysis there is a defect in the neural arch of the fifth (rarely the fourth) lumbar vertebra. There is loss of bony continuity between the superior and the inferior articular processes, the deficiency being bridged by fibrous tissue (Fig. 142). If this stretches or gives way, the consequent vertebral displacement constitutes one variety of *spondylolisthesis* (see below).

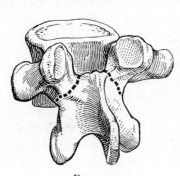

FIG. 142

Site of the defect in spondylolysis. There is lack of bony continuity at the isthmus of the neural arch (pars interarticularis) on each side.

Though the defect has hitherto been regarded as congenital it is now widely believed that it may be caused by injury ; or it may be the result of a stress fracture.

Clinically, spondylolysis (the defect without displacement) is often symptomless, but it is believed that it is sometimes a cause of deep lumbar back pain. *Radiographically*, the defect is shown clearly only in oblique projections.

Treatment. This is often unnecessary. Aching may be relieved by a surgical corset. Exceptionally, local fusion of the spine is justified.

SPONDYLOLISTHESIS
(Lumbar spondylolisthesis)

Spondylolisthesis is the term applied to spontaneous displacement of a lumbar vertebral body upon the segment next below it. Displacement is usually forwards, but may be backwards.

Cause. There are three predisposing factors : 1) spondylolysis (a defect in the pars interarticularis of the neural arch) (p. 208) ; 2) osteoarthritis of the posterior (facet) joints ; and 3) (rarely) congenital malformation of the articular processes.

Pathology. In the normal spine forward displacement of a vertebral body is prevented by engagement of its articular processes with those of the segment next below it. In spondylolisthesis there is a failure of this check mechanism, and the attachments of the intervertebral disc alone are not strong enough to hold the vertebral bodies in alignment.

In the best recognised type (' true ' spondylolisthesis) a defect in the neural arch of a vertebra (Fig. 142) allows separation of its two halves. The body, with the pedicles and superior articular processes (and the whole of the spinal column above it), slips forwards, leaving behind the laminae and inferior articular processes (Fig. 143). The fifth lumbar is the vertebra usually affected, the fourth occasionally. Displacement may increase slowly month by month or year by year, and it sometimes reaches a severe degree. Major displacement is apt to occur especially during adolescence. There may be minor irritation of one of the issuing nerves, with consequent sciatica ; but despite severe bony displacement serious interference with the nerves of the cauda equina is exceptional in this type of spondylolisthesis.

In the second type of spondylolisthesis (wrongly termed ' pseudo-spondylolisthesis ') the posterior intervertebral (facet) joints become unstable on account of osteoarthritis, with degeneration of the articular cartilage that is essential to a snug fit of the

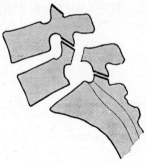

FIG. 143

Figure   143 — Spondylolisthesis
due to defect of the neural arch
(diagrammatic).   The body and
superior articular processes have
slipped   forwards,   leaving   the
spinous   process   and   inferior
articular   processes   in   normal
relationship   with   the   sacrum.
(Radiographically the defect is
seen best in oblique projections.)

Figure   144 — Spondylolisthesis
secondary to osteoarthritis. Wearing down of the cartilage of the
posterior intervertebral (facet)
joints   has   permitted   slight
forward   displacement   of   a
vertebral body.   The condition
may occur at any level in the
lumbar spine : here it is shown
at the joint between the fourth
and fifth vertebrae.

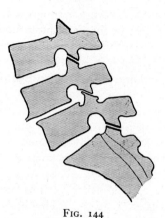

FIG. 144

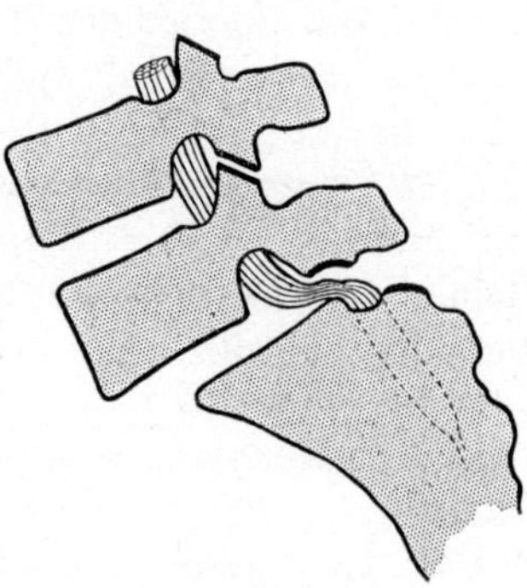

Figure   145 — Spondylolisthesis
secondary to congenital malformation of the articular processes
at the lumbo-sacral joint.   The
cauda equina is trapped between
the body of the sacrum and the
lamina of the displaced fifth
lumbar vertebra.   In this type of
spondylolisthesis   neurological
signs are to be expected.

FIG. 145

joint surfaces (Fig. 144). It may occur at any level in the lumbar spine—most commonly between the fourth and fifth lumbar vertebrae. In this type the vertebral displacement is occasionally backwards rather than forwards (Fig. 127), but in either case displacement is never severe, and neurological disturbance is unusual.

In the third and least common type the posterior intervertebral joints are unstable because the articular processes are congenitally malformed or even rudimentary; thus they form no bar to forward displacement of the spinal column. This defect occurs most often at the lumbo-sacral joint. Displacement may be severe and, since the whole vertebra is displaced complete with its neural arch, the cauda equina may be trapped, with consequent severe neurological disturbance (Fig. 145).

Clinical features. The clinical features of spondylolisthesis are inconstant: they depend to some extent upon the nature of the causative lesion and upon the degree of displacement. In some cases the deformity is entirely symptomless. When symptoms occur they take the form of chronic backache, with or without sciatica. The back pain is worse on standing. *On examination* there is often a visible or palpable ' step ' above the sacral crest, due

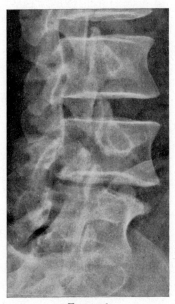

FIG. 146

Oblique radiograph of the lower lumbar region of a patient with spondylolisthesis, showing a defect of the pars interarticularis of the neural arch of the fourth lumbar vertebra (centre of illustration). Oblique radiographs such as this are essential in the differentiation of spondylolisthesis caused by a neural arch defect from the other two types of spondylolisthesis.

to the forward displacement of the spinal column; but this is obvious only when the displacement is severe. Spinal movements are restricted only slightly, if at all. *Abdomen:* When displacement is severe the spinal column is projected forwards and the lumbar vertebral bodies may be palpable through the abdomen. *Lower limbs:* Minor irritation of a sciatic root is often evidenced by impairment of straight leg raising; but severe neurological disturbance is seldom observed except in the rare cases in which congenital malformation of the articular processes allows dislocation of the whole vertebra complete with its neural arch (Fig. 145). *Radiographs* show the displacement. Oblique views will demonstrate whether or not there is a defect of the neural arch (Fig. 146).

Diagnosis. Spondylolisthesis is distinguished from other causes of back pain and sciatica by the radiographs.

Treatment. When spondylolisthesis is symptomless treatment is not required. *Non-operative treatment:* Moderate symptoms are often adequately relieved by a well fitted surgical corset, and this should be tried before operation is considered. *Operation:* This is justified only when the disability (from back pain or neurological disturbance) is severe. The operation entails the release of stretched or compressed nerves, followed by fusion of the affected segments of the spinal column by bone grafts (p. 195).

TUMOURS OF THE TRUNK AND SPINE

These tumours will be considered in two categories: 1) tumours that affect the spinal column or its contents—spinal cord or nerve roots; and 2) other tumours of the trunk.

TUMOURS IN RELATION TO THE SPINAL COLUMN, SPINAL CORD, OR NERVE ROOTS

Classification and pathology. *Tumours of the spinal cord or meninges:* These include meningioma, intradural neurofibroma and, rarely, glioma. *Tumours of nerves:* The important example is neurofibroma, which may be single or multiple. If it arises from a nerve in an intervertebral foramen it may grow inwards to compress the spinal cord and outwards towards the surface ('dumb-bell' tumour). *Tumours of bone:* Benign tumours of the spinal column are much less common than malignant tumours. They include chondroma, giant-cell tumour and vertebral haemangioma. Malignant tumours may be primary (sarcoma, multiple myeloma, chordoma), but much more often they are metastatic tumours derived usually from a carcinoma of the lung, breast, prostate, thyroid, or kidney (hypernephroma).

Clinical features. The effects of these tumours vary according to their site and character. Broadly, the effects may be placed in three groups : 1) compression of the spinal cord ; 2) local destruction of the skeleton ; 3) interference with peripheral nerves.

Compression of the spinal cord. This may occur with tumours of the spinal cord itself or of its meninges, with tumours of nerves (neurofibroma), or with tumours of the bony spinal column. The clinical manifestations depend upon the exact location of the tumour. Typically, when the spinal cord is slowly compressed, initial root pain (girdle pain in thoracic involvement, lower limb pain in lumbar) is followed by lower motor neurone paresis at the segmental level corresponding to the site of the tumour, by progressive sensory and upper motor neurone paralysis below the lesion, and often by bladder or bowel dysfunction.

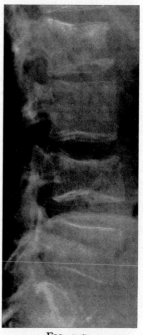

FIG. 147

Partial collapse of the second and fourth lumbar vertebrae in a patient with myelomatosis. Note that the intervertebral discs are not destroyed.

Local destruction of the skeleton. The commonest cause is a malignant tumour of the bones of the spinal column (Fig. 147)—usually a metastatic carcinoma. The predominant symptom is pain, which is constant and increases relentlessly in its severity. Frequently there are associated neurological manifestations from involvement of the spinal cord or nerve roots. The local objective signs vary from case to case. Sometimes the tumour is palpable—as, for instance, a sacral tumour. Sometimes deformity, from collapse of the bony structure, is evident clinically ; or there may be marked restriction of spinal movement, with protective muscle spasm.

Interference with peripheral nerves. Peripheral nerves—especially the nerves of the cauda equina—may be involved by tumours of the nerves themselves (neurofibroma), by tumours of the spinal column (benign or malignant), or by tumours in the peripheral course of the nerves (for example, a tumour of a rib, or a tumour arising from or within the pelvis). The clinical features depend upon the particular nerve or nerves affected and upon the extent of the involvement. Typically, there will be constant, progressive, and ultimately severe pain along the course of the affected nerve, with sensory impairment, increasing motor weakness, and depression of reflexes in the distribution of the nerve. Retention of urine is usually a prominent feature of a tumour interfering with the cauda equina.

Radiographic examination. Plain radiographs will usually help in discovering a tumour arising in the bones of the spinal column (Fig. 147), or eroding the bone from outside. In cases of vertebral destruction from tumour the adjacent intervertebral discs are typically preserved. This point helps in the distinction from erosion and collapse due to infection, in which the discs are destroyed at an early stage (compare Figs. 125 and 147). Myelography is indispensable if a tumour of the spinal cord or cauda equina is suspected. Radiographs of the chest may reveal a primary lung tumour or a metastasis; and radiographs of the rest of the skeleton may be helpful in the diagnosis of disseminated tumours such as multiple myeloma.

Diagnosis. The possibility of a tumour has to be borne in mind constantly in the differential diagnosis of back pain and lower limb pain, especially when associated with radiological signs of vertebral erosion or collapse or with neurological disturbance affecting the trunk, lower limbs or viscera. Other causes of vertebral erosion or collapse include previous trauma, pathological fracture from rarefying disease of bone, tuberculous or pyogenic infection, and syphilis. Other causes of spinal cord or cauda equina disturbance include prolapsed intervertebral disc, severe angular deformity in scoliosis or kyphosis, tuberculous or pyogenic infection, osteoarthritis, spondylolisthesis, herpes zoster, and primary neurological diseases such as disseminated sclerosis and motor neurone disease.

A history of insidious onset, with relentless increase of symptoms without remission, always suggests the possibility of tumour. Careful search should always be made for a primary tumour elsewhere in the body.

OTHER TUMOURS OF THE TRUNK

TUMOURS OF THE STERNUM AND RIBS

The sternum and ribs contain abundant red marrow, favourable to the development of blood-borne metastatic tumours or of deposits in myelomatosis. Histological examination of the sternal marrow (obtained by sternal puncture) is often of diagnostic importance in suspected metastasising tumours, for the material will often show tumour cells even in the absence of clinically evident metastases.

TUMOURS OF THE SCAPULA

The commonest tumour of the scapula is a chondroma. It grows outwards from the flat body of the bone and is therefore classed as an ecchondroma. It may attain a large size. There is a risk of malignant change, with the development of a chondro-sarcoma. For that reason a chondroma that appears to be enlarging should always be excised with an adequate margin of healthy bone. A large part of the scapula can be removed without causing serious disability.

TUMOURS OF THE PELVIC GIRDLE

The pelvic bones, like the scapula, are sometimes the seat of a chondroma (ecchondroma). It may reach a large size, and there is some risk of malignant change.

The considerable content of red marrow renders the pelvic bones liable to carcinomatous metastatic deposits, and they are also a common site of tumour deposits in myelomatosis.

CHRONIC LOWER LUMBAR LIGAMENTOUS STRAIN
(Postural back pain)

The terms chronic ligamentous strain and postural back pain are used to cover an ill defined group of affections characterised by persistent backache without demonstrable pathology. These conditions are common—in fact they form a large proportion of the cases of back pain seen in orthopaedic practice.

Cause. It is assumed that the spinal muscles fail in their function of protecting the deep ligaments in maintaining posture. Predisposing causes include childbirth, overweight, general flabbiness of muscle, and debilitating illness.

Pathology. No precise lesion is demonstrable.

Clinical features. The patient is nearly always a woman. She often dates the onset of pain from childbirth, sometimes from an operation, or from a debilitating illness ; but equally often the onset is unexplained. The pain is characteristically in the lumbar or lumbo-sacral region. It tends to be worse on activities such as stooping. *On examination* there are no abnormal physical signs. *Radiographs* are normal.

Diagnosis. This depends upon the exclusion of demonstrable pathological lesions by careful clinical and radiographic examination. A history of long-continued lumbar backache, with a total lack of clinical or radiological abnormalities, should always suggest this group of affections.

Course and prognosis. Aching often persists for many years despite treatment. Nevertheless in most cases the condition is a source of nagging discomfort rather than a serious handicap to the normal activities of life.

Treatment. Often reassurance alone is required. When treatment is called for, the three methods available are : 1) physiotherapy ; 2) manipulation ; and 3) external support. In young patients physiotherapy, in the form of active exercises to strengthen the spinal muscles, with or without heat and massage, should be tried for at least two months. If this is ineffective manipulation of the lumbar and sacro-iliac joints, usually under anaesthesia, is worth a trial : it may be followed by repeated longitudinal traction and muscle exercises. If pain persists despite these measures, fitting with a surgical corset is advised. In elderly and flabby patients physiotherapy is seldom of benefit and early resort should be had to a reinforced corset (Fig. 141).

COCCYDYNIA

In its widest sense, coccydynia includes any painful condition in the region of the coccyx. In practice, the term is restricted to the clinical entity in which persistent pain continues for many weeks or months after a local injury, despite the absence of demonstrable pathology. Eventually it is a self-limiting affection, though it may cause severe discomfort while it lasts.

Cause. Typically, coccydynia develops after an injury—usually a fall on the ' tail.' Occasionally a history of injury is lacking.

Pathology. In some cases there is probably a strain of the sacro-coccygeal joint; in others the lesion is thought to be simply a contusion of the periosteum over the lower sacrum or coccyx.

Clinical features. There is pain localised to the sacro-coccygeal area, worse when sitting. In severe cases there is also pain on defaecation. Usually the patient is free from pain when standing or lying. *On examination* there is localised tenderness over the sacro-coccygeal region. In some cases the pain can be reproduced by moving the coccyx. *Radiographs* do not show any alteration from the normal.

Diagnosis. It is important to consider other causes of pain in this area, especially infections of the sacro-coccygeal joint and tumours of the sacrum or coccyx. Investigation should include rectal examination, and radiographs must always be obtained.

Treatment. In most cases treatment is not required. All that is necessary is to exclude serious organic disease, and then to reassure the patient that the condition is harmless and that it may be expected to resolve spontaneously if left alone. Various remedies have been advocated, including short-wave diathermy, manipulation, and injections of local anaesthetic or hydrocortisone ; but none is uniformly successful. In the exceptional case of unusually severe and persistent pain the coccyx may be excised.

FIBROSITIS

The general subject of fibrositis was discussed on page 129. A loose diagnosis of ' fibrositis ' is often made in cases of thoracic or lumbar back pain, but in fact it is an uncommon condition—some even deny its existence. In many cases of supposed fibrositis the cause of the pain is more probably a ligamentous strain or an intervertebral disc lesion.

The cause of fibrositis is unknown, and there are no demonstrable pathological changes. So-called fibrositic nodules cannot be identified histologically.

Clinical features. There is aching pain in the posterior spinal muscles, of varying intensity and often influenced by climatic

8

changes. There may be ' rheumatic ' pains in other parts of the body. *On examination* there is local tenderness on palpation of the affected muscles, and small nodules may be felt. Apart from this, no clinical abnormality is found ; spinal movements are full and there is no muscle spasm. *Radiographs* show no abnormality. **Treatment.** This is by physiotherapy in the form of local heat, with or without massage or exercises.

SENILE OSTEOPOROSIS

Although the symptoms of senile osteoporosis are mainly in the back, it is strictly a general affection of the skeleton and was described as such on page 113. The spinal features are aching pain, kyphosis, liability to compression fractures of vertebral bodies, and marked rarefaction of the bones of the spinal column.

DISORDERS OF THE SACRO-ILIAC JOINTS

Sacro-iliac lesions are a rather uncommon but nevertheless important cause of back symptoms or of referred pain in the lower limb.

TUBERCULOSIS OF A SACRO-ILIAC JOINT

The patient is a child or young adult. The condition is usually confined to one side, but it may be bilateral. As in tuberculous disease of other joints, there is destruction of articular cartilage and thickening of synovial membrane, often with erosion of bone and abscess formation. *Clinically*, the main feature is pain behind the affected joint and in the iliac fossa or groin. A diffuse, ill localised pain may be referred down the lower limb. Examination shows restriction of lower spinal movements, and side-to-side compression of the pelvis aggravates the pain. An abscess is often palpable posteriorly or in the iliac fossa. *Radiographs* show local rarefaction, with loss of definition or ' fuzziness ' of the joint outline.

Treatment is like that for tuberculosis of other joints (p. 54). Constitutional treatment is by rest and chemotherapy. Local treatment is by immobilisation of the trunk and pelvis in a plaster hip spica until the disease is quiescent. Thereafter some surgeons allow the patient up in a sacro-iliac support, whereas others advise operative fusion (arthrodesis) of the affected joint as a safeguard against recrudescence of the disease.   Abscesses should be aspirated or drained.

ANKYLOSING SPONDYLITIS

Although ankylosing spondylitis usually affects a larger area of the spine it always begins in the sacro-iliac joints and the patient may present himself initially with sacro-iliac pain.   The disease was described fully earlier in this chapter (p. 195).

OTHER FORMS OF SACRO-ILIAC ARTHRITIS

Pyogenic arthritis may occur, but it is uncommon.   Its general features conform with those of pyogenic arthritis elsewhere, as described on page 43.

Rheumatoid arthritis may affect the sacro-iliac joints in common with the other joints of the spine (p. 192).

Osteoarthritis of the sacro-iliac joints is uncommon and seldom, if ever, the cause of serious disability.

SACRO-ILIAC LIGAMENTOUS STRAIN

Sacro-iliac strain was formerly a common diagnosis in cases of pain localised predominantly in the upper gluteal region.   It is now believed that in the vast majority of such cases the pain does not in fact originate in the sacro-iliac joint, but is referred to the gluteal region from a disorder in the lower lumbar spine—often an intervertebral disc lesion.   Exceptionally, however, true sacro-iliac ligamentous strain occurs.   *Clinically*, the patient is usually an adult woman.   The symptoms are often noticed first after childbirth.   The pain is accurately localised to the sacro-iliac joint, and there is a tendency also to referred diffuse aching in the thigh.   The pain is aggravated by twisting the trunk.   Examination reveals a good range of spinal movements with pain only at the extremes.   Forcible stress applied to the sacro-iliac joints by firm lateral compression of the pelvis, or by extending one hip while the other is held fully flexed, reproduces the pain. There are no neurological signs.   *Radiographs* show no abnormality.
Treatment.   Genuine sacro-iliac strain often responds well to manipulation under anaesthesia.   If this fails, recourse is usually made to physiotherapy (heat, massage, exercises) or, this failing also, to a surgical corset (Fig. 141).

EXTRINSIC DISORDERS SIMULATING
SPINAL DISEASE

ABDOMINAL DISORDERS

PEPTIC ULCER

The pain of peptic ulcer is often felt in the back as well as in the epigastrium. Exceptionally, it is felt entirely in the back or beneath the left costal margin, when it may simulate girdle pain referred along a thoracic spinal nerve.

VISCEROPTOSIS

Dragging of pendulous viscera upon the posterior abdominal wall is a contributory cause of backache. Flabbiness of the back muscles, with consequent ligamentous strain, is usually present as well. The pain from both conditions may be relieved by fitting a combined abdominal and lumbo-sacral support.

RENAL OR PERIRENAL INFECTIONS

Rarely, a carbuncle of the kidney or a perinephric abscess is confused with a back condition. The usual features are pain in the back and loin, general malaise, pyrexia, and leucocytosis.

RENAL CALCULUS

The pain may be felt chiefly in the back, though it is always towards the loin rather than in the midline. The pain is often aggravated by jarring movements—for instance, riding on a shaky bus or stepping from a pavement. There may be a history of haematuria or of attacks of colic. Spinal movements are unaffected. Radiographs will reveal the calculus.

BILIARY CALCULUS AND CHOLECYSTITIS

Pain beneath the right costal margin from a gall-bladder lesion is easily confused with girdle pain referred along an intercostal nerve from a spinal condition.

PELVIC DISORDERS

INTRAPELVIC TUMOUR

A tumour or other mass within the pelvis may interfere with the sacral plexus or its branches, causing pain which is generally of sciatic distribution. It may thus simulate sciatica arising from a spinal cause such as a prolapsed intervertebral disc or spinal tumour. A pelvic mass will usually be palpable on rectal or vaginal examination, which should form part of the routine investigation in cases of radiating lower limb pain.

GYNAECOLOGICAL DISEASE

The importance of gynaecological disorders as a cause of back pain has been exaggerated. In point of fact, there is no reasonable ground for attributing back symptoms to gynaecological causes unless a major intrapelvic disorder is demonstrable.

LOWER LIMB DISORDERS

ARTHRITIS OF THE HIP

The pain from arthritis of the hip sometimes simulates sciatic pain referred from a spinal lesion. Characteristically, hip pain is referred from the groin down the front of the thigh towards the knee. Irritation of the fourth lumbar nerve root by a spinal lesion causes pain in a somewhat similar distribution. The best safeguard against error is to examine the movements of the hip joint in every case of radiating lower limb pain.

VASCULAR DISORDERS

ARTERIAL OCCLUSION

It should always be remembered that occlusion of the aorta, of the iliac arteries or of their major branches may be associated with ischaemic muscle pain on exercise which, from its distribution in the lower back or buttocks, may easily be confused with the back pain or sciatica caused by a prolapsed intervertebral disc or other spinal lesion. The important clue to the correct diagnosis is the history of onset of pain only during exercise, with rapid relief when the exercise is stopped. In such a case the femoral or popliteal pulse will usually be weak or absent ; but it should be noted that the posterior tibial and dorsalis pedis pulses may be easily palpable even when there is complete occlusion at or near the aortic bifurcation. Plain radiographs may show calcification of the aorta or iliac vessels, and arteriography will show the site and extent of the occlusion.

References and bibliography, page 445.

CHAPTER FIVE

The Shoulder Region

THE mechanics of the shoulder are rather complex. The shoulder 'joint' in fact comprises three components—the gleno-humeral joint or shoulder joint proper, the acromio-clavicular joint, and the sterno-clavicular joint. The gleno-humeral joint allows a free range of abduction, flexion, and rotation, under the control of the scapulo-humeral muscles. The other two joints together allow 90 degrees of rotation of the scapula upon the thorax and a moderate range of antero-posterior gliding of the scapula, under the control of the cervico-scapular and thoraco-scapular muscles.

Disorders of the shoulder include most varieties of arthritis ; but it is notable that osteoarthritis—common in most joints—is rare in the gleno-humeral joint. As if to make up for this, the shoulder exhibits several affections peculiar to itself—notably tears of the musculo-tendinous cuff, the painful arc syndrome, and 'frozen' shoulder. Together these form a large proportion of shoulder disabilities.

Pain in the shoulder and arm is notoriously prone to mis-interpretation, and special care is required to differentiate intrinsic pain arising in the shoulder from extrinsic pain referred from the cervical spine, the thorax, or the abdomen.

SPECIAL POINTS IN THE INVESTIGATION OF SHOULDER SYMPTOMS

History
Characteristics of shoulder pain. It is important to find out the precise location and distribution of the pain. True shoulder pain is seldom confined to the shoulder itself. Typically, it radiates from a point near the tip of the acromion down the lateral side of the upper arm to about the level of the deltoid insertion. It is unusual for true shoulder pain to extend below the elbow.

Pain arising in the acromio-clavicular joint or sterno-clavicular joint is localised to the joint itself and does not radiate down the limb.

Referred pain in the shoulder region. The pain referred from an irritative lesion of the brachial plexus often extends from the base of the neck, over the top of the shoulder, and thence into the arm. Unlike true shoulder pain, it frequently radiates below the elbow into the forearm or

TABLE VI

ROUTINE CLINICAL EXAMINATION IN SUSPECTED
DISORDERS OF THE SHOULDER

1. LOCAL EXAMINATION OF THE SHOULDER REGION

Inspection

Bone contours and alignment
Soft-tissue contours
Colour and texture of skin
Scars or sinuses

Palpation

Skin temperature
Bone contours
Soft-tissue contours
Local tenderness

Movements

Distinguish between gleno-humeral movement and scapular movement during abduction, flexion, extension, lateral rotation, and medial rotation
? Pain on movement
? Muscle spasm
? Crepitation on movement

Power

Cervico-scapular and thoraco-scapular muscles (controlling scapular movement)—Elevation of scapula, retraction of scapula, abduction-rotation of scapula.

Scapulo-humeral muscles (controlling gleno-humeral movement)—Abduction, adduction, flexion, extension, lateral rotation, medial rotation

Acromio-clavicular joint

Examine for swelling, increased warmth, tenderness, pain on movement, and stability

Sterno-clavicular joint

Examine for swelling, increased warmth, tenderness, pain on movement, and stability

2. EXAMINATION OF POTENTIAL EXTRINSIC SOURCES OF SHOULDER SYMPTOMS

This is important if a satisfactory explanation for the symptoms is not found on local examination. The investigation should include : 1) the neck, with the brachial plexus ; 2) the thorax, with special reference to the heart and pleura ; and 3) the abdomen, for subdiaphragmatic lesions.

3. GENERAL EXAMINATION

General survey of other parts of the body.

hand, and it may be accompanied by paraesthesiae—often described as 'pins and needles' or 'a numb feeling.' Pain may also be referred to the shoulder from a lesion in the thorax or upper abdomen.

Exposure

The patient must be stripped to the waist. The examination is conducted most easily with the patient standing ; alternatively he may sit upon a high stool. For the greater part of the examination the surgeon stands behind the patient, so that he may observe more easily the position of the scapula.

Steps in Routine Examination

A suggested plan for the routine clinical examination of the shoulder is summarised in Table VI.

Movements at the Shoulder

In examining shoulder movements it is important to determine how much of the movement occurs at the gleno-humeral joint and how much is contributed by rotation of the scapula. An accurate distinction between the two types of movement can be made only by grasping the lower half of the scapula so that its movements can be detected (Fig. 148). In the normal shoulder about half the range of abduction occurs at the gleno-humeral joint and half by scapular rotation. Disorders of the shoulder generally cause restriction of gleno-humeral movement rather than of scapular movement.

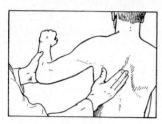

FIG. 148

Examining shoulder abduction. One hand grasps the scapula while the other steadies the elbow. In this way the proportion of the total range contributed by gleno-humeral movement and by scapular rotation can be assessed.

Stand behind the patient. *Abduction :* Instruct the patient to try to raise both arms sideways from the body so that the palms of the hands meet above the head. Measure the range, and observe what proportion of the movement takes place at the gleno-humeral joint and how much is contributed by rotation of the scapula upon the thorax. *Flexion :* Instruct the patient to raise the arms forwards towards the vertical. Again observe (by means of the hand upon the scapula) what proportion of the movement occurs at the gleno-humeral joint. *Extension :* Ask the patient to raise the elbows backwards. *Lateral rotation :* The elbows are held in to the sides and are flexed 90 degrees (Fig. 149): the forearms then serve as convenient pointers to indicate the angle of rotation (normal range = 80 degrees). *Medial rotation :* Instruct the patient to place the back of his hand in contact with his lumbar region and to carry the elbow forwards (normal range = 110 degrees).

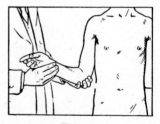

FIG. 149

Examining shoulder rotation. The elbows are flexed 90 degrees, thereby eliminating forearm rotation. The forearms serve as pointers, indicating clearly the range of rotation.

Estimation of Muscle Power

In estimating the power of the shoulder muscles two groups must be distinguished : 1) the cervico-scapular and thoraco-scapular muscles ; and 2) the scapulo-humeral muscles.

The cervico-scapular and thoraco-scapular muscles. These control movements of the scapula. Estimate the power of each group in turn and compare on the two sides. *Elevators of the scapula* (levator scapulae, upper fibres of trapezius) : Instruct the patient to shrug the shoulders against the resistance of the examiner's hands. *Retractors of the scapula* (rhomboids and middle fibres of trapezius) : Instruct the patient to brace the shoulders back. *Abductor-rotators of the scapula* (serratus anterior, with middle and lower fibres of trapezius) : Instruct the patient to push horizontally forwards with the hand against a wall (Fig. 150) or against the resistance of the examiner. If the serratus anterior is weak winging of the scapula (backward projection of its vertebral border) will be observed.

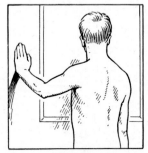

Fig. 150
Examination for weakness of the serratus anterior.

The scapulo-humeral muscles. These control movements of the gleno-humeral joint. Estimate the power of each muscle group, testing in turn the abductors, adductors, flexors, extensors, lateral rotators, and medial rotators. If the patient has lost the power to initiate active gleno-humeral movement from the dependent position, determine whether he can maintain abduction when the limb has been raised with assistance to 90 degrees. Ability to *sustain* abduction but not to *initiate* it is characteristic of isolated rupture of the supraspinatus tendon (Figs. 159-160, p. 234).

The Acromio-clavicular and Sterno-clavicular Joints

The clavicle may be regarded as a link, jointed at each end, connecting the scapula to the sternum (Fig. 151). Movement of the scapula must occur about a fulcrum at one or both ends of this link. In the normal shoulder movement of the scapula, with consequent movement at the acromio-clavicular and sterno-clavicular joints, occurs mainly 1) during elevation of the arm above 90 degrees ; and 2) when the shoulders are braced backwards or drawn forwards. To examine the acromio-clavicular and sterno-clavicular joints stand in front of the patient. Examine the joints on each side for deformity, swelling, increase of local temperature, local tenderness, and pain on movement—especially at the extremes of elevation of the arm and backward bracing of the shoulders. Observe whether there is any tendency to subluxation or dislocation of the joint on movement.

8*

Radiographic Examination

The gleno-humeral joint. The routine shoulder film is a plain antero-posterior projection with the limb in the anatomical position. When additional information is required a special axillary projection

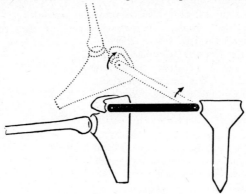

FIG. 151

The mechanics of scapular rotation. The clavicle serves as a link, jointed at each end, by which the scapula is held away from the sternum. Full rotation of the scapula entails movement both at the acromio-clavicular joint and at the sterno-clavicular joint.

with the arm abducted 90 degrees (giving a lateral view of the humerus), or stereoscopic films, should be obtained. Further films showing the upper end of the humerus in varying degrees of rotation are sometimes informative. Arthrography, after injection of radio-opaque fluid into the joint, will show whether or not the capsule is intact.

The acromio-clavicular joint and sterno-clavicular joint. Special projections are used to show each of these joints.

Extrinsic Sources of Shoulder and Arm Pain

In many cases in which the main complaint is of pain in the shoulder or arm there is no local abnormality, the symptoms being referred from a lesion elsewhere. Thus pain over the shoulder is a common symptom in affections of the neck, especially when the brachial plexus or its roots are involved. Shoulder pain is also a feature of irritative lesions in contact with the diaphragm, either in the thorax or in the abdomen. The possibility of such extrinsic lesions must always be considered in the investigation of shoulder pain. Fortunately, with careful interrogation and clinical examination there is little difficulty in distinguishing intrinsic from extrinsic lesions. The important point is that intrinsic lesions of the shoulder always give rise to local physical signs that are readily demonstrable on examination. If the shoulder is clinically normal it is improbable that it is the seat of disease, and attention should be directed towards the possible sources of referred pain.

CLASSIFICATION OF DISORDERS OF THE SHOULDER REGION

DISORDERS OF THE SHOULDER (GLENO-HUMERAL) JOINT

ARTHRITIS
   Pyogenic arthritis
   Rheumatoid arthritis
   Tuberculous arthritis
   Osteoarthritis

MECHANICAL DERANGEMENTS
   Recurrent dislocation
   Complete tear of the tendinous cuff
   Painful arc syndrome
   Rupture of the long tendon of biceps

MISCELLANEOUS
   Tenosynovitis of the long tendon of biceps.
   ' Frozen ' shoulder

DISORDERS OF THE ACROMIO-CLAVICULAR JOINT

Osteoarthritis
Persistent dislocation or subluxation

DISORDERS OF THE STERNO-CLAVICULAR JOINT

Arthritis
Persistent or recurrent dislocation

DISORDERS OF THE SHOULDER (GLENO-HUMERAL) JOINT

PYOGENIC ARTHRITIS OF THE SHOULDER

(General description of pyogenic arthritis, p. 43.)

Pyogenic arthritis of the shoulder is uncommon. It occurs most often in children, in whom infection may spread to the shoulder from a focus of osteomyelitis in the upper metaphysis of the humerus.

The clinical features resemble those of pyogenic arthritis of other joints. The onset is rapid and is accompanied by pyrexia ; and the shoulder is swollen, abnormally warm, and restricted in movement. Treatment follows the lines suggested on page 45.

RHEUMATOID ARTHRITIS OF THE SHOULDER
(General description of rheumatoid arthritis, p. 46.)

The shoulder is affected by rheumatoid arthritis less commonly than the more peripheral joints such as hands, wrists, and feet. Often both shoulders are affected simultaneously with several other joints.

As in other superficial joints, the main clinical features are local pain and stiffness, increased warmth, swelling from synovial thickening, and moderate impairment of movement.

Treatment. This is mainly that for rheumatoid arthritis in general, as described on page 49. Exercises are important in maintaining a useful range of movement. *Operative treatment :* Excision of the acromion has been recommended for painful limitation of abduction, but the results are uncertain.

TUBERCULOUS ARTHRITIS OF THE SHOULDER
(General description of tuberculous arthritis, p. 51.)

Tuberculous arthritis of the shoulder has become a rare disease in Western countries. It occurs much less commonly than tuberculosis of the spine, hip, and knee.

The pathological and clinical features correspond to those of tuberculous arthritis in any major joint, but suppuration, with formation of a tuberculous (cold) abscess, is less common in the shoulder than in other tuberculous joints. The term *caries sicca* has been used to describe this ' dry ' non-suppurative type of disease that characteristically affects the shoulder. Radiographs in the early stages show diffuse rarefaction throughout the gleno-humeral area. Later, the cartilage space is narrowed and the underlying bone may be eroded (Fig. 152). In a doubtful case synovial biopsy may be necessary to establish the diagnosis.

In a favourable case in which treatment has been begun early good recovery of function is to be hoped for, but if cartilage or bone has been destroyed permanent elimination of the joint by arthrodesis may be required (Fig. 8, p. 27).

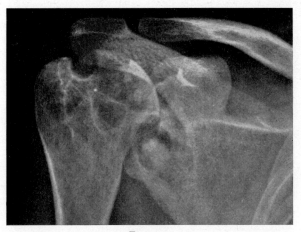

FIG. 152

Tuberculous arthritis of the shoulder. Note the loss of articular cartilage and the marked erosion of bone at the joint surfaces.

OSTEOARTHRITIS OF THE SHOULDER

(General description of osteoarthritis, p. 55.)

Unlike most other joints, the shoulder is very seldom affected by osteoarthritis. When it is affected there is usually a clear predisposing factor, such as previous injury or disease, or senility. The rarity of osteoarthritis of the shoulder is explained by its freedom from pressure stresses.

Pathology. The articular cartilage is worn away. The underlying bone becomes eburnated and at the joint margins it hypertrophies to form osteophytes.

Clinical features. The patient is usually elderly : osteoarthritis is exceptional in the shoulders of younger patients. The main complaint is of pain in the shoulder and down the upper arm. *On examination* there is no increase of local skin temperature and no synovial thickening. But a soft swelling due to effusion of fluid into the joint is common.   Movements are restricted.   *Radiographs* show narrowing of the cartilage space ; the joint outlines are clear-cut and often show some sclerosis ; there is ' spurring ' from osteophyte formation at the joint margins (Fig. 153).

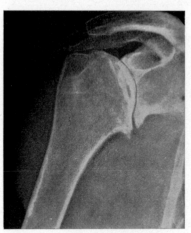

FIG. 153
Osteoarthritis of the shoulder in an old woman. Note loss of articular carti-lage, marginal osteophytes and sclerosis at the joint surfaces. Osteoarthritis is very uncommon in the shoulder.

Treatment. In many cases treatment is unnecessary once the nature of the affection has been explained.   If treatment is called for, conservative measures should usually be relied upon : short-wave diathermy, massage, and gentle exercises are often helpful.   If there is a large effusion it should be aspirated. Only exceptionally would oper-ation be justified : if it were, arthrodesis would be the method of choice.

RECURRENT ANTERIOR DISLOCATION OF THE SHOULDER

Traumatic dislocation of the shoulder is liable to cause structural changes in the gleno-humeral joint which predispose to repeated dislocations.

Pathology.   This is twofold (Figs. 154-156).   1) The capsule, and with it the glenoid labrum, is stripped from the anterior margin of the glenoid rim but retains an attachment farther down the neck of the scapula, where it becomes continuous with the periosteum.   Thus there is created an intracapsular ' pocket ' in front of the glenoid margin, into which the humeral head may be displaced (Fig. 155). 2) The articular surface of the humeral head is dented postero-laterally, probably by the initial violence (Figs. 155 and 156).   The consequent defect in the contour of the articular surface allows the head to subluxate over the front of the glenoid when the arm is in lateral rotation and abduction.   The dislocation is anterior, and it must be emphasised that the humeral head always remains within the capsule.

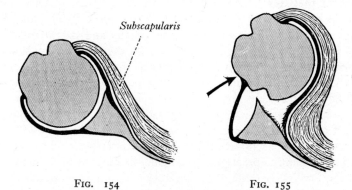

Subscapularis

FIG. 154   FIG. 155

Horizontal section of left shoulder showing the pathology of recurrent dislocation. Figure 154 shows the normal condition. In Figure 155 the humeral head is shown dislocated forwards. It has stripped the capsule from the margin of the glenoid, creating a pocket in front of the neck of the scapula into which the humeral head is displaced. Note that the humeral head has been dented by the sharp glenoid margin, producing the typical defect of the articular surface.

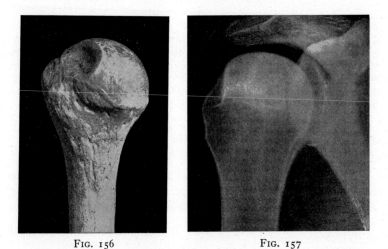

FIG. 156   FIG. 157

Figure 156—Typical defect of articular surface of humeral head, found in most cases of recurrent dislocation of the shoulder. Figure 157—Radiographic appearance with the arm in 80 degrees of medial rotation. The defect is seen at the upper and outer quadrant of the humeral head.

Clinical features. There is always a history of initial violent dislocation. Thereafter dislocation recurs with trivial violence, characteristically during combined abduction and lateral rotation (for example, in putting on a coat). *On examination* no clinical abnormality is apparent. *Radiographic examination :* Routine radiographs (with the limb in the anatomical position) do not show any abnormality, but special profile views taken with the arm in 60 to 80 degrees of medial rotation show the characteristic bony defect of the humeral head (Fig. 157).

Treatment. Conservative treatment is not effective. If dislocation recurs frequently operation is justified. The most reliable methods are the Bankart operation, in which the capsule is re-attached to the front of the glenoid margin ; and the Putti-Platt operation, in which the subscapularis tendon is shortened by overlapping or ' reefing ' in order to limit lateral rotation.

RECURRENT POSTERIOR DISLOCATION

Posterior dislocation of the shoulder is much less common than anterior dislocation. It is nevertheless prone to become recurrent. The pathology of recurrent posterior dislocation is analogous to that of recurrent anterior dislocation : 1) the capsule, glenoid labrum and periosteum are stripped from the back of the neck of the scapula ; and 2) the humeral head is dented supero-medially. Dislocation occurs on abduction and medial rotation. Repair may be effected by reefing the infraspinatus tendon on the lines of the Putti-Platt reefing of the subscapularis for anterior dislocation. An alternative method is to deepen the glenoid socket by screwing a suitably shaped block of iliac bone to the back of the neck of the scapula (bone-block operation).

COMPLETE TEAR OF THE TENDINOUS CUFF
(Torn supraspinatus)

It is important to distinguish complete tears of the tendinous cuff [1] from incomplete tears. The clinical effects are different. Whereas an incomplete tear is one cause of the ' painful arc syndrome ' (p. 235), a complete tear impairs seriously the ability to abduct the shoulder.

---

[1] The term *tendinous cuff* denotes the supraspinatus tendon together with the adjoining flat tendons that are blended with it—namely, the infraspinatus behind and the subscapularis in front. They form a cuff over the shoulder that has also been termed, inaccurately, the *rotator cuff*. Distally, the tendons forming the cuff blend with the capsule of the shoulder.

Cause. The tendon gives way under a sudden strain, usually caused by a fall. Age-degeneration of the tendon is a constant predisposing factor.

Pathology. The tear is mainly of the supraspinatus tendon, but it may extend into the adjacent subscapularis or infraspinatus

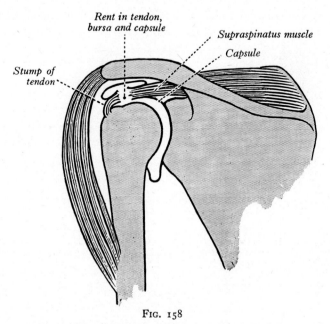

FIG. 158

Tear of supraspinatus shown diagrammatically. Note that the subacromial bursa communicates with the shoulder joint through the rent.

tendons. The tear is close to the insertion of the tendons and usually involves the capsule of the joint, with which the tendons are blended. The edges of the rent retract, leaving a gaping hole which establishes a communication between the shoulder joint and the subacromial bursa (Fig. 158).

Clinical features. The patient is usually a man over 60. After a strain or fall he complains of pain at the tip of the shoulder and down the upper arm, and of inability to raise the arm. *On examination* there is local tenderness below the margin of the acromion. When the patient attempts to abduct the arm no movement occurs at the gleno-humeral joint but a range of about 45 to 60 degrees of abduction can be achieved, entirely by scapular movement (Fig. 159). There is, however, a full range of passive movement ; and if the arm is abducted with assistance beyond 90 degrees the patient can sustain the abduction by deltoid action (Fig. 160). Thus the essential and characteristic feature in cases of torn supraspinatus tendon is inability to initiate gleno-humeral abduction. The usual explanation is that the early stages of

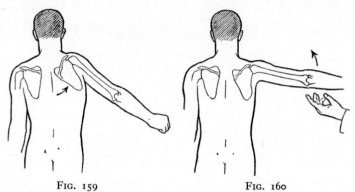

FIG. 159   FIG. 160

Complete tear of tendinous cuff (torn supraspinatus). Figure 159—Active abduction from the resting position is possible only by scapular rotation, the deltoid being unable to initiate gleno-humeral abduction without the help of the supraspinatus. Figure 160—When the limb is raised passively beyond the horizontal abduction can be sustained actively by the deltoid.

abduction demand the combined action of the deltoid muscle which supplies the main motive force, and the supraspinatus which stabilises the humeral head in the glenoid fossa (like the workman's foot against a ladder that is being raised from the ground).[1]

Diagnosis. Complete tear of the tendinous cuff must be distinguished from other causes of impaired gleno-humeral abduction, especially the painful arc syndrome and paralysis of the abductor muscles (as from poliomyelitis or nerve injury). Inability to

[1] It has been found in normal volunteers that during temporary paralysis of the supraspinatus muscle by procaine injected about the suprascapular nerve the power of abduction of the shoulder is retained, the deltoid acting successfully alone. Possibly, therefore, the actual bulk of the supraspinatus muscle is important in preventing the humeral head from riding up out of the glenoid cavity, with consequent loss of the normal fulcrum.

initiate gleno-humeral abduction, with power to sustain abduction once the limb has been raised passively, is characteristic of a widely torn supraspinatus. In the painful arc syndrome the power of abduction is retained but the movement is painful. In a case of complete tear *arthrography* will show a communication between the joint and the subacromial bursa.

Treatment. In old patients operation should usually be avoided, because the degenerate state of the tendon makes satisfactory repair impracticable : the disability tends to become gradually less noticeable, and indeed the power of active abduction (by deltoid action alone) may sometimes be regained despite the persistence of a large tear. In younger patients operation should usually be undertaken to suture the rent in the tendon. After operation the arm is rested in abduction on a splint or in plaster for three weeks, and thereafter intensive active shoulder exercises must be practised for many weeks. The results of operation are not uniformly satisfactory, probably because of the poor quality of the degenerate tendon.

PAINFUL ARC SYNDROME
(Supraspinatus syndrome)

This is a clinical syndrome characterised by pain in the shoulder and upper arm during the mid-range of gleno-humeral abduction, with freedom from pain at the extremes of the range. The syndrome is common to five distinct shoulder lesions.

Cause. The pain is produced mechanically by nipping of a tender structure between the tuberosity of the humerus and the acromion process (or coraco-acromial ligament).

Pathology. Even in the normal shoulder, the clearance between the upper end of the humerus and the acromion process is small in the range of abduction between 45 and 160 degrees. If a swollen and tender structure is present beneath the acromion it is liable to get nipped during the arc of movement in which the clearance is small (Fig. 162), with consequent pain. In the neutral position and in full abduction the clearance is greater and pain is less marked or absent (Figs. 161 and 163).

Five primary lesions can give rise to the syndrome (Fig. 164).
1) *Injury of greater tuberosity.* A contusion or undisplaced fracture of the greater tuberosity is a frequent cause.

2) *Minor tear of supraspinatus tendon.* Tearing or strain of a few tendon fibres causes an inflammatory reaction with local swelling, but power is not significantly impaired as it is after a complete tear of the tendinous cuff.

3) *Supraspinatus tendinitis.* In this condition there is believed to be an inflammatory reaction provoked by degeneration of the tendon fibres.

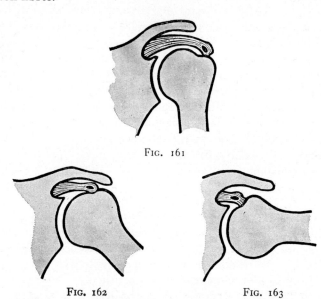

FIG. 161

FIG. 162   FIG. 163

Mechanical basis of the painful arc syndrome. The black spot represents any tender lesion near the supraspinatus insertion. Figure 161—With the arm dependent, the lesion is free from pressure. Figure 162—With the arm in mid-abduction the lesion is nipped between the humerus and the acromion. Figure 163—At full elevation the lesion is again free from pressure.

4) *Calcified deposit in supraspinatus tendon.* A white chalky deposit forms within the tendon, and the lesion is surrounded by an inflammatory reaction. The pain may begin acutely and may be extremely severe.

5) *Subacromial bursitis.* The bursal walls are inflamed and thickened from mechanical irritation.

Clinical features. Whatever the primary cause, the clinical syndrome has the same general features, though they vary in degree. With the arm dependent pain is absent or minimal. During abduction of the arm pain begins at about 45 degrees and persists through the arc of movement up to 160 degrees (Fig. 165). Thereafter the pain lessens or disappears. In descent from full elevation pain is again experienced during the middle arc of the range : often the patient will twist or circumduct the arm grotesquely in an effort to get it down with the least pain.

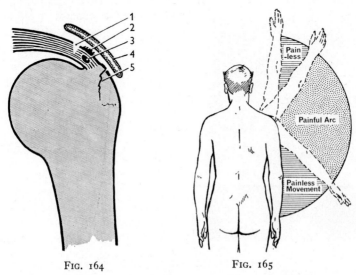

FIG. 164   FIG. 165

Figure 164—Five causes of the painful arc syndrome. The clinical features are the same in each. 1. Incomplete tear of supraspinatus. 2. Supraspinatus tendinitis. 3. Calcified deposit in supraspinatus. 4. Subacromial bursitis. 5. Crack fracture of greater tuberosity. Figure 165—Painful arc syndrome. The middle arc of abduction is painful whereas the extremes are painless.

The severity of the pain varies from case to case. In extreme cases it is so agonising that the patient is unable to face the ordeal of lifting the arm through the painful arc : a calcified deposit in the supraspinatus tendon is usually responsible for this very acute type.

Diagnosis. Painful arc syndrome is sometimes confused with arthritis of the acromio-clavicular joint, which also causes pain during a certain phase of the abduction arc. But in acromio-clavicular arthritis the pain begins later in abduction (not below 90 degrees) and increases rather than diminishes as full elevation is reached.

Differentiation between the five primary causes of the syndrome is aided by the history and by radiography. A history of injury suggests a strain of the supraspinatus tendon or a lesion of the greater tuberosity, whereas a spontaneous onset suggests tendinitis, calcified deposit or subacromial bursitis. Radiography will confirm or exclude a fracture or a calcified deposit (Fig. 166). A calcified deposit is distinguished radiologically from an avulsed fragment of bone by the fact that it is homogeneous and does not show the trabeculation character-istic of bone.

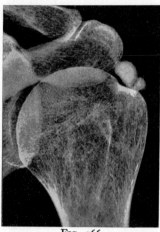

Fig. 166

To show the radiological distinction between a calcified deposit and bone. A calcified deposit has a homogeneous texture, and it differs in that respect from an avulsed fragment of bone, which would show trabeculation.

Treatment in the acute case. In mild cases treatment is often unnecessary. When treatment is called for, the method used should depend upon the primary cause of the syndrome. In most cases non-operative measures are success-ful, but operation is sometimes required.

Contusion or crack fracture of greater tuberosity : Reliance should be placed on active use and mobilising exercises. *Strain of supraspinatus, supraspinatus tendinitis,* and *subacromial bursitis :* Most of these cases respond to short-wave diathermy and mobilising exercises. *Calcified deposit in supraspinatus tendon :* In cases of moderate severity treatment is by rest in a sling and short-wave diathermy, with mobilising exercises when the pain begins to subside. If the pain is intense, as it sometimes is in these cases, immediate relief can be gained by removing the toothpaste-like deposit through an aspiration needle or through an incision into the tendon.

Treatment in the chronic case. In cases of painful arc syndrome in which severe symptoms persist despite a full trial of efficient conservative treatment operation may be required. Two methods are available. In the first and better known method the acromion process is excised back to the acromio-clavicular joint to prevent the possibility of further nipping of inflamed tissue between it and the upper end of the humerus. In the alternative method the neck of the scapula is divided and the glenoid fragment—complete with the whole gleno-humeral joint— is displaced downwards in order to widen the space between the humeral head and the acromion. This operation is still on trial.

RUPTURE OF LONG TENDON OF BICEPS

The long tendon of the biceps is one of several tendons in the body that are prone to rupture without violent stress or injury. (Others are the supraspinatus tendon and the tendon of extensor pollicis longus.)

Cause. The tendon will not rupture under ordinary stresses unless it is already weak. The predisposing factor is age-degeneration, probably accelerated by oft-repeated friction and angulation at the point where the tendon enters the bicipital groove of the humerus.

Clinical features. The patient is usually a man past middle age. While lifting or pulling with the arm he feels something give way in the region of the front of the shoulder. There is only moderate discomfort, and often the patient neglects to seek early advice. Later he may notice an unusual bulge of the muscle in front of the arm. *On examination* soon after the rupture, there is slight tenderness over the bicipital groove of the humerus. When the patient contracts the biceps muscle, as in flexing the elbow or supinating the forearm against resistance, the belly of the long head is seen to bunch up into a short round mass like a ball. There is surprisingly little weakness of elbow flexion or of supination.

Treatment. The disability is usually so slight that operation is not required. When repair is considered necessary, it is sufficient to suture the distal stump of the tendon to the walls of the bicipital groove ; the proximal stump is ignored.

TENOSYNOVITIS OF LONG TENDON OF BICEPS
(Biceps tendinitis)

This is an uncommon and rather minor affection characterised by pain and local tenderness in the region of the bicipital groove of the humerus and the long tendon of the biceps. It is generally ascribed to frictional irritation of the tendon within its groove.

Clinical features. The complaint is of pain in the front of the shoulder, worse on active use of the arm. Examination reveals local tenderness in the course of the long tendon of the biceps. The pain can often be exacerbated by moving the shoulder while the tendon is tautened by forced supination of the forearm.

Treatment. Excessive use of the shoulder should be avoided, and in severe cases a sling may be worn for part of the day. A course of short-wave diathermy to the tender area often seems to hasten recovery.

'FROZEN' SHOULDER
(Adhesive capsulitis ; periarthritis)

' Frozen ' shoulder is an ill-understood affection of the gleno-humeral joint, characterised by pain and uniform limitation of all movements, with a tendency to slow spontaneous recovery.

Cause. This is unknown. There is no evidence of infection. Injury is an inconstant factor and its significance is doubtful.

Pathology. This is not understood : it presents a baffling problem. It is believed that there is a loss of resilience of the joint capsule, but the nature of the underlying changes has not been explained. Whatever their nature, the changes are reversible, for in most cases the joint is eventually restored almost to normal.

Clinical features. The patient complains of severe aching pain in the shoulder and upper arm, of gradual and spontaneous onset. *On examination* the only finding is uniform impairment of all gleno-humeral movements—abduction, flexion, extension, rotation —which are often reduced to about a quarter or half of their normal range. In a severe case most of the shoulder movement that remains is contributed by scapular movement, which is unimpaired. *Radiographs* do not show any abnormality.

Diagnosis. Other causes of painful limitation of gleno-humeral movement, especially the various forms of arthritis, must be excluded by careful clinical and radiographic examination. The characteristic feature of 'frozen' shoulder is the uniform limitation of all gleno-humeral movements without evidence of inflammatory or destructive changes.

Course. There is a tendency towards spontaneous recovery, usually within six to twelve months. The pain subsides first, leaving gleno-humeral joint stiffness, which thereafter gradually resolves with active use of the limb. If movements are not practised deliberately some permanent restriction of movement may remain.

Treatment. In the early, acutely painful stage the arm is rested in a sling, which is removed for short periods each day to permit gentle assisted shoulder exercises. Mild analgesic drugs or phenylbutazone should be prescribed. When the pain lessens, active exercises are intensified and continued for weeks or months until full movement is regained. Short-wave diathermy is also worth a trial. If mobilisation is very slow after the pain has abated the shoulder may be manipulated gently under anaesthesia.

It is important to warn the patient at the beginning of treatment that recovery may take many months, but at the same time to give assurance that eventually recovery is likely to be complete.

DISORDERS OF THE ACROMIO-CLAVICULAR JOINT

OSTEOARTHRITIS OF THE ACROMIO-CLAVICULAR JOINT

Though not common, acromio-clavicular osteoarthritis is seen much more often than is osteoarthritis of the gleno-humeral joint. Pathologically, there are degeneration and attrition of articular cartilage, and spurs of bone (osteophytes) are formed at the joint margins.

Clinical features. There is pain, localised accurately to the acromio-clavicular joint and aggravated by strenuous use of the limb—especially by overhead work. *On examination* irregular bony thickening of the joint margins due to osteophytes can be felt. There is no soft-tissue thickening and no increase of local skin temperature. The total range of shoulder movements is not appreciably decreased, but the local acromio-clavicular pain is exacerbated at the extremes of movement. This is most easily demonstrated during abduction of the arm : the arc of movement below 90 degrees is painless, but above 90 degrees pain develops and persists throughout the remainder of the arc to full elevation (compare painful arc syndrome). *Radiographs* show narrowing of the cartilage space and marginal osteophytes.

Treatment. Often no treatment is needed. Conservative treatment is by short-wave diathermy. In severe cases operation is justified. It should take the form of excision of the lateral end of the clavicle, the conoid and trapezoid ligaments being preserved.

PERSISTENT ACROMIO-CLAVICULAR DISLOCATION OR SUBLUXATION

Persistent upward displacement of the lateral end of the clavicle is a common sequel to traumatic dislocation or subluxation of the acromio-clavicular joint. In most cases the displacement is slight and causes no symptoms. Exceptionally there is pain, worse during full elevation of the arm. *On examination* the lateral end of the clavicle is unduly prominent, and a distinct step can be felt between it and the surface of the acromion.

Treatment. Usually treatment is unnecessary. Rest in a sling for a few days is sufficient to relieve a temporary exacerbation of pain brought on by over-use of the arm. If disabling pain persists, operation is advised. A simple and effective method is to excise the lateral end of the clavicle.

DISORDERS OF THE STERNO-CLAVICULAR JOINT

ARTHRITIS OF THE STERNO-CLAVICULAR JOINT

The sterno-clavicular joint is occasionally the seat of pyogenic arthritis, rheumatoid arthritis, or tuberculous arthritis. Each of these follows the general pattern described in Chapter II, and further description is not required here. Other forms of arthritis are rarely encountered in this joint.

PERSISTENT OR RECURRENT DISLOCATION OF THE STERNO-CLAVICULAR JOINT

Forward dislocation of the medial end of the clavicle may be permanent, or it may recur on certain movements of the limb. Often, but not always, there is a history of precipitating injury.

The symptoms are slight : there is a prominence in the region of the joint, with mild local pain. Recurrent displacement of the clavicle in and out during movements of the arm may be an annoying disability. *On examination* the medial end of the clavicle, when displaced, is easily felt as a prominent forward projection. In recurrent dislocation the clavicle can be felt to click out of joint when the shoulders are braced back, and to go back into position when the shoulders are arched forwards. *Radiographs* reveal the displacement, when present. It is difficult to show the joint clearly and special projections are necessary.

Treatment. In many cases treatment is unnecessary. Non-operative treatment is ineffective. Operation is occasionally justified : the displacement is reduced and the clavicle is held in place by constructing a new retaining ligament from the tendon of the subclavius muscle or from a strip of fascia.

EXTRINSIC DISORDERS SIMULATING SHOULDER DISEASE

Pain in the shoulder or arm often has no local cause, but is referred from an extrinsic lesion. Such a possibility must always be considered in differential diagnosis.

DISORDERS OF THE BRACHIAL PLEXUS OR ITS ROOTS

The pain caused by pressure upon the brachial plexus or its roots is commonly attributed erroneously to an affection of the shoulder. Such pain varies in its precise distribution according to the site and nature of the lesion. Usually it radiates from the base of the neck, across the top of the shoulder, and down the front, side, or back of the arm ; thence it extends into the forearm, and often into the hand and fingers. Thus in its typical form the pain of a brachial plexus lesion differs from the pain of a shoulder lesion, which does not extend below the elbow.

Affections that may cause referred symptoms in the distribution of the brachial plexus include prolapsed cervical intervertebral disc, osteoarthritis of the cervical spine, cervical rib, herpes zoster, and tumours involving the spinal cord or the component nerves of the brachial plexus. These conditions were described in Chapter III.

DISORDERS WITHIN THE THORAX

ANGINA PECTORIS

In a small proportion of cases of angina pectoris the pain is felt predominantly in the shoulder region (usually on the left side). Other features are invariably present to suggest a cardiac origin, and the shoulder shows no clinical abnormality. If the history and findings are elicited with care there is little difficulty in distinguishing cardiac pain from true shoulder pain.

PLEURISY

Basal pleurisy is sometimes a cause of shoulder pain, which is explained by irritation of phrenic nerve endings, with referred pain in the distribution of the cutaneous branches of the same cervical roots (mainly C.4). The shoulder is clinically normal, and the other features of the disease are usually sufficiently clear to indicate its true nature.

DISORDERS WITHIN THE ABDOMEN

CHOLECYSTITIS

This is a cause of referred pain in the right shoulder, from irritation of the phrenic nerve endings under the diaphragm. The associated abdominal symptoms and signs, and the lack of clinical abnormality in the shoulder, should prevent diagnostic errors.

SUBPHRENIC ABSCESS

This also is an occasional cause of referred shoulder pain. Constitutional symptoms and pyrexia, with normal clinical findings in the shoulder, exonerate the shoulder from blame.

References and bibliography, page 445.

CHAPTER SIX

The Upper Arm and Elbow

APART from injury, disorders of the upper arm and elbow region are generally straightforward and present few special problems. They conform to the general descriptions of bone and joint diseases that were given in Chapter II. Thus the humerus is subject to the ordinary infections of bone, and occasionally to bone tumours—especially metastases. The elbow is liable to every type of arthritis, though none is particularly common. After the knee, it is the joint most often affected by osteochondritis dissecans and loose body formation. The ulnar nerve lies in a vulnerable position at the back of the medial epicondyle, and the possibility of impairment of nerve function complicating disease or injury of the joint should always be remembered.

SPECIAL POINTS IN THE INVESTIGATION OF UPPER ARM AND ELBOW SYMPTOMS

History

The interrogation follows the usual lines suggested in Chapter I. It is important to ascertain the exact site and distribution of the pain, and its nature. Pain arising locally in the humerus is easily confused with pain arising in the shoulder, which characteristically radiates to a point about half-way down the outer aspect of the arm. Elbow pain is localised fairly precisely to the joint, though a diffuse aching pain is often felt also in the forearm. When the ulnar nerve is interfered with behind the elbow the symptoms are mainly in the hand.

In the elbow, a history of previous injury, perhaps long ago in childhood, is often significant. Injuries in this region are notoriously liable to have late effects in the form of impaired movement, deformity, arthritis, loose body formation, or interference with the ulnar nerve.

Exposure

The whole length of the upper limb must be uncovered. The opposite limb must be similarly exposed for comparison.

Steps in Routine Examination

A suggested plan for the routine clinical examination of the upper arm and elbow is summarised in Table VII.

TABLE VII

ROUTINE CLINICAL EXAMINATION IN SUSPECTED DISORDERS
OF THE UPPER ARM AND ELBOW

---

1. LOCAL EXAMINATION OF THE ARM AND ELBOW

Inspection

Bone contours and alignment
Soft-tissue contours
Colour and texture of skin
Scars or sinuses

Palpation

Skin temperature
Bone contours
Soft-tissue contours
Local tenderness

Movements (active and passive)

Humero-ulnar joint :
Flexion
Extension
Radio-ulnar joint :
Supination
Pronation
? Pain on movement
? Crepitation on movement

Power

Flexors
Extensors
Supinators
Pronators

Stability

Lateral ligament
Medial ligament

The ulnar nerve

Sensory function
Motor function
Sweating

---

2. EXAMINATION OF POTENTIAL EXTRINSIC SOURCES
OF ARM PAIN

This is important if a satisfactory explanation for the symptoms is not found on local examination. The investigation should include : 1) the neck, with the brachial plexus ; and 2) the shoulder.

---

3. GENERAL EXAMINATION

General survey of other parts of the body. The local symptoms may be only one manifestation of a widespread disease.

Movements at the Elbow

The elbow joint has two distinct components : the hinge joint between the humerus above and the ulna and radius below, allowing flexion-extension movement ; and the pivot joint between the upper ends of the radius and ulna, allowing rotation of the forearm. It should be remembered that free rotation of the forearm is dependent not only upon an intact superior radio-ulnar joint ; it demands also free mobility between radius and ulna throughout their length, and at the inferior radio-ulnar joint. *Flexion-extension :* The normal range is from o to 150 degrees.[1] *Supination-pronation :* Rotation movements must be tested with the elbow flexed to a right angle, to eliminate rotation at the shoulder (Fig. 167). The normal range is 90 degrees of supination (palm up) and 90 degrees of pronation (palm down). If the range of rotation is restricted possible causes must be sought in the forearm and wrist as well as in the elbow.

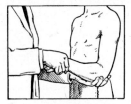

FIG. 167

Examining rotation of the forearm. The elbow is flexed 90 degrees to eliminate rotation at the shoulder.

The Ulnar Nerve

Because of the vulnerability of the ulnar nerve in its course behind the elbow, tests of ulnar nerve function should be carried out as part of the routine examination of the elbow. Examine for sensibility in the little finger and medial half of the ring finger, and test the ulnar-innervated small muscles of the hand for wasting or weakness. Note whether the skin in the territory of the ulnar nerve sweats equally with the rest of the hand.

Radiographic Examination

Radiographs of the humerus must always include antero-posterior and lateral projections, and they should take in both the shoulder joint and the elbow.

Routine radiographs of the elbow comprise an antero-posterior projection with the elbow straight and a lateral projection with the joint semi-flexed. In special circumstances additional oblique or tangential projections may be helpful. A radiograph of the forearm bones and of the inferior radio-ulnar joint is also required when rotation of the forearm is impaired.

Extrinsic Sources of Pain in the Upper Arm

Pain in the upper arm is commonly referred from a lesion elsewhere —particularly from the shoulder, and from the neck when the brachial plexus or its roots are involved. Shoulder pain usually radiates from the tip of the acromion process to about the middle of the outer aspect of the arm, but it does not extend below the elbow. In contrast, nerve pain from interference with the brachial plexus often exetnds throughout the length of the arm and forearm into the hand and fingers ; and frequently there are accompanying paraesthesiae in the form of tingling, numbness, or ' pins and needles.'

[1] o=the anatomical position, with the arm straight.

CLASSIFICATION OF DISORDERS OF THE ARM AND ELBOW

DISORDERS OF THE UPPER ARM

INFECTIONS
Acute osteomyelitis
Chronic osteomyelitis

TUMOURS
Benign tumours of bone
Malignant tumours of bone

DISORDERS OF THE ELBOW

DEFORMITIES
Cubitus valgus
Cubitus varus

ARTHRITIS
Pyogenic arthritis
Rheumatoid arthritis
Tuberculous arthritis
Osteoarthritis
Haemophilic arthritis
Neuropathic arthritis

MECHANICAL DERANGEMENTS
Osteochondritis dissecans
Loose bodies in the elbow

EXTRA-ARTICULAR DISORDERS
Olecranon bursitis
Tennis elbow
Friction neuritis of the ulnar nerve

DISORDERS OF THE UPPER ARM

ACUTE OSTEOMYELITIS

(General description of acute osteomyelitis, p. 69.)

Osteomyelitis is less common in the upper limb than in the lower. Nevertheless the humerus is a well recognised site of haematogenous infection—especially its upper metaphysis.

Pathology. Except in time of war the humerus is seldom infected directly by organisms introduced from without, for compound fractures are rare. Infection is usually haematogenous, from a focus elsewhere in the body. This type of infection occurs mainly in children, and it usually begins in the metaphysis of the bone—more often the upper metaphysis than the lower. Since both the upper and the lower metaphyses are partly enclosed within the capsule of the shoulder and the elbow respectively, a metaphysial infection is liable to spread directly to the joint, causing pyogenic arthritis (see Fig. 37, p. 71).

Clinical features. There is constitutional illness, with pyrexia. Locally, there is severe pain at the site of infection. *On examination* there is intense and well localised tenderness over the affected area— usually near one end of the bone. Later, there may be swelling and increased warmth, and a fluctuant abscess may form. The adjacent joint is commonly swollen from an effusion of fluid ('sympathetic' effusion), even if the joint itself is not involved in the infection. In the absence of joint infection, however, movements are restricted only slightly, if at all. *Radiographs* show no abnormality in the acute stage. After about two weeks there are often localised rarefaction and sub-periosteal new bone formation (Fig. 168), but these changes may be slight. *Investigations :* Blood culture is sometimes positive in the incipient stage. There is a marked polymorphonuclear leucocytosis. The erythrocyte sedimentation rate is increased.

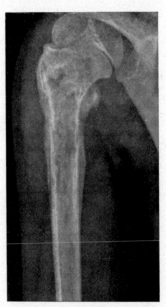

FIG. 168

Acute osteomyelitis of upper end of humerus. Radiograph four weeks after onset showing marked rarefaction of the bone, with patchy areas of destruction and much sub-periosteal new bone formation.

Treatment. This is the same as for acute osteomyelitis elsewhere. The main principles are rest and chemotherapy, with immediate drainage of the sub-periosteal abscess.

9

CHRONIC OSTEOMYELITIS
(General description of chronic osteomyelitis, p. 74.)

As in other bones, chronic pyogenic osteomyelitis of the humerus is nearly always a sequel to acute osteomyelitis that has been neglected or has responded poorly to treatment. The bone is thickened, often throughout its whole length, and there may be a persistent or intermittent purulent discharge from a sinus, or recurrent flare-ups with local pain and induration. *Radiographs* show irregular thickening with patchy areas of sclerosis and cavitation, and sometimes a sequestrum.

Treatment was described on page 75.

TUMOURS OF BONE
BENIGN TUMOURS
(General description of benign bone tumours, p. 81.)

GIANT-CELL TUMOUR (Osteoclastoma)

This is the only benign tumour of much practical importance in this region. Though it is not common at any site, it occurs relatively frequently at the upper end of the humerus, where it often extends close up to the articular surface. The tumour occurs chiefly in young adults, and its general characteristics are like those of giant-cell tumour of bone at other sites (p. 84). It should be remembered that this tumour, though usually benign, may recur after local removal and occasionally behaves in a frankly malignant fashion.

Treatment. The risk of recurrence after simple curettage or radiotherapy has to be balanced against the likely disability after radical excision of the whole of the upper end of the humerus. Each case must be considered on its merits and every factor taken into consideration.

MALIGNANT TUMOURS
(General description of malignant bone tumours, p. 86.)

Primary malignant tumours of bone are much less common in the upper limb than in the lower, and examples are seen only infrequently. Metastatic tumours, by comparison, are common, especially in the proximal part of the humerus.

OSTEOSARCOMA (Osteogenic sarcoma)

The upper metaphysis of the humerus is the favourite site in the upper limb for this highly malignant tumour. It occurs only exceptionally at the lower metaphysis. The tumour affects children or young adults and has the usual characteristics of such tumours, destroying the metaphysial region and bursting out through the cortex to invade the adjacent soft tissues. Metastasising early by the blood stream, its cells quickly take root in the lungs. Despite early treatment by amputation or massive radiotherapy the outcome is nearly always fatal (p. 88).

EWING'S TUMOUR

This occurs occasionally in the shaft of the humerus but it is very uncommon. In its behaviour it conforms to the general description given in Chapter II.

MULTIPLE MYELOMA

The tumour foci in myelomatosis develop readily in the proximal half of the humerus, which contains abundant vascular marrow.

METASTATIC TUMOURS

Carcinomatous deposits from tumours of the lung, breast, prostate, kidney, and thyroid are common in the humerus. They usually occur near the upper end of the shaft, where there is much vascular marrow. Such metastases are a common cause of pathological fracture in the upper limb. A typical example is shown in Figure 169.

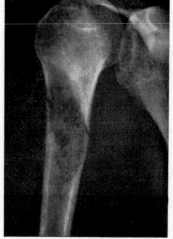

FIG. 169

Metastatic tumour in the humerus from primary carcinoma of the lung. This is a common site for metastatic tumours, which usually lead eventually to pathological fracture.

DISORDERS OF THE ELBOW

CUBITUS VALGUS

The normal elbow, when fully extended, is in a position of slight valgus—usually 10 degrees in men and 15 degrees in women. This is known as the carrying angle. If the angle is increased, so that the forearm is abducted excessively in relation to the upper arm, the deformity is known as cubitus valgus (Fig. 170).

Cause. Cubitus valgus is usually a consequence of previous disease or injury in the elbow region. The most frequent causes are : 1) previous fracture of the lower end of the humerus, with mal-union ; and 2) interference with epiphysial growth on the lateral side, from injury or infection.

Clinical features. Apart from the visible deformity there are no symptoms unless secondary effects develop.

Secondary effects. The most important sequel of cubitus valgus is interference with the function of the ulnar nerve. When valgus deformity is marked, the nerve is angled sharply round the prominent medial part of the joint, and repeated friction may lead to fibrosis of the nerve trunk. Symptoms develop insidiously over a long period : there are tingling and blunting of sensation in the ulnar distribution in the hand, with weakness and wasting of the ulnar-innervated small hand muscles (p. 263).

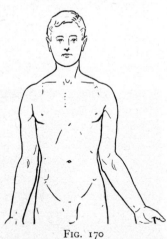

FIG. 170

Cubitus valgus. The deformity predisposes to friction neuritis of the ulnar nerve.

Long-established cubitus valgus may also lead to osteoarthritis of the elbow, especially in those who do heavy work.

Treatment. Slight uncomplicated deformity is best left alone. If angulation is severe, correction by osteotomy near the lower end of the humerus is justified. If the function of the ulnar nerve is impaired the nerve should be transposed from its post-humeral groove to a new bed at the front of the elbow.

CUBITUS VARUS

Cubitus varus is the opposite deformity to cubitus valgus. The carrying angle, or normal angle of valgus at the fully extended elbow, is decreased or reversed.

Cause. The causes are similar to those of cubitus valgus : 1) previous fracture with mal-union ; and 2) interference with epiphysial growth on the medial side.

Clinical features. There are usually no symptoms other than the visible deformity. Osteoarthritis is an occasional sequel in long-established cases.

Treatment. Minor degrees of deformity can safely be left uncorrected. If the angulation is marked it may be corrected by osteotomy through the lower end of the humerus.

PYOGENIC ARTHRITIS OF THE ELBOW
(General description of pyogenic arthritis, p. 43.)

Pyogenic arthritis is usually an acute infection with suppuration but it may occur in subacute or even in chronic form.

Pathology. As with other joints, organisms reach the elbow in three ways : 1) through the blood stream (haematogenous infection) ; 2) through a penetrating wound ; or 3) from an adjacent focus of osteomyelitis in the humerus, radius, or ulna. The last-mentioned route is the most common. There is an acute or subacute inflammatory reaction, with exudation of fluid into the joint ; the fluid is turbid or frankly purulent according to the severity of the infection. The outcome varies from complete healing, with restoration of normal function, to total destruction of the joint with fibrous or bony ankylosis.

Clinical features. The symptoms and signs correspond to those described for pyogenic arthritis elsewhere (p. 43). The onset is acute or subacute, with pain and swelling of the elbow. There is constitutional illness, with pyrexia. *On examination* the elbow is swollen, partly from fluid, partly from synovial thickening. The overlying skin is warmer than normal and it may be reddened. All movements are limited by pain and muscle spasm. *Radiographs,* normal at first, may later show diffuse rarefaction and loss of cartilage space.

Treatment. This is by aspiration or surgical drainage combined with systemic and local chemotherapy, as described on page 45.

RHEUMATOID ARTHRITIS OF THE ELBOW

(General description of rheumatoid arthritis, p. 46).

One or both elbows are commonly affected in rheumatoid arthritis, usually in conjunction with several other joints.

Pathology. The pathological changes are like those of rheumatoid arthritis elsewhere. Beginning as a chronic inflammatory thickening of the synovial membrane, it tends later to involve the articular cartilage, which may eventually be almost totally destroyed (Fig. 25, p. 48).

Clinical features. As in other joints, the main symptoms are pain, swelling from synovial thickening, abnormal warmth of the overlying skin, and impairment of movement. *Radiographic examination :* At first there are no changes. Later, there is diffuse rarefaction in the area of the joint. In long-established cases the cartilage space is lost and there may be some erosion of the bone ends (Fig. 25).

Treatment. Primary treatment is along the lines suggested for rheumatoid arthritis in general.

Operative treatment : If extensive destruction of the articular cartilage leads to persistent disabling pain operation is worth considering. Useful function, with relief of pain, can often be restored by arthroplasty of the excision type (p. 28).

TUBERCULOUS ARTHRITIS OF THE ELBOW

(General description of tuberculous arthritis, p. 51).

Tuberculous arthritis is much less common in the elbow than it is in the large weight-bearing joints such as the hip and knee.

The pathological and clinical features of joint tuberculosis were described on page 52, and further description is not required here. Biopsy may be required to establish the diagnosis.

Treatment. *Constitutional treatment* by rest and chemotherapy is required, as for other tuberculous joints. *Local treatment :* Initial treatment is by immobilisation in plaster for three to six months while the body builds up resistance against the disease. Thereafter treatment depends upon the damage sustained by the joint. If there is no evidence of destruction of articular cartilage or bone there is a reasonable chance that the disease has been arrested, and active elbow movements may be encouraged. But if cartilage is destroyed or bone eroded the joint can never be restored to normal. In these circumstances rest in plaster should be continued for as long as is necessary to allow the disease to become inactive. The resulting fibrous ankylosis often allows reasonably satisfactory function without pain, though a protective splint may have to be worn. Persisting pain or reactivation of the disease may make operative treatment necessary. *Operation :* In the elbow, unlike most other joints, simple excision of the bone ends is capable of restoring satisfactory function. The false joint so formed is rather unstable, and the arm may lack strength, but useful movement is restored. This operation is a form of arthroplasty (p. 28). The alternative is arthrodesis. The choice depends largely upon the type of work to be demanded of the limb.

OSTEOARTHRITIS OF THE ELBOW
(General description of osteoarthritis, p. 55.)

Osteoarthritis seldom occurs in an elbow that was previously normal. In nearly every case a predisposing factor has been present for several years. This is usually a damaged articular surface from previous fracture involving the joint, or from osteo-chondritis dissecans.

Clinical features. There is slowly increasing pain in the elbow, worse on heavy use of the limb. The patient may also notice that movement is impaired. In some cases there are attacks of sudden locking, suggesting the presence of a loose body in the joint. There is often a history of previous injury or disease involving the elbow. *On examination* there is palpable thickening at the joint margins, from osteophytes. Flexion and extension are impaired but rotation is often full. There is coarse crepitation on movement. *Radiographs* show narrowing of the cartilage space and pointed osteophytes at the joint margins (Fig. 171). Loose bodies (formed from detached osteophytes or from flakes of articular cartilage) may be present.

Treatment. In many cases treatment is not required once the nature of the trouble has been explained to the patient. When treatment is called for conservative measures are tried first. Physiotherapy in the form of short-wave diathermy is usually adequate, especially if heavy use of the elbow can be reduced. Exceptionally operation is advisable. Thus if a loose body has caused symptoms of locking it may be removed with excellent

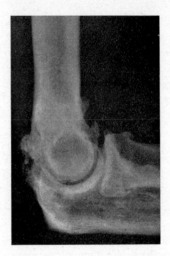

prospects of relief; and if the arthritis is predominantly in the lateral (humero-radial) half of the joint excision of the head of the radius is often helpful. Apart from these simple procedures, reliance can be placed only upon arthroplasty (by excision of the joint surfaces) or upon arthrodesis, both of them rather drastic operations that should be advised only if the disability is severe.

FIG. 171

Osteoarthritis of the elbow. Note the narrowed cartilage space and pointed osteophytes at the joint margins. In this case osteoarthritis was secondary to osteochondritis dissecans.

HAEMOPHILIC ARTHRITIS OF THE ELBOW

(General description of haemophilic arthritis, p. 60.)

Haemophilic arthritis affects the elbow more often than any other joint except the knee. As in other joints, the main feature is intra-articular haemorrhage, with consequent irritation and, later, degeneration of the joint.

The clue to the diagnosis is a history of previous bleeding or of a haemophilic tendency in the family. Haemarthrosis without major injury is suggestive and should arouse suspicion of haemophilia. A prolonged blood clotting time is an important confirmatory finding.

Treatment. General treatment is the same as that for other manifestations of haemophilia. Local treatment is by firm bandaging and rest in a plaster splint for three or four weeks, followed by gentle mobilising exercises.

NEUROPATHIC ARTHRITIS OF THE ELBOW

(General description of neuropathic arthritis, p. 62.)

In neuropathic arthritis (Charcot's osteoarthropathy) of the elbow the joint becomes disorganised in consequence of a loss of sensibility to pain. It is a rare form of arthritis.

Cause. The usual underlying cause of the disease in the elbow is syringomyelia.

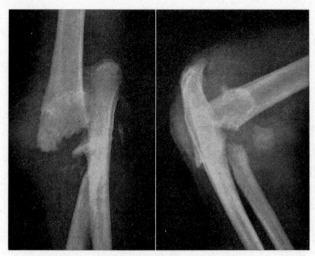

FIG. 172

Neuropathic arthritis of the elbow. There is marked absorption of bone, with pathological dislocation. The underlying cause was syringomyelia.

Pathology. The protective mechanism which prevents the normal joint from being damaged by everyday stresses fails because the ligaments are insensitive to pain. A vicious circle is established : repeated unrecognised injuries impair the stability of the joint and thereby render it more liable to further injury. The ultimate result is gross disorganisation. Basically, the changes consist in degeneration and attrition of the joint surfaces, sometimes with coincident massive hypertrophy of bone at the joint margins. Pathological dislocation may occur (Fig. 172).

9*

Clinical features. The main symptoms are swelling and a feeling of weakness due to instability. In the early stages pain may not be entirely absent, but in general lack of pain is a striking feature. *On examination* there is marked thickening and irregularity of the bone ends. The joint is abnormally lax, and lateral mobility is often pronounced. Clinical evidence of the underlying condition (usually syringomyelia) will be found. *Radiographs* show a disorganised joint, often with much destruction of bone (Fig. 172). *Investigations* should be directed towards establishing the nature of the underlying neurological disorder.

Treatment. This is mainly that of the underlying disorder. If the elbow is severely disorganised it should be protected by a right-angled splint of plastic or leather. Exceptionally, arthrodesis is justified.

OSTEOCHONDRITIS DISSECANS OF THE ELBOW

(General description of osteochondritis dissecans, p. 67.)

After the knee, the elbow is the most frequent site of osteochondritis dissecans. The disorder is characterised by necrosis of part of the articular cartilage and of the underlying bone, with eventual separation of the fragment to form an intra-articular loose body.

Cause. The precise cause is unknown. Impairment of blood supply to the affected segment of bone and cartilage by thrombosis of an end-artery has been suggested. Injury probably plays a part.

Pathology. The part of the elbow affected is nearly always the capitulum. The necrotic segment of articular surface varies in size ; commonly its surface area is about a centimetre in diameter and its depth less than half a centimetre. A line of demarcation forms between the avascular segment and the surrounding normal bone and cartilage, and after an interval of months the avascular segment separates as a loose body (sometimes two or three), leaving a shallow cavity in the articular surface which is ultimately filled with fibrous tissue. The damage to the joint surface predisposes to the later development of osteoarthritis.

Clinical features. In the early stages, before the fragment has separated, the symptoms are those of mild mechanical irritation of the joint—namely, aching after use and intermittent swelling.

On examination at this stage there is often a little swelling from effusion of clear fluid into the joint, and there is slight limitation of flexion or extension.

When a loose body has separated, the main features are recurrent painful locking of the elbow followed by effusion of fluid.

Radiographic examination : In the early stages there is an area of irregularity on the affected articular surface, usually the capitulum. Later a shallow cavity, whose margins are demarcated clearly from the bone within it, is seen (Fig. 173). Eventually the bony fragment separates from the cavity and lies free within the joint, usually in the lateral compartment.

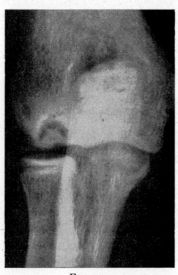

FIG. 173

Osteochondritis dissecans. A fragment of the capitulum is separating. This is the typical site of osteochondritis dissecans in the elbow.

Treatment. Operation is delayed until the fragment of bone and cartilage is ripe for separation or has actually separated. The fragment is then removed.

LOOSE BODIES IN THE ELBOW

Causes. There are four important causes of loose bodies in the elbow : 1) osteochondritis dissecans (1 to 3 bodies) ; 2) osteoarthritis (1 to 3 bodies) ; 3) fracture with separation of a fragment (1 to 3 bodies) ; and 4) synovial chondromatosis (50 to 500 bodies).

Pathology and clinical features. *Osteochondritis dissecans* was described on page 258 and *osteoarthritis* on page 255.

Loose body after fracture. A fragment may rarely be detached from the capitulum. Sometimes the medial epicondyle is detached and sucked into the joint, retaining its attachments to the flexor muscles.

Synovial chondromatosis (osteochondromatosis). This is a rare disease of synovial membrane in which numerous synovial villi become pedunculated and transformed into cartilage ; eventually they are detached to form a large number of loose bodies, many of which become calcified.

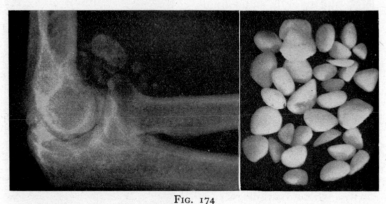

FIG. 174

Multiple loose bodies in the elbow. A case of synovial chondromatosis.

Clinical features. Many so-called loose bodies are ' silent '— that is, they cause no symptoms. Often in such cases the fragment is not in fact loose, but has soft-tissue attachments that prevent its moving about the joint.

The characteristic symptom of a freely movable loose body is sudden locking of the elbow during movement, with intense pain. The joint is usually unlocked after an interval, either spontaneously or by the patient's manœuvres. Several hours later the joint swells. The symptoms subside within a few days, but repeated attacks are to be expected. *Examination* in the stage of swelling shows the joint to be distended with fluid—a clear, pale, straw-coloured effusion. Between attacks a loose body may sometimes be felt. There is often a history or clinical evidence to suggest the cause of the loose body formation. *Radiographs* show the loose body or bodies (Fig. 174) and usually indicate the nature of the primary condition.

Treatment. Symptomless loose bodies may usually be safely left alone ; but if a loose body causes locking it should be removed by operation.

OLECRANON BURSITIS

The bursa behind the olecranon is liable to traumatic bursitis, septic bursitis, and gout.

In *traumatic bursitis* (' student's elbow ') the bursa is distended with clear fluid (Fig. 175). Treatment at first should be by aspiration, followed by the injection of hydrocortisone into the bursa. If the swelling recurs the bursa should be excised.

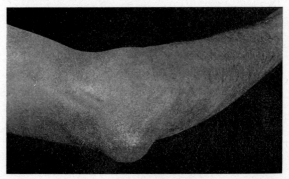

FIG. 175
Olecranon bursitis.

Septic bursitis is treated by incision to secure adequate drainage.

In *gouty bursitis* there is acute or subacute inflammation, and whitish deposits of sodium biurate (tophi) may be visible through the walls of the bursa.

TENNIS ELBOW
(Epicondylitis)

' Tennis ' elbow is a common and well defined clinical entity. It is an extra-articular affection characterised by pain and acute tenderness at the origin of the extensor muscles of the forearm.
Cause. It is believed to be caused by strain of the forearm extensor muscles at the point of their origin from the bone. Although it sometimes follows tennis, other activities are more frequently responsible.
Pathology. No pathology has been demonstrated. Hypothetically, it is assumed that there is incomplete rupture of aponeurotic fibres at the muscle origin, which is a region plentifully supplied by nerve endings. The elbow joint itself is unaffected.

Clinical features. There is pain at the lateral aspect of the elbow, often radiating down the back of the forearm. *On examination* there is tenderness precisely localised to the front of the lateral epicondyle of the humerus (Fig. 176). Pain is aggravated by putting the extensor muscles on the stretch—for example, by flexing the wrist and fingers with the forearm pronated. Movements of the elbow are full. *Radiographs* show no alteration from the normal.

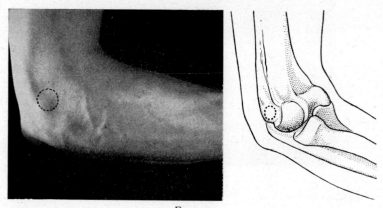

FIG. 179
In tennis elbow the point of greatest tenderness is at the front of the lateral epicondyle, not over its greatest prominence.

Course. If left alone the symptoms eventually subside spontaneously, but they may persist for as long as two years or more.

Treatment. In mild cases the patient is often willing to await spontaneous recovery once the harmless nature of the affection has been explained. Treatment is unpredictable in its results and no method can be relied upon in every case.

Conservative treatment : In the first instance treatment should be by the injection of hydrocortisone, preferably with local anaesthetic solution, into the point of greatest tenderness. This method is often successful, but only if the injection is made precisely into the tender spot. This is not always done easily, and consequently it may sometimes be necessary to repeat the injection on one or two occasions at weekly intervals. In a successful case the pain is often exacerbated for twenty-four hours or so before it begins gradually to disappear.

If local injections fail, a trial may be made of the following methods : *physiotherapy*, in the form of short-wave diathermy, deep massage to the tender area, and faradic stimulation of the extensor muscles ; *manipulation* to stretch the extensor muscles, with or without infiltration of local anaesthetic into the tender area ; *rest in plaster* for six weeks.

Operative treatment : This should be advised only in cases of severe disability not responding to conservative treatment. The extensor origin is stripped from its attachment to the lateral epicondyle and allowed to fall back into place. By the time the wound is well healed the pain will usually have disappeared.

FRICTION NEURITIS OF THE ULNAR NERVE

The ulnar nerve is vulnerable where it lies in the groove behind the medial epicondyle of the humerus. Its function may be interfered with either by constriction or by recurrent friction while in tension. Constriction is usually secondary to osteo-arthritis, with encroachment of osteophytes upon the ulnar groove. Friction under tension occurs when the carrying angle of the elbow is increased (cubitus valgus, p. 252). In both cases the nerve undergoes fibrosis, and unless the mechanical fault is relieved the changes become irreversible.

Clinical features. The patient complains of numbness or tingling in the ulnar distribution, and often of clumsiness in performing fine finger movements. *On examination* the following signs are present in the fully developed condition : *Sensory*—There is blunting or loss of sensation along the ulnar border of the hand and in the little finger and medial half of the ring finger. *Motor*— There are wasting and weakness of the ulnar-innervated small hand muscles. *Sweating*—The skin in the ulnar territory is drier than normal because sweating is impaired. *Strength-duration curves* (p. 14) plotted for the ulnar-innervated muscles may show the pattern of partial denervation before motor signs are evident clinically.

Treatment. Whenever the ulnar nerve is interfered with by a lesion at the elbow operation should be undertaken to transpose the nerve to a new bed in front of the joint, where it will be free from pressure or friction.

References and bibliography, page 445

CHAPTER SEVEN

The Forearm, Wrist, and Hand

SO much in everyday life depends upon the efficient working of the hand, and so great is the practical and economic consequence of its disablement, that the care of the diseased or injured hand has become one of the most vital branches of orthopaedic surgery. It is also one of the most fascinating.

Hand surgery is an art and a science in itself. Indeed it is fast developing as a distinct speciality, demanding a knowledge and experience not only of orthopaedics but also of plastic surgery, vascular surgery, and neurology. In America some surgeons are already devoting their whole professional career to work in this field, and there are signs of a similar trend in Great Britain.

In the treatment of hand disorders the primary emphasis should always be on restoration of function. Keen judgment is often called for in deciding between the claims of rest and of movement. It should be remembered that the hand tolerates immobilisation badly. Whereas the wrist may be immobilised for many weeks or even months with impunity, to immobilise injured or diseased fingers for a long time is to court disaster in the form of permanent joint stiffness. Although rest may be essential in the early days after a hand injury or in the acute stage of an infection, active finger exercises must be insisted upon as soon as that stage has passed. It is wise to accept it as a general rule that fingers should never be immobilised for longer than two, or at most three, weeks.

SPECIAL POINTS IN THE INVESTIGATION OF FOREARM, WRIST, AND HAND COMPLAINTS

History

It should be remembered that symptoms in the hand are often caused by disorders of the neck (with involvement of the brachial plexus) and sometimes by disorders at the elbow. Enquiry should always be made into any previous injury or other trouble with the neck or with the upper extremity as a whole.

TABLE VIII

ROUTINE CLINICAL EXAMINATION IN SUSPECTED DISORDERS
OF THE FOREARM, WRIST, AND HAND

---

1. LOCAL EXAMINATION OF THE FOREARM, WRIST, AND HAND

Inspection

Bone contours
Soft-tissue contours
Colour and texture of skin
Scars or sinuses

Palpation

Skin temperature
Bone contours
Soft-tissue contours
Local tenderness

Movements (active, passive)

At the wrist :

Radio-carpal joint — Flexion-extension ; adduction-abduction
Inferior radio-ulnar joint— Supination and pronation

At the hand :

Carpo-metacarpal joint of thumb —Flexion-extension ; adduction-abduction ; opposition

Metacarpo-phalangeal joints— Flexion-extension ; adduction-abduction
Interphalangeal joints—Flexion-extension

Power

Power of each muscle group in control of 1) wrist movement, 2) thumb and finger movement, and 3) gripping

Stability

Tests for abnormal mobility

Nerve function

Tests of sensory function, motor function, and sweating in distribution of median, ulnar and radial nerves

Circulation

Arterial pulses, warmth and colour, capillary return, cutaneous sensibility

---

2. EXAMINATION OF POSSIBLE EXTRINSIC SOURCES OF FOREARM AND HAND SYMPTOMS

This is important if a satisfactory explanation for the symptoms is not found on local examination. The investigation should include : 1) the neck and thoracic inlet, with special reference to the brachial plexus ; 2) the upper arm ; and 3) the elbow.

---

3. GENERAL EXAMINATION

General survey of other parts of the body. The local symptoms may be only one manifestation of a more widespread disease.

Exposure

For the local examination the whole forearm should be uncovered to well above the elbow. The sound limb should be exposed likewise for comparison.

Steps in Clinical Examination

A suggested routine of clinical examination is summarised in Table VIII.

Movements at the Wrist

Like the elbow, the wrist comprises two distinct components: 1) the radio-carpal joint (including the intercarpal joints), allowing flexion, extension, adduction, and abduction; and 2) the inferior radio-ulnar joint, allowing supination and pronation. The movements at each component must be examined independently.

The radio-carpal joint. The normal range of flexion is 80 degrees and of extension 90 degrees. The range of adduction, or ulnar deviation, is about 35 degrees, and of abduction, or radial deviation, about 25 degrees. It is impracticable to measure the movements of the intercarpal joints individually, and it is simplest to regard them as integral parts of the radio-carpal joint.

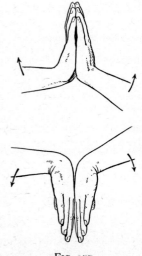

FIG. 177

A simple method of comparing the range of extension and flexion at the two wrists. Note the obvious impairment at the left wrist.

A rapid and reasonably accurate method of comparing the range of flexion-extension movement on the two sides is as follows: *To judge the range of extension:* The patient places the palms and fingers of the two hands in contact in the vertical plane and lifts the elbows as far as he can while keeping the 'heels' of the hands together (Fig. 177). The angle between hand and forearm is easily compared on the two sides. *To judge the range of flexion:* The manœuvre is reversed. The patient places the backs of the hands together, with the fingers directed vertically downwards, and lowers the elbows as far as he can (Fig. 177). The angle between hand and forearm is compared on the two sides.

The inferior radio-ulnar joint. The normal range is 90 degrees of supination and 90 degrees of pronation. To determine the range accurately the patient's elbows must be flexed to a right angle in order to eliminate rotation at the shoulder (Fig. 167, p. 247).

It must be emphasised that impaired rotation does not necessarily denote an abnormality of the wrist : it may equally well be caused by a disorder of the elbow or of the forearm.

Movements of the Hand

Movements of the hand occur mainly at three groups of joints : 1) the carpo-metacarpal joint of the thumb ; 2) the metacarpo-phalangeal joints ; and 3) the interphalangeal joints.

The carpo-metacarpal joint of the thumb. This joint allows movement in five directions : flexion, or movement of the thumb metacarpal medially in the plane of the palm ; extension, or movement of the thumb

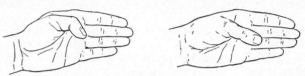

FIG 178

To show the difference between flexion of the thumb across the palm (left) and true opposition (right). In opposition the thumb metacarpal is rotated so that the thumb nail lies in a plane parallel with the palm.

metacarpal laterally in the plane of the palm ; adduction, or movement of the metacarpal towards the palm in a plane at right angles to it ; abduction, or movement of the metacarpal away from the palm in a plane at right angles to it ; and opposition, or rotation of the metacarpal to bring the thumb nail into a plane parallel with the palm (Fig. 178).

The metacarpo-phalangeal joints of thumb and fingers. These joints allow flexion-extension movement through 90 degrees (the range is variable in the thumb), and a small range of abduction from, and adduction to, the midline of the middle finger.

The interphalangeal joints of thumb and fingers. These are true hinge joints, allowing only flexion and extension.

Power

Test the power of each movement in turn. In the hand this examination demands considerable patience, for each muscle group must be tested individually. Thus in the thumb it is necessary to test the abductors, the adductor, the extensors (longus and brevis), the flexors (longus and brevis), and the opponens. In the fingers test the flexors (profundus and superficialis), the extensor digitorum and extensor indicis, the interossei and the lumbricals. *Grip :* Test the power of grip, which demands the combined action of the flexors and extensors of the wrist and the flexors of the fingers and thumb.

Nerve Function

The state of the median, ulnar, and radial nerves is determined by tests of sensory function, motor function, and sweating.

Circulation

The state of the circulation is assessed from the condition of the arterial pulses, the warmth and colour of the digits, the capillary return at the nail beds, and cutaneous sensibility. It should be remembered that sensibility to touch in the fingers is a most useful index of the adequacy of the circulation. Nerves require a blood supply to enable them to conduct impulses, and if the circulation is interrupted sensibility is quickly lost.

Extrinsic Sources of Forearm and Hand Symptoms

It is sometimes difficult to determine whether symptoms and signs in the forearm or hand are caused by a local disorder or whether they are referred from a more proximal lesion. This difficulty arises mainly in neurological conditions. For instance, the symptoms of compression of the median nerve in the carpal tunnel may be mimicked closely by a prolapsed cervical disc, and the symptoms of constriction of the ulnar nerve at the elbow may likewise be confused with those from a low cervical disc lesion or a cervical rib. When symptoms in the hand are not satisfactorily explained by the local condition a search must be made for a possible cause in the neck, upper arm, or elbow.

Radiographic Examination

Routine radiographs should include antero-posterior and lateral projections of the forearm, wrist, and hand. For detailed study of the carpal bones additional oblique projections are required.

If it is suspected that the symptoms may be referred from the neck or proximal part of the limb radiographs of the appropriate part should be obtained.

CLASSIFICATION OF DISORDERS OF THE FOREARM, WRIST, AND HAND

DISORDERS OF THE FOREARM

INFECTIONS OF BONE

Acute osteomyelitis
Chronic osteomyelitis

TUMOURS OF BONE

Benign tumours
Malignant tumours

MISCELLANEOUS

Volkmann's ischaemic contracture
Acute frictional tenosynovitis

ARTICULAR DISORDERS OF THE WRIST AND HAND

DEFORMITIES

Madelung's deformity

ARTHRITIS

Pyogenic arthritis
Rheumatoid arthritis
Osteoarthritis

MISCELLANEOUS

Kienböck's disease

EXTRA-ARTICULAR DISORDERS ABOUT THE WRIST AND HAND

INFECTIONS

Acute infections of the fascial spaces
Chronic infective tenosynovitis

TUMOURS

Tumours of bone
Tumours of soft tissue

NEUROLOGICAL DISORDERS

Compression of the median nerve in the carpal tunnel

MISCELLANEOUS

Ganglion
Dupuytren's contracture
Rupture or severance of tendons
De Quervain's tenovaginitis
Digital tenovaginitis stenosans

DISORDERS OF THE FOREARM

ACUTE OSTEOMYELITIS

(General description of acute osteomyelitis, p. 69.)

Acute osteomyelitis is rather uncommon in the forearm bones. As in other sites, the infection may be blood-borne (haematogenous) or it may be introduced from without, usually in consequence of a compound fracture. The haematogenous type occurs mainly in children. It affects the radius more often than the ulna, and the lower metaphysis rather than the upper (Fig. 40, p. 72). The upper metaphyses of both radius and ulna are partly or wholly within the capsule of the elbow ; so an infection of the metaphysis may spread directly to the joint to cause pyogenic arthritis. At the wrist, in contrast, the metaphysis of the radius is wholly outside the capsule, so direct spread of infection to the joint is unlikely. The lower metaphysis of the ulna is partly within the capsule.

The clinical features and treatment are like those of acute osteomyelitis elsewhere.

CHRONIC OSTEOMYELITIS
(General description of chronic osteomyelitis, p. 74.)

As in other bones, chronic osteomyelitis of the radius or ulna follows an acute infection.

Treatment. In most cases treatment should follow the usual lines, reliance being placed on rest and chemotherapy for non-suppurative flares of infection, and on thorough drainage operations and sequestrectomy for persistent purulent discharge. In obstinate cases the affected part of the bone may sometimes be excised without important loss of function : this applies particularly to infection of the lower end of the ulna.

BONE TUMOURS IN THE FOREARM
BENIGN TUMOURS
(General description of benign tumours of bone, p. 81.)

Any type of benign tumour may occur in the forearm bones. Only chondroma and giant-cell tumour require further mention here.

CHONDROMA
Chondromata of long bones occur chiefly in multiple form, in the condition known as dyschondroplasia, Ollier's disease, or multiple chondromatosis (p. 106). Their special significance in the forearm lies in the fact that the tumours may interfere with the normal growth of the affected bone. If growth is retarded in one bone but proceeds normally in its partner marked curvature of the bones is to be expected and it may cause ugly deformity.

Treatment. Severe deformity from uneven growth of the radius and ulna should be corrected by osteotomy, combined when necessary with excision of the lower end of the ulna.

GIANT-CELL TUMOUR (Osteoclastoma)

The lower end of the radius is one of the favourite sites in the upper limb for the development of a giant-cell tumour, which though classed as benign may show invasive tendencies. The lower end of the ulna is also susceptible. The tumour extends into the former epiphysial region close up to the articular surface (Fig. 55, p. 83).

Treatment. If the lower end of the ulna is the part affected the bone should be excised up to a point well proximal to the tumour. The resulting disability is negligible. If the tumour is in the lower end of the radius treatment is more difficult. Radical excision of the affected part of the bone is the surest safeguard against recurrence of this rather sinister tumour, and it should usually be undertaken despite the inevitable disability that it produces at the wrist. A satisfactory plan of reconstruction after removal of the lower end of the radius is to implant and fuse the lower end of the ulna into the carpus. Alternatively, the part of the radius that has been excised may be replaced by a graft, usually obtained from the fibula.

MALIGNANT TUMOURS

(General description of malignant tumours of bone, p. 86.)

The radius and ulna are seldom affected by malignant bone tumours, whether primary or metastatic. When osteosarcoma does occur in the forearm the lower end of the radius is the usual site.

VOLKMANN'S ISCHAEMIC CONTRACTURE

This is a flexion deformity of the wrist and fingers from fixed contracture of the flexor muscles in the forearm.

Cause. It is caused by ischaemia of the flexor muscles, brought about by injury to, or obstruction of, the brachial artery near the elbow.

Pathology. The effects of sudden occlusion of the brachial artery vary. In a few cases gangrene of the fingers will follow. More often, the collateral circulation is sufficient to keep the hand alive, but not to nourish adequately the flexor muscles of the forearm or the main peripheral nerve trunks. Necrosis of muscle fibres of the forearm flexor group—especially the flexor digitorum profundus and flexor pollicis longus—with subsequent fibrosis and shortening, is the essential feature of Volkmann's contracture. It is often associated with temporary or permanent ischaemic paralysis of the peripheral nerves, especially the median nerve.

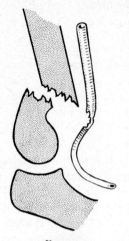

FIG. 179

To show how a supracondylar fracture of the humerus may damage the brachial artery, with risk of gangrene or ischaemic contracture. Over-tight plaster or dressings may have the same result.

Any major fracture in the elbow region or upper forearm may lead to arterial occlusion. That most commonly responsible is a supracondylar fracture of the humerus with displacement, the brachial artery being severed or contused by the sharp lower end of the main shaft fragment (Fig. 179). Contusion alone is sufficient to interrupt the flow of blood, because the artery goes into spasm and its lumen may be occluded by thrombosis.

In some cases the cause of the arterial obstruction is an over-tight plaster or bandage.

Clinical features. The condition is commonest in children. After sustaining a supracondylar fracture of the humerus or some other injury in the elbow region the child complains of pain in the forearm. *On examination* in the incipient stage, the fingers are white or blue, and cold. The radial pulse is absent. Active finger movements are weak and painful. Passive extension of the fingers is especially painful and restricted. There may or may not be evidence of interruption of nerve conductivity—namely, anaesthesia of the fingers and paralysis of the small muscles of the hand.

In the established condition, which develops gradually within a few weeks of the injury, there is a striking flexion contracture of the wrist and fingers, from shortening of the fibrotic forearm flexor muscles (Fig. 180). Sensory and motor paralysis of the hand may persist as complicating factors, but they do not form an essential feature of Volkmann's contracture as such.

Diagnosis. In the incipient stage absence of the radial pulse, with marked unwillingness to extend the fingers because of pain, should always arouse suspicion of Volkmann's contracture. If there are also anaesthesia and paralysis of the hand the diagnosis is practically certain. In the established condition the history and clinical features make the diagnosis clear.

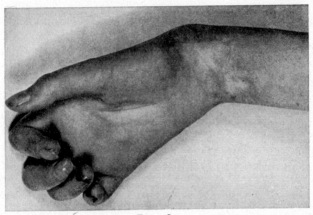

FIG. 180
Typical appearance of the hand in established Volkmann's ischaemic contracture.

Volkmann's ischaemic contracture bears no real resemblance to Dupuytren's contracture (p. 298), for it affects the wrist as well as all the joints of the fingers, and there is no palpable thickening in the palm. Moreover the contracture is demonstrably brought about by shortening of the flexor muscles, because if the wrist is flexed passively to relax the flexor tendons the range of extension at the finger joints is increased. Conversely, if the tendons are relaxed by flexing the fingers fully the range of wrist extension is increased (Fig. 181).

Treatment. In the **incipient stage** the problem is that of dealing with a sudden occlusion of the brachial artery. The case must be handled as an emergency, because the effects of occlusion become irreversible after about six hours. The following action must be taken. *First step:* All splints, plaster, and bandages that might be obstructing the circulation are removed. In the case of a fracture, gross displacement of the fragments is corrected so far as possible by gentle manipulation and a well padded plaster splint is applied. Likewise if the elbow is dislocated it must be reduced without delay. Heat cradles or hot bottles are applied over the other three limbs and trunk to promote general vasodilation. If these measures fail to bring about a return of adequate circulation within half an hour, the next step is taken. *Second step:* At operation the brachial artery is explored and the nature of the damage determined. If the occlusion is due to kinking or spasm of the artery an attempt is made to relieve it by freeing the vessel and painting the adventitia with a solution of papaverine. If the vessel is found punctured, or contused and thrombosed, the ideal treatment is to excise the damaged segment and to suture the two ends. If direct suture is impracticable an attempt should be made to restore continuity by a vein graft. Failing this, it may be necessary to ligate the ends after excision of the damaged segment.

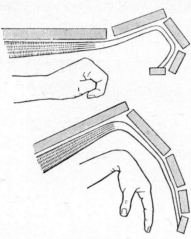

FIG. 181

In Volkmann's contracture the wrist can be partly extended if the fingers are flexed, and the fingers can be partly extended if the wrist is flexed: but the shortened fibrotic flexor muscles prevent extension of wrist and fingers together.

In the **established stage** restoration to normal is impossible: reconstructive surgery at best can only improve what function remains. The choice of treatment depends upon the circumstances of each case. In relatively mild cases the shortening of the flexor muscles may sometimes be overcome by prolonged stretching by spring splints, provided the treatment is begun early. Alternatively, the muscle shortening may be counteracted to some extent by operations such as shortening of the forearm bones or detachment and distal displacement of the flexor muscle origin (muscle slide operation). In selected cases with severe muscle infarction the best results are probably obtained by excision of the dead muscles and subsequent transfer of a healthy muscle (for example, a wrist flexor or a wrist extensor) to the tendons of flexor digitorum profundus and of flexor pollicis longus to restore active flexion of the digits. These muscle transfers may be combined, in appropriate cases, with arthrodesis of the wrist. When the median nerve is irreparably damaged by ischaemia nerve grafting is sometimes successful in restoring its function.

ACUTE FRICTIONAL TENOSYNOVITIS

(Peritendinitis ; paratendinitis)

This is an easily recognised clinical condition common in young adults whose occupations demand repetitive movements of the wrist and hand.

Cause. It is attributed to excessive friction between the tendons and the surrounding paratenon, from over-use of the hand. It is entirely distinct from infective tenosynovitis.

Pathology. The tendons most often affected are those of the deep muscles at the back of the forearm, especially the extensors of the thumb and the radial extensors of the wrist. There is a mild inflammatory reaction about the tendon and its coverings, with local swelling and oedema.

Clinical features. After unusually active use of the wrist or hand over a period of days or weeks pain is felt at the back of the wrist and lower forearm. The pain is aggravated by use of the hand. *On examination* there is localised swelling in the line of the affected tendons—usually the extensors of the thumb or wrist. If the examiner's hand is placed over the swelling while the patient flexes and extends the wrist and digits a characteristic fine crepitation is felt: it is caused by the fibrin-covered tendon gliding within the inflamed paratenon. This typical crepitation is diagnostic of frictional tenosynovitis.

Treatment. The wrist is immobilised in plaster of Paris for three weeks, the fingers being left free. This affords sufficient rest to allow the inflammation to resolve. Excessive use of the fingers and thumb should be avoided for two months.

ARTICULAR DISORDERS OF THE WRIST AND HAND

MADELUNG'S DEFORMITY

Madelung's deformity is congenital subluxation or dislocation of the lower end of the ulna. A similar deformity is more often caused by disease or injury, such as a fracture of the lower end of the radius with upward displacement of the lower fragment. The deformity varies in degree from a slight prominence of the lower end of the ulna at the back of the wrist to complete

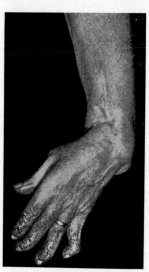

dislocation of the inferior radio-ulnar joint with marked radial deviation of the hand (Fig. 182). The more severe types of deformity may be associated with congenital absence of the radius. **Treatment.** If the disability justifies operation the lower end of the ulna should be excised. In a severe case, with marked radial deviation of the hand, it may be necessary also to fuse the radius (or ulna, if the radius is absent) to the carpus in order to gain satisfactory correction.

FIG. 182

Relative shortening of radius with subluxation of inferior radio-ulnar joint, radial deviation of the hand and prominent head of ulna (Madelung's deformity).

FIG. 182

PYOGENIC ARTHRITIS OF THE WRIST

(General description of pyogenic arthritis, p. 43.)

Pyogenic arthritis of the wrist is uncommon. Infection may be haematogenous, or it may be introduced through a penetrating wound. Spread from a focus of osteomyelitis is rare, partly because osteomyelitis itself is uncommon in the forearm bones, and partly because the lower metaphysis of the radius is entirely outside the capsule of the joint. (The lower metaphysis of the ulna is partly intracapsular.)

Clinical features. The symptoms and signs are those of

pyogenic arthritis of any superficial joint : acute onset with constitutional illness, pain and swelling about the joint, increased local warmth, and marked impairment of movement. *Radiographs in the early stages do not show any alteration from the normal* (Fig. 183). Later, if the infection persists, there is diffuse rarefaction, with loss of cartilage space and possibly some destruction of bone (Fig. 184).

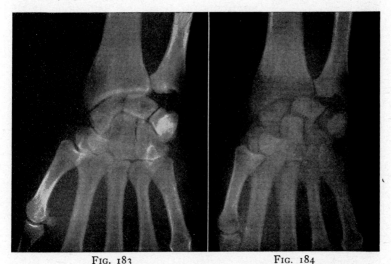

FIG. 183   FIG. 184

Pyogenic arthritis of the wrist. Figure 183—Initial radiograph, with no apparent abnormality. Figure 184—Four weeks after onset. Note the rarefaction and the slight but significant narrowing of the cartilage space, indicating destruction of articular cartilage.

Treatment. Appropriate antibiotic therapy is begun. The wrist is immobilised on a splint in a position of function—that is, in about 20 degrees of extension. The joint is aspirated or drained by incision, and the appropriate antibiotic drug is injected into it. When the infection has been overcome active wrist movements are encouraged.

PYOGENIC ARTHRITIS OF THE JOINTS OF THE HAND

Any of the small joints of the hand may be infected by pyogenic organisms. The distal interphalangeal joints of the digits are prone to infection spreading from a suppurative lesion in the adjacent pulp space, or from a penetrating wound. These infections often cause permanent damage to the joint, with impairment of movement or even rigid ankylosis.

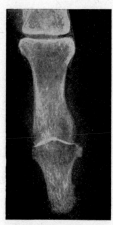

Clinical features. The affected joint is swollen, hot, and red. Movements are markedly impaired. *Radiographs* do not show any change at first, but later there are rarefaction of bone and diminution of the cartilage space (Fig. 185).

Treatment. Reliance is placed upon anti-biotic therapy, drainage and irrigation of the joint if suppuration occurs, and immobilisation during the acute stage of infection. But splintage must be discontinued and active exercises begun as soon as the infection subsides.

Fig. 185

FIG. 185
Pyogenic arthritis with destruction of the interphalangeal joint of the thumb.

RHEUMATOID ARTHRITIS OF THE WRIST AND HAND

(General description of rheumatoid arthritis, p. 46.)

Rheumatoid arthritis commonly affects the wrists and hands and is a major cause of serious loss of function and of ugly deformity. Usually many or all of the joints of the hand are affected, though occasionally the disease may begin in a single joint. Affected joints are swollen from synovial thickening, and movement is restricted. In the later stages articular cartilage and the underlying bone are eroded, and the fingers tend to deviate medially (ulnar drift) (Fig. 186). *Radiographs* do not show any abnormality at first. Later, there is diffuse rarefaction of the bones. Later still, in progressive disease, destruction of cartilage leads to narrowing of the joint space (Fig. 187).

Important though these joint changes are in rheumatoid disease of the hand, equally serious disability may be caused by involvement of the soft tissues. These soft-tissue changes may take several forms, the most important of which are as follows.

1) *Chronic tenosynovitis :* Masses of greatly thickened vascular

synovial tissue envelop the flexor or the extensor tendons over the wrist or in the hand. A secondary effect of such swelling in front of the wrist is that the median nerve may be compressed in the carpal tunnel. 2) *Rupture of tendons:* Both the extensor

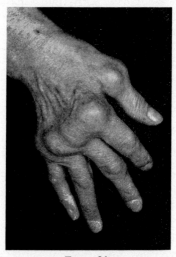

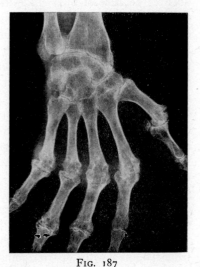

FIG. 186

Typical appearance of hand in long established rheumatoid arthritis of the metacarpo-phalangeal and inter-phalangeal joints.

FIG. 187

Long-standing ' burnt out ' rheumatoid arthritis of wrist and hand. Note the loss of cartilage space and the ulnar deviation of the fingers.

and the flexor tendons are liable to spontaneous rupture, from softening or fraying where they lie within inflamed synovial sheaths. 3) *Contracture of intrinsic muscles:* Fixed contracture of the intrinsic muscles of the hand may follow fibrosis induced by the disease. It leads to inability to flex the inter-phalangeal joints fully when the metacarpo-phalangeal joint is held extended.

Treatment. Management of these complex disabilities of the hand is difficult and often unsatisfactory. The tendency of the disease to progress during months or years of activity means often that the hand becomes seriously crippled. Nevertheless much can be done in some cases to retard the progress of the disease and to prevent deformity, either by conservative treatment **alone or by conservative treatment** combined with operation.

Conservative treatment. The general plan of treatment is like that for rheumatoid arthritis as a whole (p. 49). It will usually include the administration of drugs such as aspirin and phenyl-butazone, but cortisone and related drugs should be avoided if possible because of their undesirable side-effects. Physiotherapy is of value: it should take the form of hot paraffin-wax baths or short-wave diathermy, with mobilising exercises and encourage-ment in active use of the hand. During an acute exacerbation the wrist joint may be immobilised temporarily on a splint of plaster of Paris or of plastic, but immobilisation is never advised for the joints of the fingers.

Operative treatment. In carefully selected patients operation can be a valuable adjunct to conservative treatment, though it can never replace it. In general, operation is more rewarding when carried out in the fairly early stages of the disease, before deformity from changes in the joints and soft tissues becomes fixed and irreversible. Depending upon the nature of each individual case, operation may take one or more of the following forms.

Synovectomy. Excision of masses of thickened synovial tissue from tendon sheaths or from joints may slow down the destructive progress of the disease.

Tendon repair or replacement. Ruptured tendons may be repaired by suture or by grafting when practicable, or their lost function may be compensated by a tendon transfer operation (p. 31).

Release of tight intrinsic muscles. Impaired finger movement and grasp from fixed contracture of the intrinsic muscles can be improved by partial division of the aponeurotic insertion of the muscles into the extensor expansion at the back of each finger.

Arthroplasty. When the metacarpo-phalangeal or inter-phalangeal joints are badly disorganised arthroplasty by refashioning the joint surfaces or by the insertion of a flexible silicone-rubber ('Silastic') prosthesis may sometimes be ap-propriate. But the patient must be prepared to cooperate in a long programme of rehabilitation afterwards.

Arthrodesis. For selected joints that are painful, stiff and deformed arthrodesis in the position of most useful function is sometimes the best solution to the problem.

OSTEOARTHRITIS OF THE WRIST

(General description of osteoarthritis, p. 55.)

The degenerative changes of osteoarthritis are rather common in the wrist because of the frequency of injury to the joint and the proclivity of scaphoid fractures to non-union.

Cause. Although it is essentially a wear-and-tear process osteoarthritis seldom develops in a wrist that was previously normal.

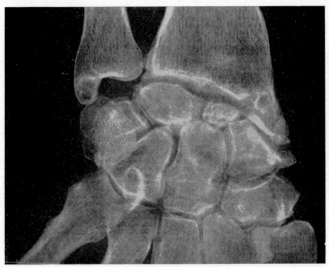

FIG. 188

Osteoarthritis of the wrist caused by an ununited fracture of the scaphoid bone. Note the diminished cartilage space, sclerosis, and spurring of bone at the joint margins, especially at the radial side of the wrist.

The wear-and-tear is nearly always accelerated by previous injury to, or disease of, the joint surfaces. The commonest predisposing factors are fracture of the scaphoid bone (especially when the fracture fails to unite and when one of the fragments suffers avascular necrosis), dislocation of the lunate bone, Kienböck's disease of the lunate bone, and ' burnt out ' rheumatoid arthritis.

Pathology. The predominant change is degeneration and wearing away of the articular cartilage lining the joint surfaces. The changes eventually involve all the carpal joints as well as the radio-carpal joint.

10

Clinical features. Months or years after one of the predisposing conditions mentioned, the patient notices gradually increasing pain and stiffness of the wrist, worse on activity. *On examination* the wrist is slightly thickened from bony irregularity, but the swelling is not marked. The skin temperature is normal. Movements are markedly limited, and painful if forced at the extremes. *Radiographs* show narrowing of the cartilage space and sharpening or spurring of the bone at the joint margins. The causative condition (for example, an ununited fracture of the scaphoid bone) is usually evident (Fig. 188).

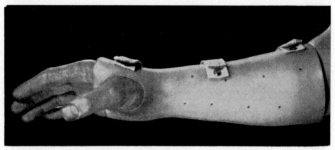

FIG. 189

Polythene wrist support. A splint such as this is sometimes used in the conservative treatment of osteoarthritis of the wrist.

Treatment. In mild cases the condition is best left alone, especially if the patient can avoid subjecting the wrist to heavy stress. When active treatment seems necessary, a choice must be made between conservative and operative methods. Conservative treatment can only diminish the symptoms ; it can never remove them. Nevertheless it is usually worth a trial. The most useful method is to combine physiotherapy, in the form of short-wave diathermy, with the provision of a firm wrist support of moulded leather or plastic (Fig. 189).

Operative treatment sometimes becomes necessary when the disability is severe. The only reliable method is by total arthrodesis of the wrist, with ablation of the radio-carpal and all the intercarpal joints. The inferior radio-ulnar joint and the triangular fibrocartilage are left undisturbed ; so rotation of the forearm is preserved.

OSTEOARTHRITIS OF THE JOINTS OF THE HAND

The metacarpo-phalangeal joints and the interphalangeal joints of the hand are frequently the site of osteoarthritis in the elderly. Such manifestations are relatively unimportant and in most cases treatment is not required. A special example demands further consideration—namely, osteoarthritis of the trapezio-metacarpal joint (carpo-metacarpal joint of the thumb).

Osteoarthritis of the Trapezio-metacarpal Joint

This is a common affection in elderly women but it may also occur in younger persons, especially when there has been previous injury such as a fracture of the base of the first metacarpal bone involving the joint. The arthritis may seriously impair the function of the thumb.

Clinical features. There is pain, localised to the trapezio-metacarpal joint, on using the thumb. The disability slowly increases over the years until activities like sewing or darning become virtually impossible. *On examination* the trapezio-metacarpal joint is prominent and slightly thickened. Active or passive movements of the thumb metacarpal cause pain. The range of movement at this joint varies widely even in normal individuals, so its measurement is of little practical value. *Radiographs* show narrowing of the cartilage space and sharpening or spurring of bone at the joint margins (Fig. 190). In many cases the joint is subluxated.

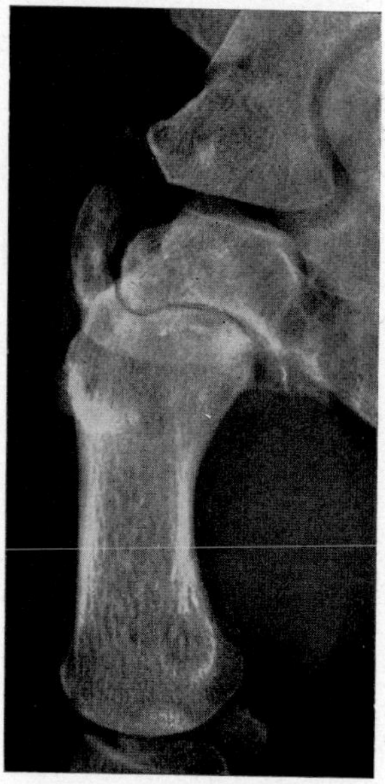

FIG. 190

Osteoarthritis of the trapezio-metacarpal joint. Note the marked narrowing of the cartilage space and the large osteophytes.

Treatment. In the early stages the condition is best left alone. For moderate symptoms a course of short-wave diathermy may be tried.

If the symptoms become disabling operation is advisable. The choice lies between arthroplasty and arthrodesis. Arthroplasty is done simply by excising the trapezium, allowing the resulting gap to fill with fibrous tissue. It gives results that are adequate for the usual elderly sufferer from this disorder. But if heavy use is to be demanded of the hand (as in the case of a labourer, for example), arthrodesis of the trapezio-metacarpal joint is to be preferred.

KIENBÖCK'S DISEASE

(Osteochondritis of the lunate bone)

Kienböck's disease is an affection of the lunate bone character-ised by temporary softening, fragmentation, and liability to deformation. It tends to give rise, later, to osteoarthritis of the wrist.

Cause. The precise cause is unknown. A disturbance of blood supply, possibly from thrombosis of a nutrient vessel, is believed to be a factor, but it is unlikely to be wholly responsible because the features of Kienböck's disease differ in certain respects from those of pure avascular necrosis. Repeated injury (for example, using the front of the wrist to drive a chisel in carpentry) is sometimes noted in the case history.

Pathology. The disease resembles osteochondritis of developing epiphysial centres in children (p. 97), such as Perthes' disease. The bone becomes granular in texture, small dense fragments being interspersed with softened areas. In this state the bone crumbles easily, and under the pressure imposed by muscle action and use of the wrist it gradually becomes squashed into a thin saucer-shaped mass. The overlying cartilage dies. After about two years the bone texture is restored to normal, but the bone remains deformed and lacks a smooth cartilaginous covering. The bone behaves like a piece of grit in a bearing and leads gradually to the development of osteoarthritis of the wrist.

Clinical features. There is pain in the wrist, most marked at the centre of the joint over the lunate area. The pain is worse during active use of the wrist. Because of the pain, the strength of grip is impaired. *On examination* there is discomfort on pressure over the lunate bone. Movements of the wrist are limited and cause pain if forced. *Radiographs* are diagnostic. In the early stages the lunate appears slightly more dense than the surrounding bones, and if its depth is compared with that of the lunate bone of the sound wrist it is seen to be reduced, though only slightly at first (Fig. 191). Later, the bone has a fragmented appearance, small areas of increased density being scattered through it, and the flattening of the bone becomes obvious. Later still, signs of osteoarthritis of the wrist are evident.

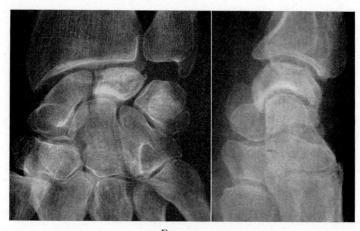

FIG. 191

Kienböck's disease of the lunate bone. Note the increased density, fragmentation, and beginning compression of the bone.

Treatment. Treatment is often rather unsatisfactory. It must depend upon the duration of the symptoms and the degree of damage to the wrist. In the earliest stage, when radiographic changes are only just perceptible, there is probably a place for immobilising the wrist in plaster for three months or so in the hope that the condition will resolve. But once the disease is clearly established surgical treatment is recommended. If the wrist is free from arthritis it is probably best simply to excise the lunate bone. The gap fills with fibrous tissue and reasonable function, with a useful range of painless movement, is usually restored. When symptoms have been present for many months osteoarthritis is usually already present. At that stage excision of the lunate is of no avail. Treatment should be the same as for osteoarthritis of the wrist (p. 282).

EXTRA-ARTICULAR DISORDERS ABOUT THE WRIST AND HAND

ACUTE INFECTIONS OF THE FASCIAL SPACES OF THE HAND

Acute infections of the hand account for a considerable proportion of the work of a casualty department or emergency room and are of great importance in industrial medicine. Unless they are treated efficiently they can lead to prolonged or even permanent disability, with impairment of working capacity.

Classification. If minor superficial infections are excluded there are six types to be considered : 1) nail-fold infection (paronychia) ; 2) pulp-space infection (whitlow, felon) ; 3) other subcutaneous infections ; 4) thenar space infection ; 5) mid-palmar space infection ; 6) tendon sheath infection.

Cause. All types are caused by infection with pyogenic bacteria. The usual causative organism is the staphylococcus aureus, but the streptococcus and occasionally other bacteria may be responsible. Minor injury such as a prick, abrasion or blister often provides the route of infection.

Pathology. The organisms reach the tissue planes by direct implantation from outside, often as the result of a trivial injury such as a prick or abrasion. They set up an acute inflammatory reaction which in many cases goes on to suppuration. Without effective treatment, infection may spread to adjacent tissue planes ; occasionally it may give rise to spreading lymphangitis or to septicaemia.

Surgical anatomy. A knowledge of the anatomy of the fascial spaces [1] of the hand is indispensable for the correct treatment of hand infections.

The nail fold and subungual space. The subcuticular plane beneath the nail fold is potentially continuous, at the base and sides of the nail, with the subungual space deep to the nail. Infection beginning in the nail fold may therefore easily spread under the nail (Fig. 192), and the resulting abscess cannot be drained effectively unless part of the nail is removed.

The pulp space. The interval between the front of the distal phalanx and the skin is traversed by tough fibrous partitions, which subdivide

---

[1] The term 'space' as used in this connection is a misnomer. It refers to the interval or plane between adjacent tissues, and in the normal hand it is only a potential space.

the space into numerous fat-filled cells (like the cells of a honeycomb) disposed at right angles to the skin surface (Fig. 192). Infection occurring in this tough tissue is virtually within a closed compartment : tissue pressure rises rapidly and accounts for early throbbing pain.

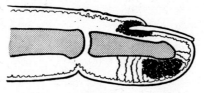

FIG. 192

Diagrammatic section showing the site of suppuration in nail-fold infection (paronychia) and in pulp-space infection (whitlow). In nail-fold infection the pus is beneath the cuticle and may extend under the nail, as shown. In pulp-space infection the pus lies in the tough fibro-fatty tissue immediately in front of the distal phalanx.

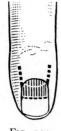 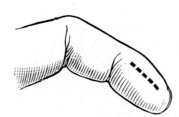

FIG. 193   FIG. 194

Figure 193—Technique of drainage of paronychial abscess. For the mildest infections it is sufficient to raise the cuticle alone without incising it ; but better drainage is secured by a vertical incision through the cuticle, on one or both sides. When pus has extended beneath the nail it is necessary also to remove the proximal half of the nail. Figure 194—Incision for drainage of pulp abscess. The incision is deepened across the pulp, in front of the phalanx, and the abscess cavity is cleared out under direct vision.

Other subcutaneous spaces. Infection may occur in the subcutaneous plane at any point in the hand. Common sites are the middle or proximal segment of a finger, and the web spaces between the digits. Less common sites are the palm of the hand and the dorsum of the hand. These superficial spaces are clearly demarcated from the deep palmar spaces next to be described, and must not be confused with them.

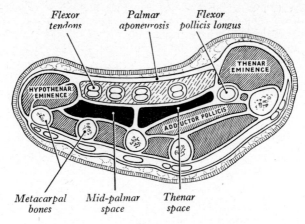

FIG. 195

The deep palmar spaces—the thenar space and the mid-palmar space—shown in diagrammatic transverse section.

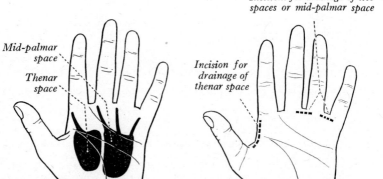

FIG. 196   FIG. 197

Figure 196—Surface marking of the deep palmar spaces. The thenar space is continuous with the first lumbrical canal and the mid-palmar space with the second, third, and fourth lumbrical canals. Figure 197—Incisions for drainage through the web spaces.

The thenar space. This lies deeply under the lateral (radial) half of the hollow of the palm. It is the interval between the adductor pollicis muscle behind and the flexor tendon of the index finger and the first and second lumbrical muscles in front. Medially it is separated from the mid-palmar space by a fibrous septum that extends deeply from the fascia on the deep surface of the flexor tendons to the fascia covering the interossei and adductor pollicis muscle (Figs. 195 and 196). The space is prolonged forwards into the delicate sheath that surrounds the first lumbrical muscle. It sometimes communicates also with the second lumbrical canal. The lumbrical canals thus provide a potential communication between the subcutaneous web spaces and the thenar space : in practice, however, it is rare for infection to spread along this route.

The mid-palmar space. This lies under the medial (ulnar) half of the hollow of the palm. It is the interval between the interossei and metacarpal bones behind and the flexor tendons (in their sheaths) of the middle, ring, and little fingers in front (Fig. 195). Laterally, it is separated from the thenar space by the fibrous septum already described. The space is prolonged forwards into the sheaths of the second, third, and fourth lumbrical muscles. Again, despite the potential communication between a web space and the mid-palmar space along the lumbrical canals, web-space infection very seldom spreads deeply to involve the palm.

The flexor tendon sheaths. Distinction must be made between the tough fibrous sheaths, which exist only in the digits, and the flimsy synovial sheaths, which line the fibrous sheaths and, in the case of the thumb and little finger, extend proximally into the palm. In acute infections of the tendon sheaths (acute infective tenosynovitis) the pus is within the synovial sheath and it is confined only by the limits of the sheath. The flexor sheaths of the index, middle, and ring fingers end proximally at the level of the transverse palmar skin crease (Fig. 198). The sheaths of the thumb and little finger extend proximally through the palm to end two or three centimetres above the level of the wrist. The proximal part of the sheath for the thumb is known as the radial bursa. The sheath for the little finger opens out proximally into the ulnar bursa, which encloses the grouped tendons of flexor digitorum superficialis and flexor digitorum profundus (Fig. 198).

Clinical features. In general, the symptoms of acute hand infections are local pain, swelling, and loss of function. There is often some degree of constitutional disturbance, with pyrexia. *On examination* there are obvious swelling, redness of the skin (except in deep infections), and marked local tenderness over the site of the infection. Special features of the individual lesions are described in the following pages.

10*

Principles of treatment.   Before suppuration has occurred, the aim of treatment is to abort the infection and avoid the need for operation.   The essentials of this expectant treatment are rest for the hand, elevation of the limb, and antibiotic drugs.   In a minor case it may be sufficient to support the hand in a sling, but in a severe case rest is best assured by a light plaster back-splint,

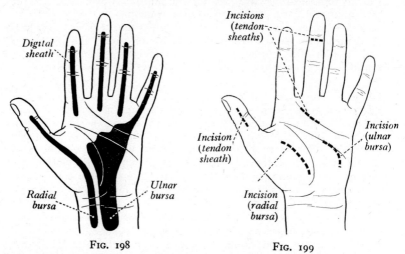

Fig. 198   Fig. 199

Figure 198—The synovial flexor sheaths.   Whereas the sheaths for the index, middle, and ring fingers end proximally at the bases of the fingers those for the thumb and little finger extend upwards to become continuous with the radial bursa and the ulnar bursa respectively.   Figure 199—Incisions for drainage and irrigation of tendon sheaths and bursae.

and elevation may be maintained by suspending the limb in a roller towel attached above the side of the bed.   The question of antibiotics is difficult because the sensitivity of the organism is not at first known.   Penicillin is usually given, often in conjunction with cloxacillin: tetracycline is an alternative.   Very few patients are seen at a stage early enough to permit success from this expectant treatment.

When suppuration has already occurred, as indicated by severe throbbing pain, intense local tenderness, pyrexia, and loss of function, the abscess should be drained surgically without further delay.   After adequate drainage has been secured the wound may be packed lightly open with vaselined gauze for two days.

Thereafter, dry dressings are used and active finger exercises are encouraged.

There has been much discussion on the technique of surgical drainage for hand infections, and there is a tendency among some surgeons to regard only their own methods as correct. It is necessary to emphasise, therefore, that success depends not so much upon an obsessional devotion to a particular method as upon the observance of certain general principles. These are as follows. Firstly, the operation must be done under favourable conditions and without undue hurry : the old method of making a hasty incision under a ' whiff of gas ' is indefensible. Anaesthesia may be general or regional (nerve block), but it should allow time for deliberate exploration of the abscess under a tourniquet, so that its full extent can be ascertained. Secondly, the incision must be adequate to allow complete emptying of the abscess. Thirdly, the incision must not endanger important underlying structures. Fourthly, the incision must be so sited that the resulting scar is innocuous. Within the limits imposed by these principles there is often more than one way of performing the actual drainage operation.

SPECIAL FEATURES OF INDIVIDUAL LESIONS

NAIL-FOLD INFECTION (paronychia). This is one of the commonest but least serious types of hand infection. *Clinical features* : There are pain, redness, and swelling at one or both sides of the nail fold and at the base of the nail. There is local tenderness over the reddened area. If suppuration has extended deep to the nail there is marked tenderness on pressure upon the nail. *Complications* : These are 1) extension to the pulp space ; and 2) chronic paronychia, following inadequate treatment of the acute infection. *Treatment* : In this type of infection conservative measures are often successful if begun within a few hours of the onset. When local suppuration has occurred the subcuticular abscess is drained by raising the cuticle from the nail or by raising it as a short flap after incising it vertically at one or both corners (Fig. 193). If pus has extended under the nail the proximal half of the nail must also be removed.

PULP-SPACE INFECTION (whitlow). This is almost as common as nail-fold infection. *Clinical features :* The pulp is swollen, tense, and tender. Severe throbbing pain, with exquisite localised tenderness, suggests that suppuration is present. *Complications* : These are 1) osteomyelitis of the terminal phalanx, often leading to necrosis and sequestration of its distal half ; 2) pyogenic arthritis of the distal interphalangeal joint ; and 3) very rarely, spread of infection to the flexor tendon sheath (suppurative tenosynovitis). *Treatment* : Conservative measures are seldom successful except in the earliest stages. Surgical drainage is effected well by a lateral incision just in front of the plane of the terminal phalanx (Fig. 194) ; it is deepened transversely across the pulp of the finger but should not extend proximally beyond a point half a centimetre distal to the terminal skin crease lest the flexor tendon sheath be inadvertently opened. An alternative method is to incise directly into the pulp over the centre of the abscess, a technique that is to be preferred if the abscess is threatening to point at the surface.

SUBCUTANEOUS INFECTIONS (other than pulp-space infections). These infections are common. *Clinical features* : The infection may arise in any part of the hand or fingers. Common sites are the middle or proximal segment of a finger, and the web spaces. There is localised swelling with redness and tenderness. In many cases the infection has spread through the skin from a subcuticular infection or blister. Care must be taken not to confuse subcutaneous infections with the deep space infections. *Complications* : These are 1) sloughing of skin over the lesion ; and 2) spread to the deep spaces or to the flexor tendon sheaths. *Treatment* : Surgical drainage is by a short incision appropriately placed to reach the abscess without harming important structures or leaving an awkward scar. In the case of a web-space infection the incision should not divide the skin fold of the web : a short transverse incision in the palm just proximal to the skin fold is adequate (Fig. 197).

THENAR SPACE INFECTION. This is a very uncommon lesion. It may arise by extension from a subcutaneous lesion or a tendon sheath infection. *Clinical features* : The radial half of the palm is ballooned out and the swelling extends to the dorsal aspect of the web between thumb and index finger. *Treatment* : Drainage is by an incision at the dorsal aspect of the first web space (Fig. 197).

MID-PALMAR SPACE INFECTION. This is also uncommon. It usually arises by extension from a subcutaneous lesion or a tendon sheath infection. *Clinical features* : The ulnar half of the palm is ballooned out. Movements of the fingers are restricted and painful. *Treatment* : Drainage can be established through the web space between the middle and ring fingers or between the ring and little fingers (Fig. 197).

TENDON SHEATH INFECTION. This is rare, but important because prompt treatment is essential if the function of the finger is to be preserved. *Clinical features* : The finger is swollen throughout its length, and acutely tender over the flexor tendon sheath. It is held semi-flexed and the patient is unwilling to extend it because of pain. *Complications* : These are 1) necrosis of the tendons and adhesions between tendon and sheath, causing permanent stiffness of the finger in semi-flexion ; and 2) spread of infection to involve the radial bursa (from the flexor sheath of the thumb), or the ulnar bursa (from the sheath of the little finger). *Treatment :* Systemic antibiotic therapy is begun immediately. The sheath is opened at its proximal end in the palm and at its distal end (Fig. 199), and irrigated with penicillin solution through a fine tube passed along the sheath ; the tube is withdrawn and the wounds are packed lightly open.

If the radial bursa or the ulnar bursa is infected it must be drained and irrigated through an additional incision in the palm (Fig. 199).

CHRONIC INFECTIVE TENOSYNOVITIS
(Including compound palmar ganglion)

Chronic inflammation of tendon sheaths in the lower forearm and hand is usually a response to low-grade infection. It is entirely distinct from acute tenosynovitis and is not preceded by it.

Cause. In most cases it is caused by infection with the tubercle bacillus. Sometimes other organisms are responsible. A similar condition may complicate rheumatoid arthritis without demonstrable bacterial infection.

Pathology. The flexor tendon sheaths in the lower forearm and hand are those most commonly affected ; less often the lesion is confined to the extensor sheaths. The affected sheaths are greatly thickened and show the changes of chronic inflammation. In most cases there is histological evidence of tuberculosis. The sheaths often contain an excess of fluid and there may be collections of small fibrinous bodies. The tendons themselves are affected only slightly.

Clinical features. There is a gradual onset of swelling, with mild aching pain, in the region of the affected tendon sheaths—usually the flexor sheaths of the lower forearm and hand. The function of the fingers and thumb is impaired. *On examination* the swelling is confined to the line of the tendon sheaths. Characteristically it affects the lowest five or six centimetres of the front of the forearm and the proximal part of the palm (Fig. 200). Sometimes the flexor sheaths of the fingers and thumb are also swollen, giving the digits a fusiform appearance. In many cases fluctuation can be elicited between the forearm swelling and the swelling in the palm. This clinical sign depends upon the presence of fluid within the tendon sheaths, and it is not always found. The fully developed condition, with swelling in forearm and palm and fluctuation between the two, constitutes *compound palmar ganglion*.

At first the range of movements of the fingers and thumb is impaired only slightly, if at all. Later, there is moderate restriction of flexion and extension of the digits, with corresponding loss of function. A tuberculous lesion may be discovered elsewhere in the body.

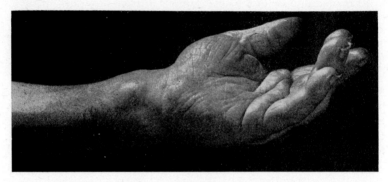

FIG. 200

Compound palmar ganglion. The swellings in the palm and at the front of the wrist are continuous deep to the flexor retinaculum.

Diagnosis. Persistent swelling of gradual onset in the line of the tendon sheaths in the lower forearm and hand always suggests chronic tenosynovitis. Fluctuation between the forearm swelling and the palmar swelling provides strong corroborative evidence. If an active tuberculous lesion is found elsewhere in the body it is reasonable to infer that the tenosynovitis is also tuberculous.

Treatment. In mild cases in which the function of the fingers and thumb is not impaired conservative treatment is advised. The wrist and forearm are immobilised in plaster of Paris for three months, the fingers being left free. In tuberculous cases a course of the appropriate antibiotic drugs is given.

In severe or intractable cases operation is recommended. It consists in excising thoroughly all the thickened and oedematous synovial sheaths. After operation finger movements are encouraged and practised daily under the supervision of a physiotherapist. A useful range of finger movement is usually restored, but permanent inability to flex the fingers fully into the palm may have to be accepted.

BONE TUMOURS IN THE HAND

BENIGN TUMOURS

(General description of benign tumours of bone, p. 81.)

The only bone tumour that requires special mention here is the benign chondroma.

CHONDROMA

A chondroma or benign cartilage tumour occurs in two forms : *enchondroma*, which grows within the bone and expands it ; and *ecchondroma*, which grows mainly outwards from the surface of the bone. Both types are prone to occur in the metacarpals and phalanges of the hand. The tumour may be solitary, but in the condition known as dyschondroplasia, multiple chondromatosis or Ollier's disease the tumours may affect many bones in the hand as well as any of the long bones, pelvic bones or scapula, and they may cause ugly swelling and deformity of the fingers (Fig. 75, p. 106). Malignant transformation is hardly known in a solitary chondroma of a bone of the hand, but it is a possibility in cases of multiple chondromatosis.

Treatment. If small, the tumour should be treated expectantly. Operation is required only if it is found to be enlarging. Large tumours should be excised, the bone substance being restored, if necessary, by grafts of cancellous bone.

MALIGNANT TUMOURS

(General description of malignant tumours of bone, p. 86.)

Malignant tumours of the bones of the hand are uncommon. CHONDROSARCOMA may arise in a previously existing benign chondroma, especially in the multiple form of chondromatosis (dyschondroplasia).

CARCINOMA, especially from the lung, rarely metastasises to a phalanx, destroying the bone. It may simulate closely an infective lesion, and the correct diagnosis may be overlooked at first.

SOFT-TISSUE TUMOURS IN THE HAND

(General description of soft-tissue tumours, p. 130.)

Special mention must be made of an unusual tumour that is seldom encountered outside the hand—namely, the giant-cell tumour of tendon sheath (localised nodular tenosynovitis).

GIANT-CELL TUMOUR OF TENDON SHEATH

This is a benign tumour, but it sometimes recurs locally unless it is removed entire. It arises from the sheath of a tendon, or from the fibrous expansion of an extensor tendon in a finger. As it enlarges it burrows between the tissue planes, taking the line of least resistance. Eventually it may form a bulky mass which almost surrounds the finger like a collar. On section the tumour is fleshy ; histologically it is composed of cells of many forms, including round cells, giant cells of foreign-body type, xanthoma cells containing cholesterol, and fibroblasts.

Treatment. The tumour should be excised entire.

COMPRESSION OF THE MEDIAN NERVE IN THE CARPAL TUNNEL
(Carpal tunnel syndrome)

Constriction of the median nerve as it passes beneath the flexor retinaculum is a common cause of discomfort in the hand, especially in middle-aged or elderly women.

Cause. Any space-occupying lesion within the carpal tunnel may be responsible. Recognised causes are chronic inflammatory thickening of the tendon sheaths, osteoarthritis of the wrist, thickening after fracture of the lower end of the radius, and myxoedema. In many cases no primary cause can be discovered.

Pathology. The median nerve lies beneath the flexor retinaculum in company with the flexor tendons of the hand. If the available space within this strong-walled tunnel is reduced the nerve is compressed against the flexor retinaculum. When the retinaculum is divided in such a case the nerve may be found constricted where it lay behind it. The ulnar nerve does not pass behind the flexor retinaculum ; so it is not liable to compression in this way.

Clinical features. The condition is commonest in women in or beyond middle life. The symptoms are sensory and motor. There is tingling, numbness, or discomfort in the radial three and a half digits (that is, in the median distribution), and there is a feeling of clumsiness in carrying out fine movements such as those concerned in sewing. Distressing tingling is often prominent during the night: the patient may have to work the fingers or shake the hand to gain relief. *On examination* the findings vary with the degree and duration of the compression. At first there are no objective findings. Later there is blunting of sensation in the median distribution. In a severe case there may eventually be evident wasting and weakness of the median-innervated small muscles of the hand. *Investigations :* Electrical tests may show decreased conduction velocity in the affected part of the median nerve.

Diagnosis. Care must be taken to exclude other causes of neurological disturbance in the hand, especially those arising in the neck from interference with the brachial plexus, and lesions of the median nerve elsewhere in its course.

Treatment. The flexor retinaculum is divided to decompress the nerve.

GANGLION
(Simple ganglion)

A ganglion is the commonest cystic swelling at the back of the wrist.

Pathology. Conflicting views have been put forward on the origin of ganglia. Some believe that they represent a degenerative

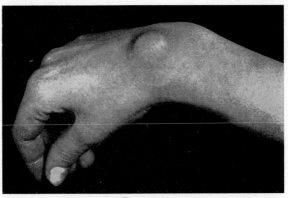

FIG. 201
A simple ganglion at the back of the wrist. This is the commonest site.

process. Others claim that they are benign tumours of tendon sheath or joint capsule. The cyst wall is of fibrous tissue and there is no true endothelial lining. It is connected at some point with a joint capsule or tendon sheath, but there is no communication between the joint cavity or tendon sheath and the interior of the cyst. The cyst may be unilocular or multilocular. The contained fluid is clear and viscous.

Clinical features. Ganglia are commonest at the back of the wrist, where they are often seen in adults of any age (Fig. 201). They also occur, less commonly, in the palm and fingers. Ordinarily there are no symptoms other than the swelling itself and, sometimes, discomfort or slight pain. *On examination* the swelling may be soft and obviously cystic, but more often it is tense. It is often mistaken for a bony prominence—but careful tests will show that it is fluctuant.

Complications. A ganglion arising deeply in the wrist or palm may interfere mechanically with the ulnar or the median nerve. There will be motor and usually sensory impairment in the distribution of the particular branch affected.

Treatment. A ganglion is harmless and in the absence of pain or complications it may safely be left alone. Sometimes the ganglion can be dispersed subcutaneously by firm local pressure. This rather dramatic treatment is harmless and temporarily effective, but the ganglion will slowly reappear. Lasting cure can be ensured only by complete excision of the ganglion—not always an easy task because the thin-walled sac often tracks deeply between the tendons, where it may be torn and a fragment left behind.

A ganglion that is interfering with a peripheral nerve demands operative excision without delay.

DUPUYTREN'S CONTRACTURE
(Contracture of the palmar aponeurosis)

This is an easily recognised condition characterised in the established phase by flexion contracture of one or more of the fingers from thickening and shortening of the palmar aponeurosis.

Cause. This is unknown. There is a hereditary predisposition. In a predisposed person injury possibly plays a part but its exact significance is uncertain. There is an increased incidence of the disorder among epileptics.

Pathology. The palmar aponeurosis (palmar fascia) is normally a thin but tough membrane whose fibres radiate from the termination of the palmaris longus tendon at the front of the wrist to gain insertion into the proximal and middle phalanges of the fingers. It lies immediately beneath the skin. In Dupuytren's contracture the aponeurosis, or part of it, becomes greatly thickened (often to half a centimetre or more), and it contracts,

drawing the fingers into flexion at the metacarpo-phalangeal and
proximal interphalangeal joints. The medial half of the aponeurosis

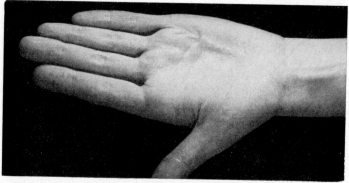

FIG. 202

Early Dupuytren's contracture. There is a nodule of thickened aponeurosis
in the palm, with slight puckering of the skin ; but so far there is no flexion
contracture of the fingers.

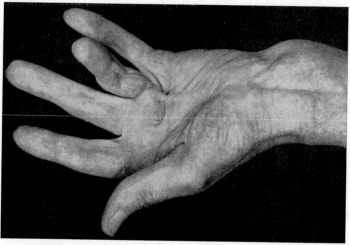

FIG. 203

A typical example of Dupuytren's contracture of the palmar aponeurosis
in which the ring finger has been drawn down into flexion.

is affected most, and serious flexion deformity is usually confined
to the ring and little fingers, with only moderate deformity of the
middle finger. The joints themselves are unaffected at first, but

in long-established cases secondary capsular contractures occur. The plantar aponeurosis in the foot is occasionally affected, but in the foot the lesion usually takes the form of a firm nodule under the instep rather than of an actual contracture involving the toes. **Clinical features.** The affection is much more common in men than in women. Often both hands are affected. The earliest sign is a small thickened nodule in the mid-palm opposite the base of the ring finger (Fig. 202). The area of thickening gradually spreads from this point, giving rise eventually to firm cord-like bands that extend into the ring or little finger, or both, and prevent full extension of the metacarpo-phalangeal and proximal inter-phalangeal joints (Fig. 203). The skin is closely adherent to the fascial bands, and is often puckered. The flexion deformity becomes progressively worse in the course of months or years.

In some cases these changes in the palm are accompanied by thickenings over the dorsum of the interphalangeal joints (knuckle pads). The feet may also show nodules in the sole.

Treatment. The only effective treatment is by operation. That does not imply, however, that operation is necessary in every case : a contracture that is not progressing rapidly is often better left alone, especially in an elderly patient. Operation entails excision of the thickened part of the palmar aponeurosis by painstaking dissection. Simple division of the taut contracted bands is un-satisfactory, because the contracture tends to recur.

RUPTURE OR SEVERANCE OF TENDONS IN THE HAND

Most tendon divisions in the hand are caused by cuts with sharp objects such as glass or knives. Certain tendons are prone to rupture : thus the extensor tendon of a finger is easily torn from its insertion into the distal phalanx by sudden forced flexion of the finger ; and the extensor pollicis longus tendon is liable to rupture spontaneously after fractures of the lower end of the radius in consequence of its becoming frayed where it crosses the roughened bone.

Clinical features and diagnosis. Loss of function of a tendon is obvious clinically. When the findings are correlated with the history the diagnosis is usually clear.

Treatment. This varies according to the tendon affected and the site of severance or rupture (see next page and Figs. 204-205).

Sometimes treatment is unnecessary or undesirable, but more often operative reconstruction is to be advised: the tendon is

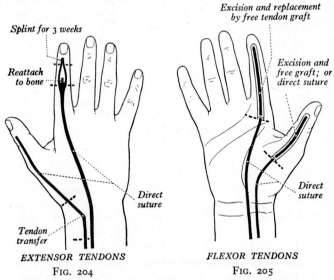

Splint for 3 weeks

Reattach to bone

Excision and replacement by free tendon graft

Excision and free graft; or direct suture

Direct suture

Direct suture

Tendon transfer

EXTENSOR TENDONS
FIG. 204

FLEXOR TENDONS
FIG. 205

Treatment of tendon injuries at various sites. Figure 204—Extensor tendons. Figure 205—Flexor tendons. For details, see text.

either sutured directly or replaced by a free tendon graft or by a tendon transfer, according to circumstances.

SPECIAL FEATURES OF INDIVIDUAL LESIONS

INJURIES OF EXTENSOR TENDONS

AVULSION OF EXTENSOR TENDON from distal phalanx of a finger. This is known as 'mallet' or 'baseball' finger. It is caused by sudden forced flexion of the distal interphalangeal joint—for instance, by a blow on the tip of the finger from a cricket ball. In a few cases a small fragment of bone is avulsed with the tendon. The patient is unable fully to extend the distal interphalangeal joint (Fig. 206). *Treatment:* Immediate treatment is to splint the finger for three weeks with the distal interphalangeal joint fully extended and the proximal interphalangeal joint flexed 90 degrees—a position which ensures that the distal part of the extensor expansion is

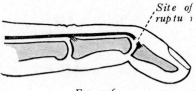

Site of ruptu 1

FIG. 206

Mallet finger. The extensor tendon is avulsed from its insertion. The terminal joint cannot be extended fully.

relaxed. The avulsed tendon always unites to the bone, but often with lengthening, in which case the deformity persists. The choice then lies between accepting the disability, which is slight, or operation. Operation entails shortening the extensor tendon by excision of a short section at the level of the middle phalanx.

RUPTURE OF THE MIDDLE SLIP OF THE EXTENSOR EXPANSION. This is caused by sudden forced flexion of the proximal interphalangeal joint, the middle slip of the extensor expansion being torn from its attachment to the middle phalanx. The patient is unable to extend the proximal interphalangeal joint fully. The distal joint becomes hyperextended. *Treatment :* The choice lies between immobilisation on a splint in the straight position for three weeks, or operative repair. In a fresh case simple splintage probably gives the better results.

SEVERANCE OF EXTENSOR TENDONS AT THE BACK OF THE HAND. This injury has a good prognosis. There is a tendency to spontaneous union with recovery of normal function. *Treatment :* Primary suture should be undertaken if the injury is recent. Failing this, expectant treatment may be adopted for two or three months, during which spontaneous restoration of function can be hoped for. If disability persists, freshening and direct suture of the divided ends is advised.

RUPTURE OF EXTENSOR POLLICIS LONGUS TENDON complicating fracture of lower end of radius. The tendon gives way after becoming frayed

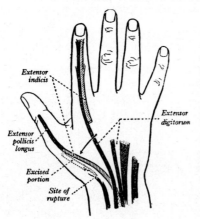

FIG. 207

Transfer of extensor indicis to replace a ruptured extensor pollicis longus. The tendon of extensor indicis is divided opposite the neck of the second metacarpal, re-routed towards the thumb, and sutured to the freshened distal stump of the extensor pollicis longus. This transfer is to be preferred to direct suture when the ends of the ruptured tendon are frayed.

by repeated movement over the roughened lower end of the radius. The extensive fraying makes direct suture unsatisfactory. *Treatment :* The tendon of extensor indicis is divided at the level of the neck of the second metacarpal bone, re-routed towards the thumb, and sutured to the freshened distal stump of the extensor pollicis longus (Fig. 207).

INJURIES OF FLEXOR TENDONS

DIVISION WITHIN A FIBROUS FLEXOR SHEATH OF A FINGER. Severance at this site presents the most difficult problem of all tendon injuries. The results of operative repair are unpredictable, and in many cases the operation fails to restore a useful range of active finger movement.

Treatment : If a flexor superficialis tendon alone is divided and the flexor profundus is intact treatment is not required, for there is virtually no disability.

If a flexor profundus tendon alone is divided, the flexor superficialis being intact, the loss of active flexion at the distal interphalangeal joint can often be accepted. Attempted repair of the tendon is usually better avoided because of its uncertain results. Arthrodesis of the distal

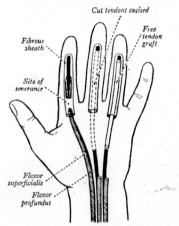

FIG. 208

Tendon graft for reconstruction of severed flexor tendons in the digital sheath. Successive stages of the operation are shown in the index, middle, and ring fingers. The use of a free graft eliminates the need for a tendon junction within the sheath.

interphalangeal joint in slight flexion reduces the disability to a negligible level.

If both tendons are divided operative reconstruction of the flexor profundus (not the superficialis) is advised. Except when the wound is exceptionally clean and ideal conditions for immediate definitive repair are available, the reconstruction should be deferred until the skin wound is healed and the joints are mobile.

Technique : Direct suture of the severed ends is seldom satisfactory except when conditions are especially favourable for immediate primary repair—that is, when the tendon has been divided cleanly by a sharp instrument and when facilities for skilled definitive repair are immediately available. Even then there is a risk that the tendon will stick to the narrow sheath at the site of suture. In the more usual type of case in which repair of the tendon is delayed until the skin wound is healed, the most satisfactory method is to remove the flexor superficialis tendon entire (to make more room in the sheath) and to replace the whole of the digital part of the flexor profundus tendon by a free tendon graft (from the palmaris longus or from a toe extensor) sutured proximally to the profundus tendon in the palm, and inserted distally into a drill hole in the distal phalanx (Fig. 208). This method eliminates the need for a tendon junction within the sheath.

In a recent two-stage modification of this technique a new synovial sheath is prepared in advance by laying in a flexible silicone-rubber ('Silastic') rod for four weeks before the tendon graft is inserted.

DIVISION OF FLEXOR POLLICIS LONGUS IN THE THUMB. The problem is less difficult than that presented by division of both flexor tendons in a finger. Repair may be attempted either by direct suture, or by replacement of the digital part of the tendon by a free graft as described for the fingers.

DIVISION OF FLEXOR TENDONS IN THE PALM OR WRIST. Direct suture is advised. It may be done primarily if the wound is clean. The prognosis is good if a single tendon is affected but it is uncertain in cases of multiple tendon divisions at the front of the wrist, especially if the nerves are also injured.

DE QUERVAIN'S TENOVAGINITIS
(Tenovaginitis of the abductor pollicis longus
and extensor pollicis brevis)

This is a common and well recognised condition characterised by pain over the styloid process of the radius and a palpable nodule in the course of the abductor pollicis longus and extensor pollicis brevis tendons.

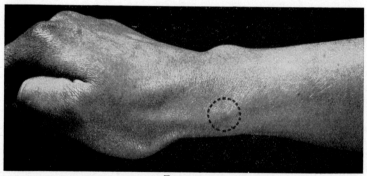

FIG. 209
Site of tenderness in de Quervain's tenovaginitis.

Cause. The precise cause is unknown. Excessive friction from over-use may be a factor, because the condition seems prone to follow oft-repeated actions such as wringing clothes.

Pathology. The fibrous sheaths of the abductor pollicis longus and extensor pollicis brevis tendons are thickened where they cross the tip of the radial styloid process. The tendons themselves appear normal. The condition is possibly analogous to that other common form of tenovaginitis, ' trigger ' finger (see below).

Clinical features. The condition is commonest in middle-aged women. The main symptom is pain on using the hand, especially when movement tenses the abductor pollicis longus and extensor pollicis brevis tendons (as in lifting a teapot). *On examination* there is local tenderness at the point where the tendons cross the radial styloid process (Fig. 209) ; the thickened fibrous sheaths are usually palpable as a firm nodule. Passive adduction of the wrist or thumb causes the patient to wince with pain.

Diagnosis. The clinical picture is so characteristic that, provided the condition is borne in mind, its diagnosis presents little difficulty.

Treatment. There is a tendency to very slow natural recovery with rest, or after the local injection of hydrocortisone. But operation provides so certain a cure that it should always be advised if the disability is severe. All that is necessary is to slit or ' de-roof ' the offending tendon sheaths.

DIGITAL TENOVAGINITIS STENOSANS
(' Trigger ' finger ; snapping finger)

In this rather common condition thickening and constriction of the mouth of a fibrous digital sheath interfere with the free gliding of the contained flexor tendons.

Cause. This is unknown.

Pathology. The proximal part of the fibrous flexor sheath at the base of a finger or thumb is thickened and the mouth of the sheath is constricted. The contained tendons become ' waisted ' opposite the constriction, and swollen proximal to it. The swollen segment enters the mouth of the sheath only with difficulty when an attempt is made to straighten the finger from the flexed position (Fig. 210).

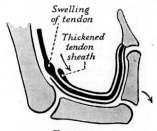

FIG. 210

Mechanism of ' trigger ' finger. The swollen part of the tendon is reluctant to enter the constricted mouth of the fibrous sheath. When sufficient force is exerted it enters with a snap. The thickening forms a palpable nodule at the base of the finger.

Clinical features. The condition occurs 1) in the fingers of the middle-aged (especially women), and 2) in the thumb in infants or young children.

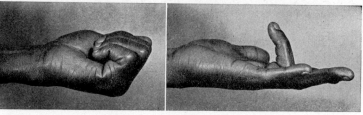

FIG. 211

' Trigger ' finger. The fingers can be flexed without difficulty, but when the patient attempts to straighten them the affected finger sticks in the position shown.

The adult type. There is complaint of tenderness at the base of the affected finger and of locking of the finger in full flexion (Fig. 211). The locking can be overcome either by a supreme effort or by extending the finger passively with the other hand, when the flexion is released with a distinct snap. *On examination* there is a palpable nodule, usually slightly tender, at the base of the affected finger or thumb—that is, over the mouth of the fibrous flexor sheath. The snapping cannot be reproduced on passive movements ; it can be demonstrated only when the patient flexes the finger fully with its own muscles.

The infantile type (contracted thumb of infants). The infant is unable to straighten the thumb, which is locked in flexion. *On examination* it may or may not be possible to extend the thumb passively. A palpable nodule is present at the base of the thumb in the position of the mouth of the fibrous flexor sheath. It should be noted that this condition in infants is often mistaken for a dislocated thumb or for a congenital deformity.

Treatment. Both the adult and the infantile type can be cured by the simple operation of incising the mouth of the fibrous flexor sheath longitudinally.

EXTRINSIC DISORDERS SIMULATING DISEASE OF THE FOREARM OR HAND
DISORDERS OF THE NECK

Certain disorders of the neck interfere with the brachial plexus or its roots, and thereby produce their predominant symptoms—or even their only symptoms—in the lower arm or hand. By far the commonest of such disorders are prolapse of a cervical inter-vertebral disc and osteoarthritis of the cervical spine (cervical spondylosis). Less common as causes of peripheral symptoms are cervical rib, tumours of the spinal column or of the spinal cord, and soft-tissue tumours involving nerves. All these conditions were described in Chapter III.

Rarely, neck disorders affect the lower arm or hand by inter-fering with the subclavian artery. Examples are occasionally seen in cases of cervical rib, or when the artery is obstructed by a tumour or aneurysm.

TUMOUR AT THE THORACIC INLET

A mass at the thoracic inlet is an occasional cause of peripheral symptoms in the upper limb. The commonest cause is an apical tumour of the lung (Pancoast's tumour) involving the nerves of the brachial plexus.

DISORDERS OF THE UPPER ARM

Rarely, a disorder of the upper arm may produce its chief effects in the lower arm or hand, usually through the medium of the major nerve trunks. A well known example is crutch palsy, in which there is weakness or paralysis of the extensor muscles of the wrist, fingers, and thumb from repeated pressure of a crutch upon the radial nerve in the axilla. Occasionally the axillary artery has been injured in the same way, with consequent ischaemic manifestations in the digits.

DISORDERS OF THE ELBOW

Affections of the elbow may be associated with vague referred pain in the forearm. This is especially true of tennis elbow, in which the pain extends along the extensor aspect of the forearm, often to the hand. Almost always, however, the local symptoms in the elbow overshadow the referred symptoms ; so mistakes in diagnosis are unlikely.

In the condition of friction neuritis of the ulnar nerve, however, the symptoms and signs are predominantly in the hand, and one might suspect a local disorder of the hand itself if the possibility of a lesion at the elbow were not considered and investigated.

References and bibliography, page 445.

CHAPTER EIGHT

The Hip Region

THE hip presents some of the most fascinating problems in the whole field of orthopaedic surgery. Practically and economically, its injuries and diseases are important because they so often cause prolonged suffering and serious disablement. Academically, the region is of interest for several reasons : the mechanics of the joint are complex ; it is one of the most difficult joints to examine with accuracy ; and—of special significance to students—cases of hip disease are often presented as tests of clinical acumen in the examinations in surgery. Time spent on learning how to examine the hip correctly will usually be very well rewarded.

SPECIAL POINTS IN THE INVESTIGATION OF HIP COMPLAINTS

History
The characteristics of hip pain. Pain in the region of the hip is notoriously misleading, for often it is referred from the spine or pelvis and has no connection with the hip joint itself. Therefore one must always

TABLE IX

USUAL AGE INCIDENCE OF COMMON HIP DISORDERS

Age at Time of Diagnosis (Years)	Disease
0 to 2	Congenital dislocation
2 to 5	Tuberculous arthritis ; transient arthritis
5 to 10	Perthes' disease ; transient arthritis
10 to 20	Slipped upper femoral epiphysis
20 to 50	Osteoarthritis (secondary to previous injury or disease)
50 to 100	Osteoarthritis (primary)

be cautious in attributing such pain to a hip lesion without first investigating the possibility of an extrinsic cause.

Pain arising in the hip is felt mainly in the groin and in the front or inner side of the thigh. Pain is often referred also to the knee ; indeed pain in the knee is sometimes the predominant feature. In contrast, the 'hip' pain that is referred from the spine is felt mainly in the gluteal region, whence it often radiates down the back or outer side of the thigh.

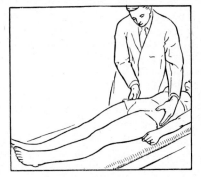

True hip pain is made worse by walking, whereas gluteal pain referred from the spine is aggravated by activities such as stooping and lifting, and it is often eased by walking.

Age incidence of hip disorders. Many of the important disorders of the hip occur in childhood, and often at a particular period of childhood. So true is this with some disorders

FIG. 212

First step in the clinical examination of the hip : determining the lie of the pelvis.

that the age of the patient at the onset of symptoms affords some indication of the likely nature of the trouble, as shown in Table IX.

Exposure

For the proper examination of the hip the patient should be stripped except for a pelvic slip or underpants and, in women, a brassiere. The first part of the examination is conducted with the patient lying ; afterwards he is examined standing and walking.

Steps in Clinical Examination

A suggested routine for clinical examination of the hip is summarised in Table X.

Setting the Pelvis Square

This is an important preliminary step. Determine from the position of the anterior superior iliac spines whether or not the pelvis is lying square with the limbs (Fig. 212). If it is not, an attempt is made to set it square. If this is impossible it means that there is incorrectible adduction or abduction at one or other hip : in that event the fact that the pelvis is tilted should be noted and borne in mind during the subsequent steps of the examination.

Measuring the Length of the Limbs

Methods of measuring the lower limbs are often confusing to the uninitiated, but it is important that they should be properly understood. Accuracy in measurement is of more than academic

TABLE X

ROUTINE CLINICAL EXAMINATION IN SUSPECTED DISORDERS
OF THE HIP

1. LOCAL EXAMINATION OF THE HIP REGION

(Patient recumbent)

Position of pelvis

Determine the lie of the pelvis and set it square with the limbs if possible

Inspection

Bone contours and alignment
Soft-tissue contours
Colour and texture of skin
Scars or sinuses

Palpation

Skin temperature
Bone contours
Soft-tissue contours
Local tenderness

Measurements of limb length

Real or true length :

Anterior superior iliac spine to medial malleolus. (Angle between pelvis and limbs to be equal on each side)

If discrepancy found, determine site of shortening :

(a) Above trochanter (Bryant's triangle; Nelaton's line; Schoemaker's line)
(b) Below trochanter (measure each bone)

'Apparent' or false discrepancy :

Xiphisternum to medial malleolus. (Limbs to be parallel and in line with trunk)

Examination for fixed deformity

Including Thomas's manœuvre for detection and measurement of fixed flexion deformity

Movements (active and passive)

Flexion
Abduction ; abduction in flexion
Adduction
Medial rotation ; lateral rotation
Extension (with patient prone)

Power (tested against resistance of examiner)

Estimate strength of each muscle group

Examination for abnormal mobility

Test for longitudinal (telescopic) movement
Click test (in new-born)

(Patient standing)

Examination for postural stability

Trendelenburg's test

Gait

2. EXAMINATION OF POTENTIAL EXTRINSIC SOURCES OF HIP SYMPTOMS

This is important if a satisfactory explanation for the symptoms is not found on local examination. The investigation should include : 1) the spine and sacro-iliac joints ; 2) the abdomen and pelvis ; and 3) the major blood-vessels.

3. GENERAL EXAMINATION

General survey of other parts of the body. The local symptoms may be only one manifestation of a widespread disease.

significance ; it is of practical importance when corrective operations or adjustments to the shoes are contemplated.

It is necessary to measure, first, the real or *true length* of each limb. Secondly, it is necessary to determine whether there is any ' *apparent* ' or *false discrepancy* in the length of the limbs from fixed pelvic tilt (Figs. 213-214). Whereas it is always necessary to measure the true length, it is necessary to measure ' apparent ' discrepancy only when there is an incorrectible pelvic tilt.

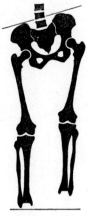 

FIG. 213   FIG. 214

' Apparent ' or false discrepancy in limb length is caused entirely by incorrectible lateral tilting of the pelvis (Fig. 213). If the pelvis is square with the limbs there can be no ' apparent ' discrepancy in limb length (Fig. 214).

Measurement of true length. Ideally it would be desirable to measure from the normal axis of hip movement—that is, the centre of the femoral head—but since there is no surface landmark at that point it is impracticable to do so. The measurement is therefore taken from the nearest convenient landmark—namely, the anterior superior spine of the ilium. Distally, measurement is usually made to the medial malleolus.

The anterior superior spine, be it noted, is well lateral to the axis of hip movement. This makes no matter if the angle between limb and pelvis is the same on each side. But it will render the measurements fallacious if the angle between limb and pelvis is not the same on each side. This will be understood best by reference to Figure 215. It will be seen that abduction of a limb brings the medial malleolus nearer to the corresponding anterior superior spine, whereas adduction of the limb carries the medial malleolus away from the anterior superior spine. Thus if measurements are made while the patient lies with one hip adducted and the other abducted (a common posture in cases of hip disease) inaccurate readings will be obtained : the length will be exaggerated on the adducted side and belittled on the abducted side.

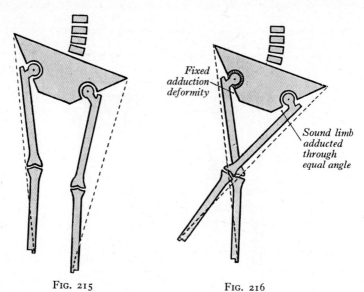

Fixed adduction deformity

Sound limb adducted through equal angle

FIG. 215   FIG. 216

Figure 215—Since the anterior superior spine is lateral to the hip joint abduction approximates the foot to it and adduction carries the foot away from it. For this reason measurements of true length are inaccurate if the angle of abduction or adduction is not equal on the two sides. Figure 216—Correct way of measuring true length when there is a fixed adduction deformity of one hip. The other hip must be adducted through an equal range. (Position of tape-measure shown by interrupted lines.)

The rule is, therefore, that *to obtain an accurate comparison of their true length by surface measurement the two limbs must be placed in comparable positions relative to the pelvis*. Thus if one limb is adducted and cannot be brought out to the neutral position the other limb must be adducted through a corresponding angle by crossing it over the first limb before the measurements are taken (Fig. 216). Similarly, if one hip is in fixed abduction the other must be abducted through the same range before the measurements of true length are made.

Fixing the tape-measure at the anterior superior spine. A flat metal end (as found on the ordinary tailor's measure) is essential. The metal end is placed immediately *distal* to the anterior superior spine and is pushed up against it. The thumb is then pressed firmly backwards against the bone and the tape-end together (Fig. 217). This gives rigid fixation of the tape-measure against the bone.

Taking the reading at the medial malleolus. The tip of the index finger is placed immediately distal to the medial malleolus and pushed up against it. The thumb nail is brought down against the tip of the index finger so that the tape-measure is pinched between them (Fig. 218). The point of measurement is indicated by the thumb nail.

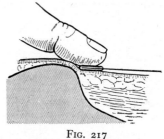

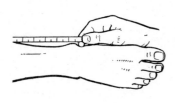

FIG. 217	FIG. 218
Fixing the tape-measure at the anterior superior spine.	Taking the measurement at the medial malleolus.

Determining the site of true shortening. If measurements reveal real shortening of a limb it is necessary to determine whether the shortening is above the trochanteric level (suggesting an affection in or near the hip), or below the trochanteric level (suggesting an affection of the limb bones).

SHORTENING ABOVE THE GREATER TROCHANTER.[1] Tests for shortening above the trochanteric level are : 1) the measurement of Bryant's triangle ; 2) the construction of Nelaton's line ; and 3) the construction of Schoemaker's line.

Bryant's triangle : In principle, this is nothing more than a method of comparing the distance between the greater trochanter and the wing of the ilium on the two sides.[2] With the patient lying supine, a perpendicular is dropped from the anterior superior spine of the ilium towards the couch. A second line is projected upwards from the tip of the greater trochanter to meet the first line at a right angle (Fig. 219). This is the important line of the triangle : it is measured and compared on the two sides. (The third side of the triangle is unimportant. It joins the anterior superior spine to the tip of the greater trochanter.)

Measurement of Bryant's triangle gives a comparison between the pelvis-to-trochanter distance on each side. Relative shortening on one

[1] The measurements to be described under this heading are seldom carried out in practice because the information that they give is more easily obtained from the radiographs. Nevertheless the student should know the principles of the tests for examination purposes.

[2] A simpler and equally informative method is to measure, on each side, the distance between the tip of the greater trochanter and the highest point of the iliac crest.

side indicates that the femur is displaced upwards in consequence of a lesion in or near the hip. But if there is a possibility that both sides are abnormal measurement of Bryant's triangle is not helpful.

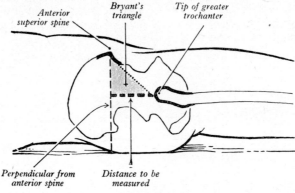

FIG. 219

Bryant's triangle, which indicates whether the greater trochanter is higher on one side than the other. The side of the triangle shown as a heavy interrupted line is measured.

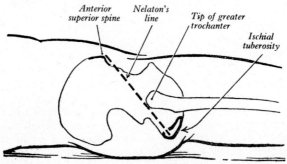

FIG. 220

Nelaton's line, which indicates approximately whether the greater trochanter is at the normal level. Normally the tip of the trochanter lies on or just below a line joining the anterior superior spine and the tuberosity of the ischium.

Nelaton's line : With the patient lying on the sound side, a tape-measure or string is stretched on the affected side from the tuberosity of the ischium to the anterior superior spine of the ilium (Fig. 220). Normally the greater trochanter lies on or below that line. If the trochanter lies above the line the femur has been displaced upwards.

Schoemaker's line : This is a similar test. A line is projected on each side of the body from the greater trochanter through and beyond the anterior superior spine. Normally the two lines meet in the midline above the umbilicus (Fig. 221). If one femur is displaced upwards owing to shortening above the greater trochanter the lines will meet away from the midline on the opposite side. If both femora are displaced upwards the lines will meet at or near the midline but below the umbilicus

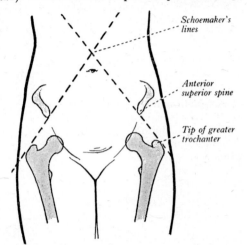

Schoemaker's lines

Anterior superior spine

Tip of greater trochanter

FIG. 221

Schoemaker's line in a normal subject. When the femur is displaced upwards the line passes below the umbilicus.

SHORTENING DISTAL TO THE TROCHANTER. True shortening is sometimes caused by an abnormality below the trochanteric level, such as a congenital defect of development, impaired epiphysial growth, or a previous fracture with overlapping of the fragments. To investigate this possibility individual measurements should be made of the femur (tip of greater trochanter to line of knee joint) and of the tibia (line of knee joint to medial malleolus) on each side.

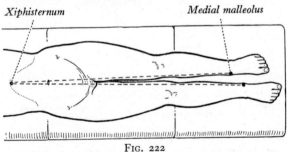

Xiphisternum   *Medial malleolus*

FIG. 222

For correct measurement of 'apparent' discrepancy in limb length the limbs must be parallel and in line with the trunk.

Measurement of 'apparent' discrepancy in limb length. 'Apparent' or false discrepancy in limb length is due entirely to incorrectible sideways tilting of the pelvis (Fig. 213). The usual cause is a fixed adduction deformity at one hip, giving an appearance of shortening on that side, or a fixed abduction deformity, giving an appearance of lengthening. Exceptionally, fixed pelvic obliquity is caused by severe lumbar scoliosis.

To measure apparent discrepancy the limbs must be placed parallel to one another and in line with the trunk. Measurement is made from any fixed point in the midline of the trunk (for example, the xiphisternum) to each medial malleolus (Fig. 222).

If there is a discrepancy of true length it must be allowed for when 'apparent' discrepancy is determined.

Examination for Fixed Deformity

Contracture of the joint capsule or of muscles may cause fixed deformity at the hip, preventing its being placed in a neutral position. Fixed flexion, fixed adduction, and fixed lateral rotation are common in some forms of arthritis.

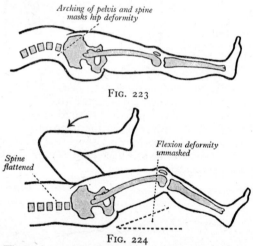

Arching of pelvis and spine masks hip deformity

FIG. 223

Spine flattened

Flexion deformity unmasked

FIG. 224

Thomas's test for fixed flexion deformity. Figure 223—Flexion deformity masked by arching of spine and pelvis. Figure 224—Deformity revealed by flexing the sound hip and, by continuing the flexion force, correcting the arching of spine and pelvis.

Fixed adduction deformity. This is detected by judging the relationship between pelvis and limbs. It will already have been noted at an earlier stage of the examination. If fixed adduction is present the transverse axis of the pelvis (as indicated by a line joining the two anterior superior spines) cannot be set at right angles to the affected limb, but lies at an acute angle with it.

Fixed abduction deformity. The angle between the transverse axis of the pelvis and the limb is greater than 90 degrees.

Fixed flexion deformity. This is determined by a manœuvre known as Thomas's test. *Principle of Thomas's test :* If a patient has a fixed flexion deformity at the hip he compensates for it, when lying on his back, by arching the spine and pelvis into exaggerated lordosis (Fig. 223). This allows the affected limb to lie flat on the couch. To measure the angle of fixed flexion deformity it is necessary to correct the lumbo-pelvic lordosis. This is done by flexing the pelvis (and with it the lumbar spine) by means of the fully flexed sound limb (Fig. 224).

Technique of the manœuvre : One hand is placed behind the lumbar spine (between it and the couch) to assess the degree of lumbar lordosis. If there is no lordosis when the affected limb lies flat on the couch there can be no fixed flexion deformity and there is no need to proceed with the test. If there is excessive lordosis, as indicated by arching of the back, it is corrected in the following way : The *sound* hip is flexed to the limit of its range. The limb is then pushed further into flexion, thereby rotating the pelvis on a horizontal transverse axis until the arching of the spine is obliterated. During this manœuvre the dis-ordered limb, if in fixed flexion, is automatically lifted from the couch as the lumbar lordosis is reduced (Fig. 224). The angle through which the thigh is raised from the couch is the angle of fixed flexion deformity.

Fixed lateral rotation. The most reliable index of the rotational position of the thigh is the patella, which normally points forwards when the hip is in the neutral position. If there is fixed lateral rotation the limb cannot be rotated to the neutral position. The angle by which it falls short of the neutral when rotated medially as far as possible is the angle of fixed lateral rotation deformity.

Movements

The accurate determination of hip movements demands much care, because restriction of hip movement is easily masked by movement of the pelvis. It is therefore essential to place one hand upon the pelvis to detect any movement there, while the other guides and supports the limb. *Flexion :* Movement of the pelvis is best detected by grasping the crest of the ilium (Fig. 225). Only in this way is it possible to differentiate between true hip movement and the false flexion imparted by rotation of the pelvis. The normal range of true hip flexion is about 120 degrees, but it varies according to the build of the patient. *Abduction :* The limb to be tested is supported by one hand while the other hand bridges the pelvis from anterior superior spine to anterior superior spine (Fig. 226). In this way true abduction at the hip can be differentiated from the false abduction that is imparted by tilting of the pelvis. The normal range of true abduction at the hip is 30 to 40 degrees (more in children). *Abduction in flexion :* This is often the first movement to suffer restriction in arthritis of the hip. The patient flexes his hips and knees by drawing the heels towards the buttocks. He then allows the knees to fall away from one another towards the couch. The normal range is about 70 degrees (90 degrees in young children). *Adduction :* The limb to be examined is crossed over the other limb. Again care must be taken to differentiate between true

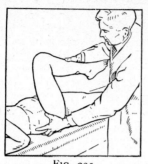

FIG. 225

Testing hip flexion. The right hand supports the limb while the left grips the ilium to detect pelvic rotation.

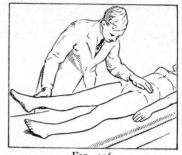

FIG. 226

Testing abduction of the hip. The right hand supports the limb while the left, bridging the two anterior superior spines, is ready to detect tilting of the pelvis.

adduction and the false movement imparted by tilting of the pelvis. The normal range of adduction is about 30 degrees. *Lateral rotation and medial rotation :* Judge the range by an imaginary pointer thrust axially into the patella, not by the position of the foot. The normal range both of medial and of lateral rotation is about 40 degrees. *Extension :* Contrary to what has often been written, the range of extension at the hip is virtually nil—5 or 10 degrees at the most. Seeming backward movement of the thigh is in fact contributed almost entirely by rotation of the pelvis and extension of the spine, not by extension at the hip joint proper.

Examination for Abnormal Mobility

In cases of marked instability of the hip longitudinal movement or ' telescoping ' can sometimes be demonstrated—especially in children with congenital dislocation of the hip. To carry out the test the limb is grasped firmly in one hand and alternately pushed and pulled in its long axis, the trunk being steadied by the examiner's other hand upon the iliac crest.

In infants it is important to examine for dislocation by the click test of Ortolani and others. This is described on page 323.

Examination for Postural Stability: the Trendelenburg Test

The Trendelenburg manœuvre is a test of the stability of the hip, and particularly of the ability of the hip abductors (gluteus medius and gluteus minimus) to stabilise the pelvis upon the femur. *Principle of the test :* Normally, when one leg is raised from the ground the pelvis tilts upwards on that side, through the action of the hip abductors of the standing limb (Fig. 227). (This automatic mechanism allows the lifted leg to clear the ground in walking.) If the abductors are inefficient they are unable to sustain the pelvis against the body weight and it tilts downwards instead of rising on the side of the lifted leg (Fig. 228). *Technique :* Stand behind the patient. Instruct him first to stand upon the sound limb and to raise the other from the ground. Having thus got the idea of what he is required to do, he should now stand on the affected limb and lift the sound leg from the ground. By inspection, or by palpation with a hand upon the iliac crest, observe whether the pelvis rises or falls on the lifted side. Remember that the limb upon which the patient stands is the one under test. If the pelvis rises on the opposite side (normal) the test is negative (Fig. 227). If it

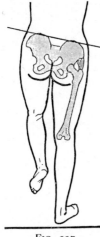

Figure 227—Negative Trendelenburg test. The hip abductors are acting normally, tilting the pelvis upwards when the opposite leg is raised from the ground.

Figure 228—Positive Trendelenburg test. The hip abductors are unable to control the dropping of the pelvis when the opposite leg is raised.

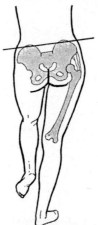

FIG. 227   FIG. 228

falls, the test is positive (Fig. 228) ; in other words the abductor muscles are incapable of stabilising the pelvis upon the femur.

Causes of positive Trendelenburg test : There are three fundamental causes : 1) paralysis of the abductor muscles (example—poliomyelitis) ; 2) marked approximation of the insertion of the muscles to their origin by upward displacement of the greater trochanter, so that the muscles are slack (examples—severe coxa vara ; congenital dislocation of the hip) ; 3) absence of a stable fulcrum (example—ununited fracture of the femoral neck). Sometimes two of these factors may operate together : for instance, in a case of upward dislocation of the hip there may be an unstable fulcrum as well as approximation of the origin of the abductor muscles to their insertion.

Gait

Watch how the patient stands and observe his gait on walking. Note that a patient with an unstable or painful hip prefers to use a stick in the *opposite* hand.

Extrinsic Causes of Pain in the Hip Region

If examination of the hip itself fails to reveal abnormalities sufficient to account for the patient's symptoms, possible causes outside the hip must be investigated. Attention should be directed particularly to the spine and sacro-iliac joints (including a neurological survey of the lower limbs), to the abdomen and pelvis (including rectal or bimanual examination if necessary), and to the vascular system (state of the peripheral pulses).

Radiographic Examination

Routine radiographs should include an antero-posterior projection showing the whole pelvis with both hips, and lateral films of each hip.

In special cases there is a place for stereoscopic films and for arthrography (that is, radiography after the intra-articular injection of radio-opaque fluid). When there is a possibility that the symptoms may be referred from the back additional radiographs of the spine and sacro-iliac joints must be obtained.

CLASSIFICATION OF DISORDERS IN THE HIP REGION

ARTICULAR DISORDERS OF THE HIP

CONGENITAL DEFORMITIES
Congenital dislocation of the hip

ARTHRITIS
Transient arthritis of children
Pyogenic arthritis
Rheumatoid arthritis
Tuberculous arthritis
Osteoarthritis

OSTEOCHONDRITIS
Perthes' disease

MECHANICAL DISORDERS
Slipped upper femoral epiphysis

EXTRA-ARTICULAR DISORDERS IN THE REGION OF THE HIP

DEFORMITIES
Coxa vara

INFECTIONS
Tuberculosis of the trochanteric bursa

MECHANICAL DISORDERS
Snapping hip

ARTICULAR DISORDERS OF THE HIP
CONGENITAL DISLOCATION OF THE HIP

This is a spontaneous dislocation of the hip occurring either before or during birth or shortly afterwards. In Western races it is one of the commonest of the congenital deformities : it is also of special importance because neglect or inefficient treatment incurs the penalty to the patient of lifelong crippling.

Cause. Much remains to be learnt, but it is becoming clear that a number of factors are concerned in the causation. 1) *Genetically determined joint laxity.* Generalised ligamentous laxity is found in a proportion of the patients, and may also be present in the parents. 2) *Hormonal joint laxity.* In females a ligament-relaxing hormone (' relaxin ') may be secreted by the foetal uterus in response to oestrone and progesterone reaching the foetal circulation. Laxity of the hip ligaments from this cause might be responsible for the greater incidence of dislocation in girls. 3) *Breech malposition.* The incidence of hip dislocation is slightly greater after breech delivery than after normal delivery. It is possible that the sudden full extension of the hips entailed in breech delivery may be the factor that precipitates dislocation, especially in the presence of ligamentous laxity. 4) *Genetically determined dysplasia of the hip.* In the past, congenital under-development of the component parts of the hip was thought to be important, but it is no longer regarded as a major primary cause of dislocation because in the new-born infant with a dislocated hip the acetabulum and the femoral head have usually been found to be normal in size and shape. There is no doubt, however, that defective development of the acetabulum does occur occasionally as a distinct entity, probably genetically determined and always bilateral. In the infant it predisposes to dislocation, and in the event of dislocation it increases the difficulty of restoring stability. In the adult who has escaped dislocation in infancy it leaves the acetabula unduly shallow, with a tendency to subluxation and osteoarthritis of the hip.

Of these various factors in causation, ligamentous laxity (factors (1) and (2)) is probably the most important.

Pathology. *The femoral head :* In a case of persistent dislocation the bony nucleus appears late and its development is retarded. The femoral head is dislocated upwards and laterally from the

11*

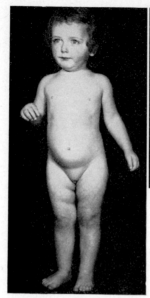

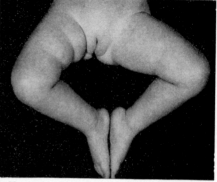

FIG. 230

Congenital dislocation of the right hip. The right lower limb was slightly shorter than the left, as suggested here by the typical extra skin folds in the thigh. Figure 230 shows the reduced range of abduction of the affected hip—another typical feature in children beyond the first few months of life, though not in the new-born.

FIG. 229

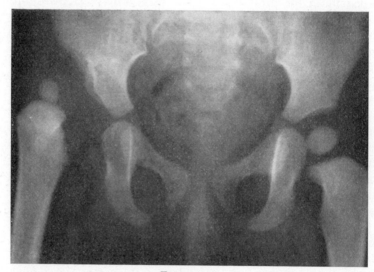

FIG. 231

Congenital dislocation of the right hip in a child of 2. The three points to note are the retarded development of the capital epiphysis, the steeply sloping acetabular roof, and the lateral and upward displacement of the upper end of the femur.

acetabulum.   *The femoral neck:* In most cases the neck is anteverted beyond the normal angle for infants of 25 degrees. *The acetabulum:* The ossific centre for the roof of the acetabulum, like that for the femoral head, is late in developing.   The bone slopes upwards at a steep angle instead of forming a nearly horizontal roof for the acetabulum.   The cartilaginous part of the roof is fairly well formed at first, but if the dislocation is allowed to persist development does not proceed normally, and the socket assumes a shallow contour with steeply sloping roof. *The fibrocartilaginous labrum:* The labrum or ' limbus ' is often folded into the cavity of the acetabulum and may impede complete reduction of the dislocation.   *The capsule:* This is gradually elongated as the femoral head is displaced upwards.

Clinical features. Girls are affected five times as often as boys. In one-third of all cases both hips are affected.   Unless it is specially looked for, abnormality may not be noticed until the child begins to walk.   Walking is often delayed, and there is a limp or a waddling gait.   *On examination* at that time, the main features in unilateral cases are asymmetry (notably of the buttock folds) and shortening of the affected limb (Fig. 229).   In bilateral cases the striking features are widening of the perineum and marked lumbar lordosis.   The range of joint movements is full except for abduction, which is characteristically slightly restricted (Fig. 230). In most cases the affected limb is abnormally mobile in its long axis (telescopic movement).   *Radiographic examination:* In the established state there are three important radiographic features (Fig. 231) : 1) The ossific centre for the head of the femur is late in appearing and its development is retarded ;   2) the bony acetabular roof has a pronounced upward slope ;   and 3) the femoral head (as judged by the position of the ossific centre) is displaced upwards and laterally from its normal position in the centre of the acetabulum.   *Arthrography* (radiography after the injection of opaque fluid into the joint) is useful in showing the outline of the cartilaginous elements of the joint.

Diagnosis. *In the new-born :* Nearly always, dislocation of the hip may be detected in the first few days of life by a diagnostic man-œuvre resembling that described by Ortolani (1937).   The surgeon faces the child's perineum and grasps the upper part of each thigh between fingers behind and thumb in front, the child's knees being fully flexed and the hips flexed to a right angle (Fig. 232). While each thigh in turn is steadily abducted towards the couch the middle finger applies forward pressure behind the greater trochanter. An easily palpable click caused by the femoral head slipping into the acetabulum denotes that the hip was dislocated.

In older children: Delay in beginning to walk or abnormality of gait in early childhood should always arouse suspicion, and radiographic examination should be insisted upon.

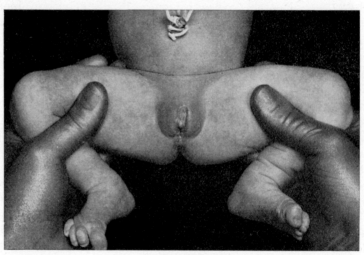

FIG. 232

Examining the hips of a new-born infant for instability. While the hip is abducted through the full range forward pressure is applied by the middle finger behind the greater trochanter. For details, see text.

Course and prognosis. The earlier the dislocation is reduced the better the prognosis. Even under the best conditions only about half or two-thirds of the patients treated after the first year of life can be expected to remain permanently free from trouble. Gradual redislocation is all too frequent, and pain from secondary degenerative changes often develops in middle adult life.

It is therefore important that, through careful examination of every new-born infant, congenital dislocation be detected within the first week of life, when simple treatment can nearly always assure normal development of the hip.

Treatment. This varies according to the age of the patient when advice is sought.

NEONATAL CASES (within six months of birth). The dislocation is reduced by abduction of the hip. Abduction is maintained by a splint or by a plaster, usually for three months. In these early cases this simple treatment is usually all that is required. Periodical radiographic checks up to the age of a year should however be insisted upon.

AGE 6 MONTHS TO 3 YEARS. This still forms a large group, though with more frequent diagnosis at birth the proportion of patients treated neonatally should gradually increase.

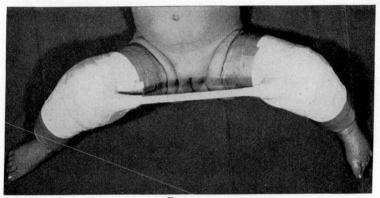

FIG. 233

A method of holding the hips in abduction and medial rotation.

Conservative treatment. Treatment may sometimes be conservative throughout, but in many cases—probably in most—timely operation reduces the risk of relapse : it also shortens the period of immobilisation. The dislocation is reduced by weight traction followed, if necessary, by gentle manipulation. The purpose of traction is gradually to stretch the soft tissues and to bring the femoral head down to the level of the acetabulum. If while traction is continued the limb is gradually abducted (a little more each day until 90 degrees of abduction is reached), reduction will often take place without further manipulation, especially in a young child. If reduction has not occurred after traction for four weeks gentle manipulation under anaesthesia will usually succeed in putting the femoral head back into place. Reduction is maintained by immobilising both hips in plaster in 80 degrees of abduction. It is a common practice now to hold the hips medially rotated [1] at first (Fig. 233), but many surgeons still prefer to hold the hips in lateral rotation. The plaster is retained for one to one and a half years, to allow the acetabulum to develop adequate depth. Free mobilisation is then permitted, and further treatment is not required unless dislocation or subluxation is found gradually to be recurring.

Operative treatment. The indications for operation in children of this age are as follows.

1) Failure to secure perfect reduction of the dislocation, usually from obstruction of the acetabulum by interposed soft tissue (notably an infolded acetabular labrum or ' limbus '). In this event operation is undertaken to clear the acetabulum and to secure perfect reduction.

2) Excessive anteversion of the femoral neck. The increased angle of anteversion that is a common feature of congenital dislocation of the hip may predispose to gradual redislocation. Most surgeons therefore advise that excessive anteversion be corrected by rotation osteotomy—that is, by dividing the femur below the greater trochanter and twisting the femoral shaft laterally in relation to the upper end of the femur. This is usually done about a month after the dislocation has been reduced.

3) Recurrence of dislocation or subluxation after removal of the plaster. Gradual redislocation sometimes occurs if the acetabulum fails to develop well while the hip is held reduced in plaster. It should be treated by operation designed to improve the shape and depth of the acetabulum, or to alter the disposition of the acetabulum as a whole (by osteotomy of the innominate bone), so that it faces more directly downwards. Only three of the several methods available need be mentioned here : 1) acetabuloplasty ; 2) capsular arthroplasty (Colonna's operation) ; and 3) osteotomy of the innominate bone (Salter's operation).

Acetabuloplasty. In the simplest form of acetabuloplasty a rim of bone and cartilage is levered down from the ilium to widen the acetabular roof and make it more horizontal (Fig. 234). The wedge-shaped space thus produced above the osteo-cartilaginous flap is propped open with a bone graft. This procedure is sometimes known as the shelf operation.

---

[1] There is some evidence that immobilisation of the hips in medial rotation leads to increase in the angle of anteversion of the femoral neck : those who rely upon splintage in medial rotation should therefore be prepared to correct anteversion by rotation osteotomy in a high proportion of cases.

Capsular arthroplasty (Colonna's operation). The acetabulum is deepened by gouging out its cartilaginous floor, and a layer of capsule and synovial membrane is interposed between the femoral head and the acetabulum to serve as a lining for the remodelled joint (Fig. 235).

Osteotomy of the innominate bone (Salter's operation). The innominate bone is divided completely just above the acetabulum, the cut emerging at the greater sciatic notch. The whole of the lower half of the bone, bearing the intact acetabulum, is then sprung downwards and outwards, hinging at the symphysis pubis (Fig. 236). In this way the acetabulum is redirected to face more directly downwards, with consequent increased stability of the hip.

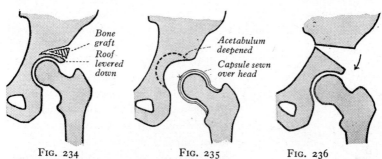

FIG. 234   FIG. 235   FIG. 236

Three methods of improving the stability of the hip. Figure 234—Shelf operation.   Figure 235—Capsular arthroplasty (Colonna operation).   Figure 236—Osteotomy of the innominate bone.

COMMENT

Although few would dispute the soundness of the general principles of treatment outlined above, controversy still exists as to how strictly the criteria for operation should be applied. It is probably true to say that the present trend is towards more frequent operation in the early stage, not only to ensure perfect reduction of the dislocation but also (a few weeks later) to correct the excessive anteversion that is almost constantly present. It seems likely that after operative reduction and rotation osteotomy the period of immobilisation may safely be reduced to as little as three or six months. This in itself may be regarded as a worth-while advantage of operative treatment, and sometimes indeed a full justification for it.

In neglected cases, or when dislocation or subluxation threatens to recur after primary treatment, it will be generally agreed that recourse should be had to one of the several reconstructive operations that are available. Three have been mentioned above, but there are other alternative techniques (see bibliography). At present there are no sure criteria upon which to base a choice between these various methods, and the decision is largely a matter of personal opinion.

References and bibliography, page 445.

AGE 4 TO 8 YEARS. After the age of 3 years conservative treatment is unlikely to be successful. If reduction is to be attempted [1] it should therefore be by open operation. In these late cases the acetabulum is nearly always poorly developed ; so at the time of operative reduction the opportunity should be taken to improve stability by one of the reconstructive operations already described. Rotation osteotomy will also be necessary if there is found to be excessive anteversion of the femoral neck, as is nearly always the case. Thereafter the limb is held in plaster in the neutral position for two months.

AGE 9 YEARS ONWARDS. After the age of 9 years treatment of freshly diagnosed congenital dislocation of the hip is not advised unless secondary degenerative changes lead to severe pain. If increasing pain justifies operative treatment, the choice of method depends largely upon whether the dislocation affects one or both hips. If only one hip is affected arthrodesis often offers a satisfactory solution. If both hips are affected abduction osteotomy at the level of the ischial tuberosity (Schanz) should usually be advised (Fig. 237). This operation helps to stabilise the hip by preventing abduction of the pelvis on the femur, thereby eliminating the Trendelenburg 'dip' on walking. At the same time the adducted upper fragment lying close to the side wall of the pelvis affords it greater support, and stability is further improved by the medial shift of the femoral shaft.

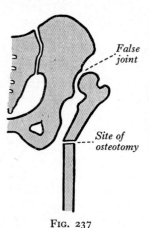

False joint

Site of osteotomy

FIG. 237

Low abduction osteotomy (Schanz) for painful unreduced congenital dislocation in adults.

TRANSIENT ARTHRITIS OF THE HIP
(Traumatic synovitis of the hip ; observation hip)

The so-called transient arthritis of childhood is a short-lived affection of the hip of uncertain pathology, characterised clinically by pain, limp, and limitation of hip movements.

[1] There are some who advise against any attempt at reduction in children towards the upper limit of this age group—say over the age of 5 or 6. The decision is often a difficult one and must depend upon the circumstances of each individual case.

Cause. This is unknown. Injury is possibly a factor but the evidence in support of it is slender.

Pathology. This is unknown. Possibly there is a mild inflammation of the synovial membrane, initiated by minor injury.

Clinical features. The condition is virtually confined to children under 10, especially boys. The child complains of pain in the groin and thigh and he is noticed to limp. *On examination* the only physical sign is limitation of hip movements. *Radiographs* do not show any alteration from the normal.

Diagnosis. Transient arthritis of the hip is important only because it resembles clinically the earliest stages of tuberculous arthritis or of Perthes' disease, before the characteristic radiographic features have become apparent. Transient arthritis should be diagnosed only after the hip has recovered—never while the symptoms and signs are present. While the symptoms and signs last the case should be regarded as one of suspected tuberculous arthritis and the child placed under observation in bed ; full recovery within a few weeks excludes tuberculous arthritis and justifies a retrospective diagnosis of transient arthritis.

Course. Full recovery, with return of a normal range of hip movements, invariably occurs within four or six weeks.

Treatment. Rest in bed until the pain has settled and full movements are restored is the only treatment required.

PYOGENIC ARTHRITIS OF THE HIP
(General description of pyogenic arthritis, p. 43.)

Pyogenic arthritis of the hip is uncommon. It occurs mostly in children, in whom it is often secondary to osteomyelitis of the upper end of the femur. The disease has special characteristics in young infants.

Pathology. Organisms (usually staphylococci or streptococci) may reach the joint directly through the blood stream, or the infection may spread from an adjacent focus of osteomyelitis. Rarely a penetrating wound is responsible. In new-born babies the infection may enter through the umbilicus. There is an acute imflammatory reaction in the joint tissues, with an effusion of turbid fluid or pus. In favourable cases healing with restoration to normal can occur, but often the joint is permanently destroyed or damaged. In infants bony ankylosis does not occur because the femoral head and the acetabulum are composed almost entirely of cartilage rather than of bone, but there may be total destruction of the developing femoral head with secondary dislocation of the hip (pathological dislocation). The femur may remain short, from destruction of the upper femoral growth cartilage. Additional shortening will occur if the dislocation is allowed to persist and the femur to slide upwards on the ilium ; so the discrepancy may be marked by the time adolescence is reached.

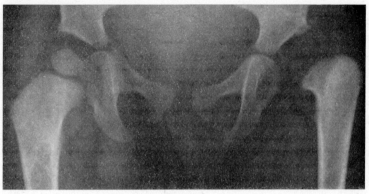

FIG. 238

Old pyogenic arthritis of the hip in an infant. The epiphysis of the head of the femur has been destroyed and the hip is dislocated. Note the normal appearance of the acetabular roof, which distinguishes this from a congenital dislocation.

In older children and adults pyogenic arthritis may be followed by either bony or fibrous ankylosis.

Clinical features. The clinical features differ so much in infants and in older subjects that separate descriptions are required.

PYOGENIC ARTHRITIS OF INFANTS. The onset is within the first year of life. Often there has been a known septic lesion somewhere on the body (for example, umbilical sepsis), but it may have caused little anxiety. Then the child becomes unwell and pyrexial. *On examination* it is not always apparent at first that the hip is the seat of the trouble. But careful examination will show thickening in the hip area, and movements of the joint are restricted. Sometimes an abscess points at the skin surface in the buttock or thigh. *Radiographic examination :* In the early stages there is no alteration of the bone shadows, but the soft-tissue shadows may suggest swelling about the hip. If the infection progresses to the stage of destroying the capital epiphysis of the femur the ossific nucleus fails to appear as it should at about the age of one year. In such a case subsequent radiographs may show gradual dislocation of the hip. This 'pathological' dislocation is distinguished from congenital dislocation by the facts that the acetabular roof is of normal shape and that the capital epiphysis is permanently absent (Fig. 238). *Investigations :* Aspiration of the hip yields pus from which the causative organism may be identified.

PYOGENIC ARTHRITIS IN OLDER CHILDREN AND ADULTS. The onset is acute or subacute, with pain in the hip made worse by attempted weight-bearing, and severe limp. There is constitutional disturbance with pyrexia.

On examination there is a fullness about the hip region from swelling of the joint. All movements of the hip are markedly restricted, and painful if forced. *Radiographic examination :* There may be no change in the early stages, but sometimes the space between the acetabulum and the femoral head is widened on account of distension of the joint with pus. Later, if the infection persists, the bone is rarefied and the cartilage space is narrowed. Finally, there may be bony ankylosis of the joint (Fig. 239). *Investigations :* The erythrocyte sedimentation rate is raised. There is

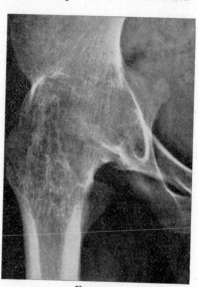

FIG. 239

Bony ankylosis of the hip caused by pyogenic arthritis. The infection spread to the hip from a focus of osteomyelitis in the upper metaphysis of the femur.

a polymorphonuclear leucocytosis. Aspiration of the joint yields pus from which the causative organism may be identified.

Treatment. *Constitutional treatment* is by rest and administration of appropriate antibiotics—for instance ampicillin and cloxacillin. *Local treatment :* Rest for the joint and relief of muscle spasm are best ensured by weight traction through adhesive skin strapping applied to the leg. The joint is aspirated daily until pus ceases to re-form ; after each aspiration a solution of penicillin or other appropriate antibiotic is injected into the joint. In severe cases more effective drainage may be obtained by incision into the joint. When the infection has been overcome active movements are encouraged.

Pathological dislocation complicating pyogenic arthritis of infants, with total destruction of the upper femoral epiphysis. Definitive treatment of this crippling condition must await adolescence. In childhood the aim of treatment is to prevent progressive upward displacement of the femur and thereby to minimise shortening. Provided the infection has settled, operation should be undertaken to deepen the acetabulum, to place the upper end of the femur within it, and, if necessary, to lever down a ' shelf ' of ilium over it. In adolescence, when the bones are nearing full development, arthrodesis may be recommended if the hip is painful.

RHEUMATOID ARTHRITIS OF THE HIP
(General description of rheumatoid arthritis, p. 46.)

The hip joints often escape in cases of rheumatoid arthritis. But when they are affected the consequent disability is serious. **Clinical features.** The changes may affect one or both hips, in common with several other joints. The main symptoms are pain and limitation of movement, aggravated by activity. *On examination* swelling is not obvious because the joint is so deeply situated ; for the same reason the temperature of the overlying skin is not increased as it is in rheumatoid affection of the more superficial joints. The range of all hip movements is impaired and movement is painful if forced. Fixed flexion deformity or adduction deformity may develop. The gluteal and thigh muscles are wasted. *Radiographic examination :* At first there are no radiographic changes. Later, there is diffuse rarefaction in the area of the joint. Later still, destruction of articular cartilage leads to narrowing of the cartilage space between femur and acetabulum (Fig. 240). *Investigations :* The erythrocyte sedimentation rate is increased during the active phase. The latex fixation test and the Rose-Waaler test may be positive.

Course. The disease becomes inactive after months or years,

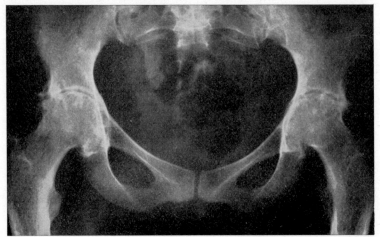

FIG. 240

Long-established rheumatoid arthritis of the hips, with destruction of the cartilage space. The marginal osteophytes indicate that osteoarthritis is becoming superimposed upon the old rheumatoid disease.

but the hip is seldom restored to normal. In long-established cases degenerative changes are superimposed upon the original inflammatory condition, giving rise to secondary osteoarthritis.

Treatment. Constitutional treatment is the same as that for rheumatoid arthritis in general. Local treatment for the hip joints depends upon the activity and severity of the inflammatory reaction. In the worst cases rest in bed is required, but when the reaction is moderate or mild exercises and active use within the limits of pain are encouraged. Intra-articular injections of hydrocortisone have sometimes given relief. Various physiotherapeutic methods may be given a trial in attempts to reduce discomfort and hasten resolution. For a deep joint such as the hip short-wave diathermy is the most effective of these measures.

Operative treatment : When pain is severe and walking is limited to a few yards operation is justified. Since many other joints are usually affected as well as the hips, conditions are seldom suitable for arthrodesis of the hip. Arthroplasty, by the insertion of a metal cup (cup arthroplasty), by replacing the femoral head or the whole joint with a metal prosthesis (replacement arthroplasty), or by excision of the head and neck of the femur, offers reasonable hope of a painless joint with useful movement (Figs. 246-248).

TUBERCULOUS ARTHRITIS OF THE HIP
(General description of tuberculous arthritis, p. 51.)

The hip is one of the joints most frequently affected by tuberculosis. In Western countries, however, its incidence has declined sharply in the past two decades and it is now uncommon.

Clinical features. The patient is usually a child—often 2 to 5 years old—or a young adult. There is often a history of contact with a person with active pulmonary tuberculosis. The symptoms are pain and limp. The general health is usually impaired. *On examination* a thickening is often palpable in the region of the hip. All movements of the hip are limited, often markedly, and attempts to force movement provoke pain and muscle spasm. The gluteal and thigh muscles are wasted. A ' cold ' abscess is sometimes palpable in the upper thigh or buttock. A tuberculous lesion may be apparent elsewhere in the body.

Radiographic examination: The earliest sign is diffuse rarefaction in the area of the hip. This is detected most easily when the bones are compared with those of the sound side, taken on the same film (Fig. 241). At first the changes are slight, but it must be emphasised that even slight rarefaction is significant. In the more fully developed stage the rarefaction is obvious ; and later there are fuzziness of the joint margins and narrowing of the cartilage space, indicating erosion of the articular cartilage (Fig. 242). Later still, bone may also be eroded ; but in a favourable case the disease is arrested before these later changes occur.

Diagnosis. This is mainly from transient arthritis, Perthes' disease (osteochondritis), low-grade pyogenic arthritis, and rheumatoid arthritis. In the early stages, before radiographic changes are evident, distinction from transient arthritis is not always possible until progress has been observed for three or four weeks. Important features supporting a diagnosis of tuberculosis are : a history of contact with tuberculosis (often parental) ; the presence of a tuberculous lesion elsewhere ; a positive Mantoux reaction in children ; a ' cold ' abscess ; the characteristic radiographic changes ; a high sedimentation rate ; and the typical histological appearance on biopsy of the synovial membrane.

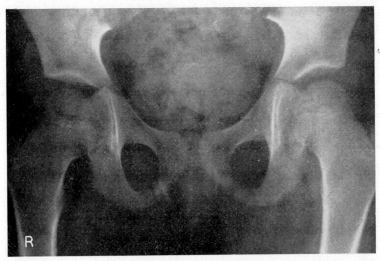

FIG. 241

Early stage of tuberculous arthritis of the right hip.   The bone is rarefied but
the cartilage space is not reduced.   The joint might be saved.

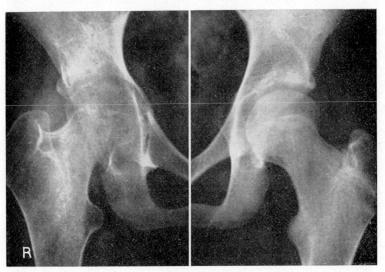

FIG. 242

Tuberculous arthritis of right hip in a more advanced stage.   The cartilage has
been destroyed and the articular surfaces of the bones have lost their sharp
definition.   The joint is permanently destroyed.

Course and prognosis. In a reasonable proportion of cases, especially in children, the lesion is aborted by treatment and a sound joint is preserved, provided there has been no destruction of cartilage or bone when treatment is begun. If cartilage and bone are eroded the joint is permanently damaged and often totally destroyed, with eventual fibrous ankylosis. Unless this is converted by operation to bony fusion there is some risk that the disease may become active again later.

Treatment. In its essentials treatment is the same as that for other tuberculous joints. *Constitutional treatment* is by rest in airy surroundings, and chemotherapy with streptomycin, para-amino-salicylic acid (PAS), and isonicotinic acid hydrazide (INAH). The drugs are continued for six months unless signs of toxicity appear.

Local treatment is initially by rest for the hip, usually in plaster, for a first period of six months. The subsequent treatment depends upon the progress made. If radiographs after six months show no destruction of cartilage or bone, if the general health is good, and if the erythrocyte sedimentation rate has shown steady improvement, the hip is left free for a clinical trial. Joint movements are practised in bed for a further month, and if there is no evidence of deterioration full activity is gradually resumed.

On the other hand, if at the end of the first six months' treatment radiographs show destruction of cartilage or bone (Fig. 242) all hope of preserving a movable joint is abandoned and sound bony fusion becomes the ultimate objective. To that end immobil-isation (not necessarily in recumbency) is continued until the lesion becomes quiescent, as judged from the general health, the erythrocyte sedimentation rate, and improved radiographic appearance. Finally, the joint is fused by operation, preferably by one of the extra-articular techniques (ilio-femoral or ischio-femoral arthrodesis) (Fig. 9, p. 27). In children arthrodesis should be deferred until the age of 12 years.

OSTEOARTHRITIS OF THE HIP

(General description of osteoarthritis, p. 55.)

Osteoarthritis of the hip is a common cause of severe disablement, especially in the elderly.

Cause. It is caused by wear and tear. Any injury or disease that damages the joint surfaces accelerates the wear-and-tear process and thus predisposes to the development of osteoarthritis. Common examples are fracture of the acetabulum, Perthes' osteochondritis, and slipped upper femoral epiphysis. In another group a developmental imperfection (dysplasia) or congenital sub-luxation or dislocation is responsible. In other cases the changes are simply a consequence of age degen-eration.

Pathology. The articular cartilage is worn away, especially where weight is transmitted. The under-lying bone becomes hard and eburnated. Hypertrophy of bone at the joint margins leads to the formation of osteophytes.

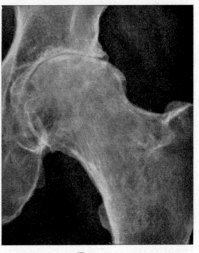

FIG. 243

Osteoarthritis of the hip. The character-istic features are narrowing of the carti-lage space, sclerosis of the bone surfaces, and osteophytes at the joint margins.

Clinical features. The patient is usually elderly; but when osteoarthritis is secondary to previous hip disease or to injury it often arises in middle life. There is pain in the groin and front of the thigh ; often also in the knee. The pain is made worse by walking and eased by rest. Later, there may be complaint of stiffness, which manifests itself in everyday life by inability to reach the foot to tie the shoe laces or cut the toe nails. The symptoms tend to increase progressively month by month and year by year until they eventually cause severe painful limp and incapacity for normal activities. *On examination* all hip movements are impaired. Limitation of abduction, adduction, and rotation is marked, but a good range of flexion is often preserved. Forced movements are painful. Fixed deformity (flexion, adduction or lateral rotation, or a combination of these) is common (Fig. 244). *Radiographic examination :* The changes are characteristic. There is diminution of the cartilage space,

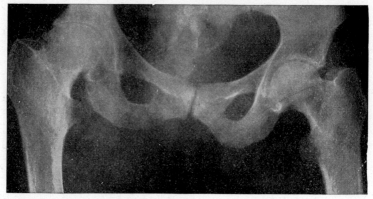

FIG. 244

Advanced osteoarthritis of right hip. Note the adduction deformity—a
common feature that causes apparent shortening of the limb.

with a tendency to sclerosis of the surface bone (Figs. 243-244).
Hypertrophic spurring of bone (osteophyte formation) is usually
seen at the joint margins.

Treatment. The treatment required depends upon the severity
of the disability. Mild osteoarthritis is best left untreated ; in
cases of moderate severity conservative treatment suffices ; in
severe cases operation is often advisable.

Conservative treatment. Clearly no form of conservative treatment
can possibly influence the distorted anatomy of the joint. At best
such treatment is only palliative ; it may alleviate but cannot
abolish the pain. Five methods will be mentioned. 1) *' Relative '
rest :* By this is meant a modification of the patient's mode of life
by change of occupation or adjustment of duties so that the work
thrown upon the hip is reduced. 2) *Drugs :* Mild analgesics are
often helpful, especially when the pain disturbs sleep. 3) *Physiotherapy :* Local deep heat by short-wave diathermy, with exercises
to strengthen the muscles and to preserve mobility, often produces
temporary relief. 4) *Injections into the joint:* The injection into
the joint of hydrocortisone, with or without a local anaesthetic
solution, has been tried, and in a few cases temporary relief has
been claimed. 5) *Radiotherapy :* This is occasionally worth a
trial in severe cases when operation is considered inadvisable.

Operative treatment. Operation may be required if pain is severe—especially if it hinders sleep and interferes seriously with the patient's capacity for walking or work. Five types of operation are in use.

1) *Denervation :* Severance of the obturator nerve and the nerve to the quadratus femoris cuts off a large part (but not all) of the sensory nerve supply of the hip. The relief obtained is incomplete and usually only temporary.

2) *Muscle release :* It has been claimed that division of the muscles about the hip relieves the pain of osteoarthritis, perhaps by eliminating muscle tension. The muscles that are usually divided are the psoas, the tensor fasciae latae, the rectus femoris and the adductors : the front of the capsule may also be incised. Walking is resumed within one or two weeks of the operation. Relief of pain is sometimes claimed but it is usually incomplete and temporary.

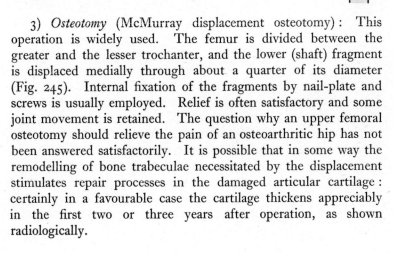

FIG. 245

Displacement osteotomy of the femur (McMurray). The femur is divided between the greater and the lesser trochanter, and the shaft fragment is displaced medially through a distance equal to about a quarter of its diameter. The fragments have been fixed with a nail-plate.

3) *Osteotomy* (McMurray displacement osteotomy) : This operation is widely used. The femur is divided between the greater and the lesser trochanter, and the lower (shaft) fragment is displaced medially through about a quarter of its diameter (Fig. 245). Internal fixation of the fragments by nail-plate and screws is usually employed. Relief is often satisfactory and some joint movement is retained. The question why an upper femoral osteotomy should relieve the pain of an osteoarthritic hip has not been answered satisfactorily. It is possible that in some way the remodelling of bone trabeculae necessitated by the displacement stimulates repair processes in the damaged articular cartilage : certainly in a favourable case the cartilage thickens appreciably in the first two or three years after operation, as shown radiologically.

4) *Arthrodesis :* The joint is fused in a position of 15 to 20 degrees of flexion (Fig. 9, p. 27). There is complete relief of pain, and good function is possible so long as the other hip and the knees are normal.

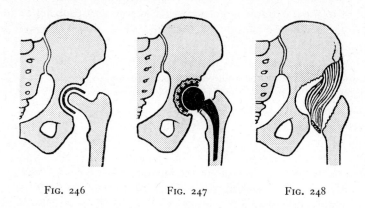

FIG. 246   FIG. 247   FIG. 248

Three methods of arthroplasty of the hip. Figure 246—Cup arthroplasty. Figure 247—Total replacement arthroplasty. Figure 248—Excision arthroplasty (Girdlestone pseudarthrosis).

5) *Arthroplasty :* A new joint may be fashioned by one of three methods. In *cup arthroplasty* the femoral head and the acetabulum are smoothed, and a highly polished metal cup is placed between them to serve as a new lining for the joint. The cup is designed to move freely upon the femoral head and in the acetabulum (Fig. 246). In *replacement arthroplasty* the femoral head is excised and replaced by a metal prosthesis which is designed to remain permanently fixed in the femoral shaft. At the same time the acetabulum may be deepened to receive a metal or plastic socket which is anchored in place by a long stem or by acrylic ' cement ' (total replacement arthroplasty) (Fig. 247). In *excision arthroplasty* (Girdlestone pseudarthrosis) a false joint is created by excising the head and neck of the femur and the upper half of the wall of the acetabulum, and suturing a mass of soft tissue (such as the gluteus medius muscle) in the gap thus created, to act as a cushion between the bones (Fig. 248).

Choice of Method. Neurectomy is seldom effective and should be used only in exceptional circumstances, if at all. The muscle release operation has also proved disappointing and is falling into disfavour.

The four operations that form the mainstays of surgical treatment are displacement osteotomy, arthrodesis, cup arthroplasty and total replacement arthroplasty. A fifth operation, excision arthroplasty, is used occasionally as a salvage procedure. In recent years total replacement arthroplasty (replacement of both the femoral head and the acetabulum) has achieved such spectacular success and acclaim that the other operations have been largely overshadowed. It is necessary therefore to emphasise that it is not a panacea, and that there is still a place for each of the other operations mentioned, even though the indications for them have been considerably narrowed since total replacement arthroplasty was introduced.

*Displacement osteotom*y is suitable for relatively young patients (say under 60) with moderately early osteoarthritis, a reasonably spherical femoral head well centred in the acetabulum, and a fair range of movement still preserved. If these criteria are fulfilled it can give good and lasting relief of pain in over 80 per cent of patients. So long as displacement does not exceed about a quarter or at most a third of the diameter of the femoral shaft the operation does not preclude the undertaking of total replacement arthroplasty later, should the result of the osteotomy prove disappointing. *Arthrodesis* has a very limited application. It may be appropriate as an alternative to other methods in young patients (under 40) with severe, strictly unilateral osteoarthritis, especially when the anatomy is much distorted and hip movement already greatly restricted. Arthrodesis is accepted very reluctantly in countries where squatting is the normal habit; and in general it is not favoured in North America. *Cup arthroplasty* is uncertain in its results : the operation entails temporary dislocation of the hip, which jeopardises the blood supply to the femoral head and may cause collapse of the bone from avascular necrosis. The failure rate is therefore high. Nevertheless a successful cup arthroplasty is probably better and more durable than any other type of hip reconstruction ; so it should not be entirely discarded. It is to be considered in young patients (under 40) with severely painful osteoarthritis, especially when conditions are unsuitable for displacement osteotomy or arthrodesis. *Total replacement arthroplasty* gives excellent results in a high proportion of cases, with full relief of pain and a reasonable range of movement. It also offers the advantage of rapid convalescence. It is by far the most satisfactory solution to the problem of osteoarthritis in the elderly patient, no matter whether it is unilateral or bilateral. It is still necessary, however, to exercise caution in recommending it for younger patients, because it is not yet known to what extent a good result is lasting, and what are the risks of loosening or breakdown of the prosthesis in the long term. The risk of complications has also to be borne in mind—particularly of infection, a catastrophe that virtually destroys any chance of success from replacement arthro-plasty. In these younger patients, therefore, it is necessary to weigh the likely advantages and possible hazards of the operation against the degree of disability that is imposed by the diseased hip.

Excision arthroplasty (Girdlestone pseudarthrosis) is best regarded as a salvage operation, to be resorted to only if other methods are inappro-priate or fail. It is the only operation available in the event of irretriev-able failure of a total replacement arthroplasty. It can give a painless hip with reasonable movement, but at the cost of appreciable shortening and instability, usually necessitating the permanent use of a stick.

PERTHES' DISEASE
(Legg-Perthes' disease; coxa plana; pseudocoxalgia; osteochondritis of the femoral capital epiphysis)

Perthes' disease is osteochondritis of the epiphysis of the femoral head. The general features of osteochondritis were described in Chapter II (p. 97). Like most examples of osteo-chondritis, Perthes' disease is an affection of childhood. The femoral head is temporarily softened and may become deformed. The main importance of the condition is that it may lead to the development of osteoarthritis of the hip in later life.

Cause. This is unknown. A local disturbance of blood supply is believed to play a part.

Pathology. The bony nucleus of the epiphysis undergoes necrosis and loses its trabecular structure. While in this state it is liable to become flattened, especially if it is subjected to pressure such as that entailed by weight-bearing. Eventually the bone is revascularised and hardens again, but if it has been deformed it never regains its normal shape. The whole cycle of necrosis and revascularisation occupies two years or more.

Growth at the epiphysial cartilage is often impaired, and consequently the femoral neck may be permanently shorter than normal, though the head itself is usually enlarged.

Clinical features. The disease is almost confined to children of 5 to 10 years. It usually affects only one hip. The child com-plains of pain in the groin or thigh, and is noticed to limp. There is no disturbance of general health. *On examination* the only striking sign is moderate limitation of all hip movements, with pain and spasm if movement is forced. *Radiographic examination :* The earliest radiographic changes are usually present by the time advice is sought. There is a slight decrease in the depth of the

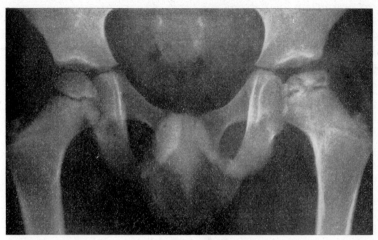

FIG. 249

Perthes' disease of the left hip. Note the shrunken appearance of the
bony nucleus of the femoral epiphysis, the corresponding increase in depth
of the cartilage space, the patchy changes of density, and the suggestion
of fragmentation.

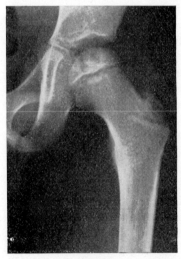

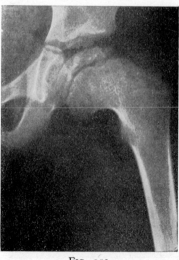

FIG. 250

Same patient as above, after two
years' relief from weight-bearing.
The shape of the head is virtually
normal, and the femoral neck is of
normal length. There is little risk
of osteoarthritis.

FIG. 251

In this patient, despite prolonged
relief from weight-bearing, the femoral
head is markedly flattened and the
femoral neck is short. The deformity
of the femoral head predisposes to
osteoarthritis.

ossific nucleus of the femoral head, whereas the clear cartilage space is often increased in depth : in other words the bony nucleus seems to have shrunk within its surrounding bed of cartilage (Fig. 249). The nucleus becomes denser than that of the normal side, and later it takes on a fragmented or granular appearance, areas of increased density being interspersed with areas of relative porosis. In severe cases the nucleus becomes progressively more flattened. Eventually the texture of the bone returns to normal (Fig. 250), but if flattening has occurred the femoral head is permanently deformed (Fig. 251).

Diagnosis. Perthes' disease is distinguished from tuberculous arthritis, which it resembles clinically, mainly by the radiographs. The normal erythrocyte sedimentation rate and blood count, and the good general health, are other distinguishing features.

Prognosis. The disease has no direct adverse effect upon the general health. The main risk is to the future function of the affected hip joint, because if the femoral head suffers permanent severe deformity the later development of osteoarthritis—

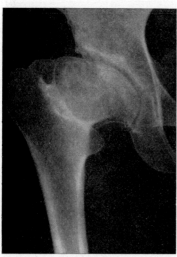

Fig. 252

Old untreated Perthes' disease. The severe flattening of the joint surface is already causing osteoarthritis.

often between the ages of 30 and 50—is almost inevitable (Fig. 252).

The outcome in a particular case is difficult to predict at the beginning. It depends to some extent on whether only part of the femoral epiphysis is involved (favourable prognosis) or whether the whole epiphysis is affected. In the most favourable cases the head is restored almost perfectly to normal and there is little or no impairment of growth of the femoral neck (Fig. 250) ; whereas in other cases, despite the strictest management, the final state of the femoral head and neck leaves much to be desired (Fig. 251).

In general, the outlook is rather more favourable in the younger children than in the older.

Treatment. It has to be admitted that the treatment of Perthes' disease is often disappointing : no universally satisfactory method has yet been evolved. Until recently it was generally taught that the hip should be protected from weight-bearing throughout the period when the bony nucleus is soft, as the best safeguard against severe deformity of the femoral head. In the past, prevention of weight-bearing was ensured by keeping the child in bed, usually with weight traction on the affected limb. This treatment might have to be continued for as long as two years before the femoral head was revascularised. It usually entailed the child's being admitted to a long-stay hospital where facilities for education were available. Most surgeons now believe that such drastic disruption of the child's home life is not justified, especially since the results are often imperfect. An alternative method of conservative treatment is to keep the child in bed for only a relatively short period—perhaps two months—in order to allow pain and irritability of the hip to subside, and thereafter to protect the hip by a caliper which transmits the body weight through the ischial tuberosity instead of through the hip joint. This allows the child to be up and about and usually to attend an ordinary school. At many centres this method is now the method of choice. Like prolonged recumbency, however, it fails to ensure results that are consistently satisfactory, much variability in the final shape of the femoral head being observed from case to case.

Operative treatment. Because of the unpredictable and often indifferent outcome of conservative treatment attempts to improve the results by operation have repeatedly been made. The operation that is currently favoured is known as varus osteotomy of the upper end of the femur. The femur is divided below the greater trochanter and the upper fragment—that is, the head and neck—is tilted downwards and medially so that the neck-shaft angle is reduced. The idea behind this is to bring the whole of the upper femoral epiphysis co-axially within the acetabulum, which it is hoped will serve as a mould to maintain the spherical shape of the femoral head while it is in the softened state. At operation the bone fragments are fixed with a nail-plate, and the child is allowed to walk after four weeks. This operation is still on trial, and it is not known to what extent, if any, it will give improved results in so far as the final shape of the femoral head is concerned. In the meantime it may be said

12

that the operation offers the advantage of a more rapid return to normal life, without the encumbrance of an unsightly caliper.

SLIPPED UPPER FEMORAL EPIPHYSIS
(Adolescent coxa vara ; epiphysial coxa vara)

This is an affection of late childhood in which the upper femoral epiphysis is displaced from its normal position upon

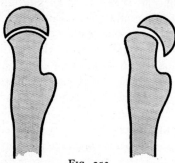

FIG. 253

Upper end of child's femur seen from the side. *Left*—Normal position of epiphysis. *Right*—Slipped epiphysis. The displacement is always backwards and downwards.

the femoral neck. The displacement occurs at the epiphysial line.

Cause. This is unknown.

Pathology. The junction between the capital epiphysis and the neck of the femur loosens. With the downward pressure of weight-bearing and the upward pull of muscles on the femur the epiphysis is displaced from its normal position. Displacement is always downwards and backwards, so that the epiphysis comes to lie at the back of the femoral neck (Fig. 253). The displacement usually occurs gradually, but occasionally a sudden displacement is caused by injury, such as a fall. Left undisturbed, the epiphysis fuses to the femoral neck in the abnormal position. The consequent deformity of the articular surface then predisposes to the later development of osteoarthritis.

Clinical features. The patient is between 10 and 20 years of age. In about half the cases there is evidence of an endocrine disturbance leading to a plump ' fat-boy-of-Dickens ' type of build ; but in other examples the child is of normal development. In about half the cases both hips are affected, one after the other. Typically, there is a gradual onset of pain in the hip, with limp. Sometimes the pain is predominantly in the knee, which may confuse the diagnosis. Rarely, these symptoms develop acutely after an injury.

On examination the physical signs are characteristic, for there is selective limitation of certain hip movements, the other movements being full or even increased.   The movements that are

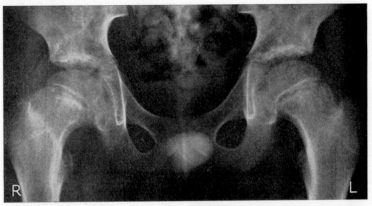

FIG. 254

This radiograph shows how a slipped epiphysis may easily be overlooked if antero-posterior films alone are examined.   The only indications that the right femoral epiphysis is displaced are a slight reduction of its vertical depth and slight rounding of the upper corner of the femoral neck.   Now see the lateral radiograph in Figure 255.

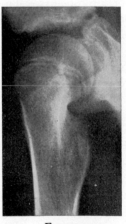

Figure   255 — Lateral radiograph of the right hip shown in Figure 254.   Slight backward slipping of the epiphysis is clearly revealed.

Figure   256 — Another patient.   Slipped epiphysis of severe degree.

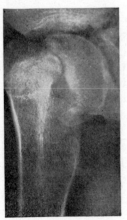

FIG. 255

FIG. 256

limited are flexion, abduction, and medial rotation.   Lateral rotation and adduction are often increased, and the limb tends to lie in lateral rotation.

Radiographic examination: Even a slight displacement of the epiphysis is recognisable, provided good *lateral* radiographs are obtained. It must be stressed that a slight displacement is easily overlooked if antero-posterior films alone are examined (Fig. 254.) Lateral radiographs are essential. In the lateral film the epiphysis is seen to be tilted over towards the back of the femoral neck,[1] the posterior 'horn' being lower than the anterior (Figs. 253-256).

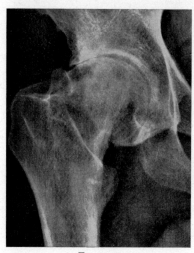

FIG. 257

Osteoarthritis developing twenty years after uncorrected slipped epiphysis.

Diagnosis. Slipped upper femoral epiphysis should be suspected in every patient of 10 to 20 who complains of pain in the hip or knee. The characteristic clinical features, together with the radiographic evidence of epiphysial displacement, are conclusive. The condition is nevertheless often missed, simply because lateral radiographs are not obtained (Fig. 254).

Complications. Avascular necrosis and consequent collapse of the epiphysis may occur if its blood supply is damaged. This complication is usually a consequence of manipulation or operation, but it may occur spontaneously.

If severe displacement is allowed to remain uncorrected osteoarthritis always develops in later life (Fig. 257).

Treatment. The treatment depends upon the degree of displacement.

Slight displacement. When displacement is slight (less than one centimetre as measured on the radiograph) (Fig. 255) the position may be accepted and all that is necessary is to prevent further displacement. This is achieved by driving threaded wires or a

---

[1] Students often have difficulty in determining in lateral radiographs of the upper end of the femur which is the back and which is the front of the bone. The key is the bony projection formed by the trochanters : this is always posterior.

screw along the neck of the femur into the epiphysis (Fig. 258). A three-flanged nail may be used for fixation as an alternative to threaded wires, but it does not easily penetrate the rather hard epiphysis and may damage its blood supply.

Severe displacement. When displacement is severe (Fig. 256) the position cannot be accepted because of the certainty that painful osteoarthritis will develop in adult life. The position must therefore be improved. Three methods are available : manipulation, operative replacement of the epiphysis at the site of slipping, and compensatory osteotomy at a lower level.

Manipulation, with or without preliminary weight traction, is only occasionally successful; it is worth trying in cases of recent displacement, especially if caused by injury. Manipulation should be carried out very gently lest the blood supply to the epiphysis be damaged. After successful manipulative reduction further slipping should be prevented by inserting threaded wires or a screw.

Operative replacement of the epiphysis, with fixation by wires or a screw, may be considered when symptoms have been present for less than three months. At such a relatively early stage the operation can restore the hip virtually to normal. Its disadvantage—and that a serious one—is that it may impair the blood supply of the epiphysis, thereby leading to avascular necrosis of the femoral head and precipitating the onset of osteoarthritis.

Compensatory osteotomy is an alternative method that is preferred by most surgeons, especially when the symptoms have been present for more than three months. By that time adaptive changes have occurred in the bone and they preclude the restoration of a normal joint by operative replacement of the epiphysis. The osteotomy is done just below the trochanteric level (Fig. 259). A wedge of bone is removed so that the shaft of the femur is angled into flexion and abduction relative to the

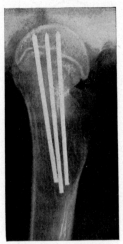

FIG. 258

Slipped epiphysis with only slight displacement. Threaded wires have been inserted to prevent further slipping.

upper fragment; at the same time the shaft is rotated medially·
The operation thus compensates for the downward and backward
tilting of the epiphysis; correction should be sufficient to bring
the epiphysis once more into the weight-transmitting segment of the acetabulum. The operation entails no risk of damage to the blood supply of the femoral head, but it leaves the articular surface of the upper end of the femur deformed, and therefore does not altogether remove the risk of secondary osteoarthritis in later years.

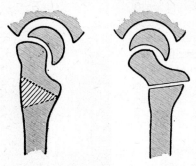

FIG. 259

Sub-trochanteric osteotomy for slipped
femoral epiphysis (diagrammatic). By
removal of an appropriate wedge of
bone (shown outlined in the left-hand
drawing), the epiphysis is restored to
proper relationship with the acetabulum. The operation has the advantage that the blood supply of the
epiphysis is not endangered.

COMMENT

There is general agreement that when the displacement is slight it is best to accept the position and to prevent further slipping by inserting threaded wires.

There is still much discussion on the treatment to be adopted when
the displacement is too great to be accepted, and yet cannot be
corrected by gentle manipulation. At present most surgeons are
more cautious than they were in undertaking direct operative replacement of the epiphysis, because of the serious risk of damaging its
blood supply and causing avascular necrosis. There is a general
tendency to rely upon the safer operation of compensatory osteotomy
at the sub-trochanteric level.

EXTRA-ARTICULAR DISORDERS IN THE REGION OF THE HIP

COXA VARA

The general term coxa vara includes any condition in which
the neck-shaft angle of the femur is less than the normal of about
125 degrees. The angle is sometimes reduced to 90 degrees or
less. The deformity is caused mechanically by the stress of body
weight acting upon a femur that is defective or abnormally soft.

Causes. The most important causes of coxa vara are: 1) *Congenital.* Part of the femoral neck remains as unossified cartilage, which gradually bends during childhood (congenital coxa vara; infantile coxa vara). This type is uncommon. 2) *Slipped upper femoral epiphysis* (epiphysial coxa vara). This was described on page 346. 3) *Fracture.* Coxa vara is common after fractures in the trochanteric region with mal-union, and in ununited fractures of the neck of the femur. 4) *Softening of bone*, in general affections such as rickets, osteomalacia, or parathyroid osteodystrophy.

Effects. Coxa vara leads to true shortening of the limb. Approximation of the greater trochanter to the ilium impairs the efficiency of the hip abductors, leading in severe cases to a Trendelenburg ' dip ' and consequent limp (p. 318).

Treatment. The treatment is mainly that of the underlying condition. In appropriate cases the neck-shaft angle can be corrected by osteotomy just below the greater trochanter.

TUBERCULOSIS OF THE TROCHANTERIC BURSA

The extensive bursa between the greater trochanter and the gluteal aponeurosis is occasionally the site of tuberculous infection. This type of bursitis has now become uncommon in Britain.

Pathology. The tubercle bacilli presumably reach the bursa through the blood stream from a focus elsewhere. There is a chronic inflammatory reaction in the walls of the bursa, usually with the formation of a tuberculous abscess. The abscess may burst through the skin to form a chronic discharging sinus. Later, the surface of the greater trochanter is sometimes eroded.

Clinical features. The patient is usually a young adult. He complains of a swelling in the trochanteric region, with local discomfort and sometimes a persistent discharge of pus. *On examination* the trochanteric area is thickened, warmer than normal, and perhaps reddened. Often there is a palpable abscess or a discharging sinus. Movements of the hip are not impaired. *Radiographs* typically show no abnormality, but in long-standing cases there is sometimes a superficial roughening or erosion of the lateral aspect of the greater trochanter. *Investigations :* The erythrocyte sedimentation rate is increased. Biopsy of the walls

of the bursa shows the typical histological features of tuberculosis.
Complications. Secondary involvement of the hip joint, with
the usual features of tuberculous arthritis, has hitherto been a
common late complication. Probably its frequency will be reduced
by effective treatment of the primary bursitis.

Treatment. After a preliminary one month period of rest and
systemic chemotherapy, with aspiration as required, the bursa
should be excised entire.

SNAPPING HIP

Snapping hip is a harmless condition in which a distinct
snap is heard and felt on certain movements of the joint. It
does not denote any underlying injury or disease and it is of no
practical significance. The snap is attributed to slipping of a
tendinous aponeurosis—probably that of the gluteus maximus—
over the bony prominence of the greater trochanter. It is heard
easily when the patient flexes the hip actively, but it is not
reproduced by passive movement with the muscles relaxed.
Treatment is not required.

EXTRINSIC DISORDERS SIMULATING DISEASE OF THE HIP

As has already been mentioned, it frequently happens that a
patient complains of symptoms in the region of the hip or thigh
when in fact they arise at a distance. The conditions that may
confuse the diagnosis in this way fall into three main groups :
1) disorders of the spine or sacro-iliac joints ; 2) disorders of the
abdomen or pelvis ; and 3) occlusive vascular disease.

DISORDERS OF THE SPINE AND SACRO-ILIAC JOINTS
PROLAPSED INTERVERTEBRAL DISC

The pain of a prolapsed or strained lumbar intervertebral
disc is often referred to the gluteal region or lateral aspect of the
thigh : indeed this is the commonest clinical feature in cases of
intervertebral disc injury of slight or moderate degree. The
patient himself, and often his doctor, may ascribe the symptoms
to a lesion of the hip. But the history is unlike that of a hip
affection. On examination other evidence of a spinal disorder

will usually be found, whereas the hip itself is normal clinically and radiographically.

SACRO-ILIAC ARTHRITIS

The pain caused by arthritis of a sacro-iliac joint—whether it be tuberculous, pyogenic, or the early stages of ankylosing spondylitis—spreads diffusely over the gluteal area and may simulate an affection of the hip. Mistakes should be prevented by careful clinical examination and by routine radiography of the whole pelvis in cases of alleged hip complaints.

DISORDERS OF THE ABDOMEN AND PELVIS

PELVIC OR LOWER ABDOMINAL INFLAMMATION

Inflammation involving the side wall of the pelvis may mimic a hip lesion very closely; indeed even experienced surgeons have been deceived. The condition responsible is usually a subacute suppurative lesion such as a deep peri-appendicular abscess or a pyosalpinx. The hip symptoms arise partly from irritation of the obturator nerve, causing referred pain in the thigh, and partly from irritative spasm of the hip muscles that have their origin within the abdomen or pelvis—namely the psoas, iliacus, pyriformis, and obturator internus. The muscle spasm may cause marked restriction of hip movements, with pain if movement is forced. Differentiation from an intrinsic lesion of the hip depends upon a careful history and a complete physical examination, including an investigation of the abdomen and pelvis. It is always important to bear in mind the possibility of abdominal or pelvic inflammation when the nature of an alleged hip complaint remains in doubt after clinical and radiographic examination of the joint.

OCCLUSIVE VASCULAR DISEASE

THROMBOSIS OF LOWER AORTA OR MAIN BRANCHES

Ischaemic pain in the muscles of the buttock or thigh, from occlusion of the lower abdominal aorta or its main branches, may occasionally simulate disease of the hip. Distinction should not be difficult: in occlusive vascular disease the pain is brought on by activity and is quickly relieved by rest; the femoral pulses will be weak or absent even though the pulses in the foot may be strong; and the hip will show a full range of painless movement.

References and bibliography, page 445.

12*

CHAPTER NINE

The Thigh and Knee

THE knee depends for its stability upon its four main ligaments and upon the quadriceps muscle. The importance of the quadriceps cannot be over-emphasised. So efficiently can a powerful quadriceps control the knee that it can maintain stability despite considerable laxity of the ligaments. In many injuries and diseases of the knee the quadriceps wastes strikingly, and to some extent the condition of the muscle is an index of the state of the knee : if it is wasted it is probable that there is an abnormality within the joint.

Apart from its vulnerability to injury, the knee is also particularly prone to almost every kind of arthritis. Moreover, it is the joint most commonly affected by osteochondritis dissecans and intra-articular loose body formation.

The region of the knee is the zone of most active bone growth in the lower limb (contrast the upper limb, where most growth occurs towards the shoulder and wrist). Perhaps partly for this reason the metaphyses near the knee are common sites of osteomyelitis and of primary malignant bone tumours.

The knee is, in fact, a region where nearly every kind of orthopaedic disorder may be represented.

SPECIAL POINTS IN THE INVESTIGATION OF THIGH AND KNEE COMPLAINTS

History

The history is of particular importance in the diagnosis of disorders of the knee. In a case of torn meniscus, for instance, the history is often the most important factor in the diagnosis. When there has been a previous injury to the knee, the exact sequence of events at the time of the injury and afterwards must be ascertained. Inquiry is made into the mechanism of the injury; what the patient was doing at the time ; whether he was able to carry on afterwards. Was he able to finish the game ? If not, was he carried from the field or was he able to walk ? How soon after the injury did the knee swell ? Was he able to straighten the knee fully ? If not, how did he eventually get it straight ? Was he able to bend it ? These and many other details must be elicited by careful questioning because they are so important in building up a

TABLE XI

ROUTINE CLINICAL EXAMINATION IN SUSPECTED DISORDERS OF THE THIGH AND KNEE

1. LOCAL EXAMINATION OF THE THIGH AND KNEE

Inspection

  Bone contours and alignment
  Soft-tissue contours
  Colour and texture of skin
  Scars or sinuses

Palpation

  Skin temperature
  Bone contours
  Soft-tissue contours
  Local tenderness

Measurement of thigh girth

  Comparative measurements at precisely the same level in each limb. (Note particularly the bulk of the quadriceps muscle)

Movements (active and passive, against normal knee for comparison)

Flexion
Extension
? Pain on movement
? Crepitation on movement

Power (tested against resistance of examiner)
Flexion
Extension

Stability

  Medial ligament
  Lateral ligament
  Anterior cruciate ligament
  Posterior cruciate ligament

Rotation tests (McMurray)

  (Of value only when a torn cartilage is suspected)

Stance and gait

2. EXAMINATION OF POTENTIAL EXTRINSIC SOURCES OF THIGH OR KNEE SYMPTOMS

This is important if a satisfactory explanation for the symptoms is not found on local examination. The investigation should include : 1) the spine ; and 2) the hip.

3. GENERAL EXAMINATION

General survey of other parts of the body. The local symptoms may be only one manifestation of a widespread disease.

picture of what exactly happened to the knee. Caution is necessary in accepting the patient's story of ' locking ' at its face value. Many patients speak of ' locking when the knee simply feels stiff and painful, or when it causes momentary jabs of pain on movement. True locking from a torn meniscus means simply that the knee cannot be straightened fully; it can usually be flexed freely. In locking from a loose body within the joint the knee may be jammed so that it will neither flex nor extend, but this is rather uncommon and the knee usually unlocks itself after an interval.

Exposure

For proper examination the whole length of the limb must be uncovered. In the case of male patients it is essential that the trousers (and long underwear) be removed. It is impossible to examine a knee adequately when the thigh is half covered by tightly rolled trousers or underpants. The sound knee must also be exposed for comparison. The patient must be recumbent upon a couch—not just sitting with his foot propped on a stool.

Steps in Clinical Examination

A suggested routine for clinical examination of the thigh and knee is summarised in Table XI.

Determining the Cause of a Diffuse Joint Swelling

The knee exemplifies better than any other joint the different types of diffuse articular swelling. That the joint is in fact swollen should be obvious from inspection : comparison of the two knees will show that the concavities normally present at each side of the patella have been filled out on the affected side.

A diffuse swelling of the knee can arise only from three fundamental causes : 1) thickening of bone ; 2) fluid within the joint ; and 3) thickening of the synovial membrane (in practice it is found that this is the only soft tissue about the knee that swells appreciably). Determination of the particular cause or combination of causes in a given case depends entirely on careful palpation.

Thickening of bone. Thickening of bone is detected without difficulty by deep palpation if the affected side is compared with the normal. There may be a general enlargement, caused perhaps by a bone infection or by an expanding tumour or cyst ; or there may be simply a local prominence, caused usually by osteophytes at the joint margin or by an exostosis.

Fluid within the joint. With practice, it is easy to detect even a small fluid effusion. It must be emphasised, however, that the widely used ' patellar tap ' test is unreliable. The test is negative in the presence of fluid in two circumstances : first, when there is insufficient fluid to raise the patella away from the femur ; and secondly, when there is a tense effusion. If used at all, the ' patellar tap ' test should be used only as a supplementary method. A fluid effusion is best detected by the fluctuation test. The palm of one hand is placed upon the thigh immediately above the patella—that is, over the suprapatellar pouch.

The other hand is placed over the front of the joint, with the thumb and index finger just beyond the margins of the patella (Fig. 260). Pressure of the upper hand upon the suprapatellar pouch drives fluid from the pouch into the main joint cavity, where it bulges the capsule at each side of the patella and imparts an easily detectable hydraulic impulse to the finger and thumb of the lower hand. Conversely, by pressure of this finger and thumb the fluid can be driven back into the suprapatellar pouch, the hydraulic impulse being clearly received by the upper hand. In this way an unmistakable sense of fluctuation can be elicited between the two hands.

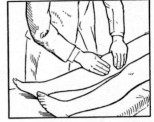

FIG. 260

Fluctuation test for intra-articular fluid. Fluctuation is elicited between the two hands. One hand compresses the suprapatellar pouch, while the thumb and fingers of the other receive the impulse at either side of the patella.

Distinction between effusions of blood, serous fluid, and pus is made partly from the history, partly from the clinical examination. An effusion of blood (haemarthrosis) appears within an hour or two of an injury and rapidly becomes tense. An effusion of clear fluid develops slowly (twelve to twenty-four hours) and is never so tense as a blood effusion. An effusion of pus is associated with general illness and pyrexia.

Thickening of synovial membrane. A thickened synovial membrane is always a prominent feature of chronic inflammatory arthritis. The thickening is often most obvious above the patella, where the reduplicated membrane forms the suprapatellar pouch. It has a characteristic boggy feel on palpation, rather as if a sheet of sponge rubber had been placed between the skin and the underlying bone. It is worth noting that since it is highly vascular a thickened synovial membrane is always associated with increased warmth of the overlying skin.

Movements

Accurate assessment of the range of movement is particularly important in the knee, because even a slight impairment of movement is significant. It is important to note also whether movement is painful and whether it is accompanied by crepitation.

Flexion. The normal range varies with the build of the patient. Thin patients can flex more than fat patients—usually enough to bring the heel in contact with the buttock. The range of the sound knee must be taken as the normal for the individual.

Extension. There is a fairly wide variation in the normal range of extension : it is wrong to accept o degrees as the starting-point of movement.[1] Most normal women can hyperextend their knees whereas some normal men cannot extend quite to the straight position. It is important to

[1] o degrees = the anatomical position, with the knee straight.

detect even a slight impairment of knee extension : therefore the range on the sound side must be taken as the yardstick of normal extension and a very careful comparison must be made between the two sides.

Tests for Stability

The integrity of each of the four major ligaments is tested in turn. *Testing the medial and lateral ligaments.*   For this test the joint must be

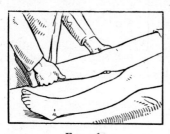

FIG. 261
Testing the medial ligament.

in full extension and the quadriceps must be relaxed.   Normally the ligaments are taut only when the knee is fully extended : if the knee is slightly flexed the ligaments will be slack even though they are undamaged. *Technique :* Support the limb by a hand gripping the ankle region.   Instruct the patient to relax the muscles so that the limb drops back into full extension. See that the quadriceps muscle is relaxed.   Using the free hand as a fulcrum at the side of the knee, apply first an abduction force to the leg to test the medial ligament (Fig. 261) and next an adduction force to test the lateral ligament.   If the ligament is torn, the joint will open out when stress is applied.   If the ligament is strained but not torn, the joint will remain stable but stress applied to the ligament will cause pain.

Testing the anterior and posterior cruciate ligaments.   The knee must be flexed 90 degrees, the foot must be fixed on the couch, and the quadriceps must be relaxed. The *anterior* cruciate ligament prevents *anterior* glide of the tibia on the femur : the *posterior* cruciate ligament prevents *posterior* glide. *Technique :* The patient's knee being flexed to a right angle and the foot placed firmly on the couch, sit lightly on the foot to prevent it from sliding (Fig. 262).   With the interlocked fingers of the two hands form a sling behind the upper end of the tibia, and clasp the sides of the leg between the thenar eminences.   Place the tips of the thumbs one upon each femoral condyle. Alternately pull and push the upper end of the tibia to determine the amount of antero-posterior movement.   Normally there is an antero-posterior glide of up to half a centi-

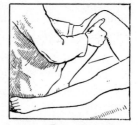

FIG. 262

Testing the cruciate ligaments.   The patient's foot is steadied by sitting upon it.   Pulling the tibia forwards tenses the anterior ligament ;   pushing it backwards tenses the posterior ligament.

metre ; but since the normal is variable it is wise to use the patient's sound limb for comparison.   Excessive glide in one or other direction indicates damage to the corresponding cruciate ligament.

Rotation Test for Pedunculated Tag of Meniscus

In this manœuvre, often known as McMurray's test, the tibia is rotated upon the femur with the knee in various positions of flexion and extension. Its object is to demonstrate mobile pedunculated tags of meniscus, and the test is important only when a torn meniscus is suspected. By manœuvring the knee it is hoped to cause the pedunculated tag, if present, to become temporarily jammed between the bone ends, so that a loud click or 'clonk' will be produced when the tag is disengaged by straightening the knee. *Technique* : The limb is grasped firmly by the ankle region so that the examiner has control of rotation of the tibia and of flexion-extension movements of the knee. The free hand is placed over the knee to feel for clicks. The rotation tests are started with the knee fully flexed and repeated with the knee in progressively less flexed positions. The first test : The knee being flexed fully, rotate the tibia laterally upon the femur to the full extent. Now straighten the knee slowly while the rotation is maintained : listen and feel for a click. Repeat the test in exactly the same way but with the tibia rotated medially instead of laterally. Then repeat, alternately with lateral and medial rotation, with the knee in less degrees of flexion—for example, at 120 degrees, 105 degrees, 90 degrees, 75 degrees, and 60 degrees. A loud click, distinct from the normal patellar click and usually associated with pain, suggests a tag tear (not a 'bucket-handle' tear) of a meniscus. *Caution* : Loud clicks can often be produced in normal knees. Most of them arise from movements of the patella, and they are not accompanied by pain. Discretion must be used in interpreting a click as an abnormal finding.

Extrinsic Causes of Pain in the Thigh and Knee

In most cases symptoms felt in the knee have their origin locally in or near the joint. But there are exceptions that may trap the unwary. Most important, pain in the knee may be the predominant feature of a lesion of the hip, such as arthritis or slipped upper femoral epiphysis. Less commonly sciatic pain, perhaps from a prolapsed intervertebral disc, has its greatest intensity at the level of the knee. In the investigation of pain in the knee we must therefore recognise the possibility that it may be referred from the spine or hip, and extend the examination to those regions if a satisfactory explanation for the trouble is not found on local examination.

Radiographic Examination

In the routine radiographic examination of the knee plain antero-posterior and lateral films are sufficient. They should include a reasonable length of the femur and of the tibia and fibula. Tangential projections of the femoral condyles with the knee flexed are sometimes helpful, especially when osteochondritis dissecans is suspected. When it is suspected that the knee symptoms might be referred from a lesion of the hip or spine appropriate radiographs of those regions should be obtained.

CLASSIFICATION OF DISORDERS OF THE THIGH AND KNEE

DISORDERS OF THE THIGH

INFECTIONS
Acute osteomyelitis
Chronic osteomyelitis
Syphilitic infection

TUMOURS
Benign bone tumours
Malignant bone tumours

ARTICULAR DISORDERS OF THE KNEE

ARTHRITIS
Pyogenic arthritis
Rheumatoid arthritis
Tuberculous arthritis
Osteoarthritis
Haemophilic arthritis
Neuropathic arthritis
Syphilitic hydrarthrosis
Chondromalacia of the patella

MECHANICAL DISORDERS
Tears of the menisci
Cysts of the menisci
Discoid lateral meniscus
Osteochondritis dissecans
Intra-articular loose bodies
Recurrent dislocation of the patella
Habitual dislocation of the patella

EXTRA-ARTICULAR DISORDERS IN THE REGION OF THE KNEE

DEFORMITIES
Genu varum and genu valgum

INJURIES
Rupture of the quadriceps apparatus
Apophysitis of the tibial tubercle (Osgood-Schlatter's disease)

CYSTIC SWELLINGS
> Prepatellar bursitis
> Popliteal cysts

POST-TRAUMATIC OSSIFICATION
> Pellegrini-Stieda's disease of the medial femoral
> condyle

DISORDERS OF THE THIGH

ACUTE OSTEOMYELITIS

(General description of acute osteomyelitis, p. 69.)

The femur is one of the bones most commonly affected by pyogenic osteomyelitis. The infection is carried to the femur either through the blood stream (haematogenous osteomyelitis), when it usually affects the lower metaphysis; or it is introduced through an external wound, especially in cases of compound fracture. The pathological and clinical features of osteomyelitis were described on p. 69.

Treatment. This is the same as for acute osteomyelitis elsewhere. In acute haematogenous osteomyelitis the urgent essentials are, first, to begin chemotherapy with the appropriate antibiotic or combination of antibiotics; and secondly, to evacuate pus, preferably by incision of the periosteum and, if thought advisable, by drilling holes in the bone. The skin wound may usually be sutured primarily. A careful watch should be kept for evidence of involvement of the hip or knee.

In osteomyelitis complicating an open fracture the essential principle of treatment is to secure free drainage.

CHRONIC OSTEOMYELITIS

(General description of chronic osteomyelitis, p. 74.)

Chronic pyogenic osteomyelitis is nearly always a sequel to acute infection that has been neglected or has responded poorly to treatment. As with the acute disease, the lower end of the femur is affected more often than the upper; but in many cases the infection spreads to involve a large part or even the whole of the shaft. The bone is thickened irregularly, and whereas parts of it are sclerotic it is often honeycombed with small or large cavities containing pus or granulation tissue.

Clinically, there may simply be a chronic discharge from a sinus, or there may be recurrent flares of infection with intervening periods of quiescence. *Radiographs* show the irregular thickening of the bone, with areas of sclerosis and cavitation. Sometimes a sequestrum is seen lying loose within a cavity : it has a clear-cut irregular margin, and may appear denser than the surrounding bone. **Treatment.** This is the same as for chronic osteomyelitis elsewhere. Recurrent flares of infection will often subside with systemic chemotherapy and rest alone. If there is persistent profuse discharge from a sinus, operation is required. The objects are to remove all dead bone and to eliminate bone cavities by de-roofing them and allowing the soft tissues to fall in.

SYPHILITIC INFECTION

(General description of syphilis of bone, p. 79.)

Syphilitic disease of bone is now rare in the West, but it is still seen occasionally and the possibility of its occurrence should be borne in mind. The femur is one of the commonest sites of syphilitic gumma and of diffuse syphilitic osteoperiostitis.
Clinical features. The complaint is of a gradually enlarging swelling, with moderate pain. The swelling feels hard or firm, and it may reach large proportions. *Radiographs* may show a diffuse thickening of the femoral shaft, sometimes with a more localised area of destruction.

BONE TUMOURS IN THE THIGH

The femur is one of the commonest sites of the important bone tumours.

BENIGN TUMOURS

(General description of benign bone tumours, p. 81.)

Of the four main types of benign bone tumour—osteoma, chondroma, osteochondroma, and giant-cell tumour—only the giant-cell tumour requires further consideration here.

GIANT-CELL TUMOUR (Osteoclastoma)

The lower end of the femur is a particularly frequent site for this tumour. The upper end is affected much less often. The tumour usually arises in young adults. It begins in what was the metaphysial region, but since the epiphysis is fused there is no obstacle to its spread into the articular end of the bone (Fig. 56, p. 84). The bone is gradually 'expanded,' the cortex becoming very thin. Pathological fracture may occur. Though classed with the benign tumours, a giant-cell tumour tends to recur after inadequate removal and in some cases it has the character of a sarcoma, metastasising through the blood stream.

Treatment. Radiotherapy is no longer recommended because of the uncertain outcome and the risk of its inducing malignant transformation. Thorough curettage of the tumour and filling the resultant cavity with bone grafts has been widely used but it is attended by a high incidence of recurrence. Most surgeons now prefer to excise the tumour-bearing lower end of femur entire, and to fuse the knee by means of bone grafts, stability being maintained in the meantime by a long intramedullary nail driven down the femur and across the gap into the tibia.

MALIGNANT TUMOURS

(General description of malignant bone tumours, p. 86).

The femur is a common site for all of the four main types of malignant bone tumour.

OSTEOSARCOMA (Osteogenic sarcoma)

This is usually a tumour of childhood or early adult life ; when it occurs in patients beyond middle age it is often a complication of Paget's disease. Typically it arises in the metaphysis of a long bone, and the lower metaphysis of the femur is the favourite site. The tumour is highly malignant, and despite treatment it usually causes death from pulmonary metastases.

EWING'S TUMOUR

This also occurs mainly in children. Unlike most bone tumours, it affects the shaft of the bone, which it expands in a fusiform manner. Over it, layer upon layer of new bone is laid down, giving a typical 'onion-peel' appearance as seen in the radiograph. Although the tumour responds dramatically to radiotherapy for a while it is ultimately fatal from blood-borne metastases.

MULTIPLE MYELOMA (Myelomatosis)

This is a tumour of later life. There are multiple tumour foci scattered through several bones, especially those containing abundant red marrow. The upper half of the femur is a favourite site (Fig. 60, p. 87). The tumour responds temporarily to radiotherapy but it is eventually fatal.

METASTATIC (SECONDARY) TUMOURS

Metastatic tumours of bone are much more common than any of the primary malignant tumours. The femur is commonly affected, especially in its proximal half (Fig. 263).

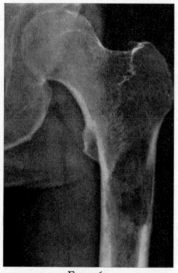

FIG. 263

Metastatic tumour in the femur—a common site. The primary tumour was in the lung.

Pathology. The tumours that metastasise most readily to bone are carcinomas of the lung, breast, prostate, kidney, and thyroid. The bone structure is destroyed by the tumour (except in the occasional osteoblastic or bone-forming metastasis from the prostate). Pathological fracture is common.

Clinical features. Pain is the predominant symptom, but sometimes the tumour causes little disturbance until a pathological fracture occurs.

Treatment. Radiotherapy often affords temporary relief: metastases from thyroid carcinoma may respond to radio-active iodine. Hormone therapy is worth trying in metastases from the breast, prostate and thyroid, and in some cases adrenalectomy may be worth considering. Most pathological fractures of the femur lend themselves well to internal fixation with a nail-plate or a long medullary nail. This facilitates nursing and greatly increases the patient's comfort, because external splints can be dispensed with.

ARTICULAR DISORDERS OF THE KNEE

PYOGENIC ARTHRITIS OF THE KNEE
(General description of pyogenic arthritis, p. 43.)

Pyogenic arthritis is commoner in the knee than in most other joints, partly because the knee is so exposed to injury and partly because of the close relationship of the joint cavity to the lower metaphysis of the femur, which is one of the commonest sites of acute osteomyelitis. The onset is acute or subacute, with pain, swelling, and loss of function. *Radiographs* do not show any abnormality in the early stages.

Treatment. *Constitutional treatment* is by rest and chemotherapy. Whenever possible the causative organism must be identified and its sensitivity to antibiotic drugs determined, so that the most effective drug may be given. *Local treatment :* The joint is rested in a plaster or on a Thomas's splint in a position 20 degrees short of full extension. In severe cases weight traction may help to relieve pain and spasm. The purulent effusion is removed daily by aspiration so long as it re-forms, and a solution of the appropriate antibiotic drug is injected into the joint. Rest is continued until the infection has been overcome ; thereafter active movements are encouraged.

RHEUMATOID ARTHRITIS OF THE KNEE
(General description of rheumatoid arthritis, p. 46.)

The knees are among the joints most frequently affected by rheumatoid arthritis, and they often suffer severe permanent disability. Both knees are often affected simultaneously with several other joints.

The knees are painful, swollen from synovial thickening, and warm to the touch. Movements are impaired, and painful if forced. *Radiographs* do not show any abnormality at first. Later there is diffuse rarefaction in the area of the joint. In long-established cases destruction of articular cartilage leads to narrowing of the cartilage space (Fig. 264), and there may be clear-cut erosions of bone.

Course and prognosis. The inflammation dies down after months or years, but the knee is seldom restored to normal. The joint surfaces are usually damaged and wear out sooner than those of a normal joint. Thus osteoarthritis is liable to be superimposed upon the original rheumatoid condition.

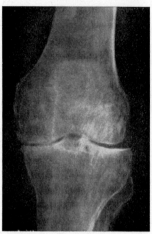

FIG. 264

Long-established rheumatoid arthritis of the knee. The bone is rarefied and the cartilage space is narrowed.

Treatment. In the active stage the treatment is that for rheumatoid arthritis in general (p. 49). Local treatment for the knees depends upon the severity of the inflammatory reaction. If it is severe, rest in bed or even temporary immobilisation in plaster is advisable. When it is moderate or slight, activity within the limits of pain is encouraged. Physical treatment is worth a trial. The most effective methods are exercises to preserve muscle power and joint movement, and local heat in the form of short-wave diathermy. Injections of hydrocortisone into the joint have sometimes given relief. *Operative treatment.* Four types of operation are employed in suitable cases: 1) synovectomy; 2) upper tibial osteotomy; 3) arthroplasty; and 4) arthrodesis. In deciding between them each case must be considered on its merits, and no hard-and-fast rules can be laid down.

Synovectomy : When there is persistent boggy thickening of the synovial membrane but when the articular cartilage is well preserved the operation of synovectomy (excision of the synovial membrane) is worth considering. Comfort may be much improved and the advance of the disease is possibly slowed.

Upper tibial osteotomy : Tibial osteotomy aims to relieve pain arising from the articular surfaces, and also to correct deformity. It is especially valuable when destruction of articular cartilage has proceeded more in one half of the joint than in the other. For instance, if the medial half of the joint has become markedly narrow through destruction of cartilage while the lateral compartment remains relatively intact, there will be obvious bow-leg deformity and pain is likely to be prominent in the diseased medial compartment of the joint, which is forced by the mal-alignment to take most of the weight (Fig. 265). Correction of the mal-alignment by removal of a wedge of bone, based laterally, transfers the weight-bearing thrust towards the more healthy lateral compartment and is often effective in relieving pain. The osteotomy is done about a centimetre below the upper articular surface of the tibia, and to permit early walking the fragments are usually fixed together at operation by metal staples (Fig. 265).

Arthroplasty of the knee has not reached anything like the state of development that has been achieved in the hip. In a favourable case pain is relieved and moderate function is restored ; but the outcome is uncertain, and even at the best the knee is unlikely to stand up indefinitely to really vigorous activity. Arthroplasty therefore tends to be reserved for elderly patients with severe disorganisation of both knees, especially when disease of other joints makes it unlikely that heavy demands will be made on the reconstructed knee. Several techniques of knee arthroplasty are available : most rely upon a metal hinge, the elongated upper and lower arms of which are jammed or cemented into the shafts of the femur and tibia respectively (Fig. 266) ; or upon polished metal inserts that replace the articular surface of the tibia or femur.

Arthrodesis is by far the most reliable operation for the disorganised rheumatoid knee, for it ensures total abolition of pain and good stability. The joint is usually fused in about 15 or 20 degrees of flexion. A stiff knee is, of course, an awkward handicap, but it is a price that is often acceptable to a patient who has been incapacitated by relentless pain over a long period.

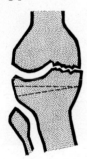 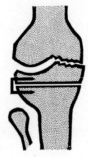 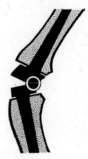

FIG. 265   FIG. 266

Figure 265. *Left*—Bow-leg deformity from uneven destruction of articular cartilage, that of the medial compartment being much thinner than that of the lateral. Body weight is now transmitted mainly through the diseased medial half of the joint. Interrupted line indicates wedge of bone to be excised for correction of deformity. *Right*—After corrective osteotomy and fixation with staples the line of weight transmission is shifted towards the more healthy lateral compartment. Figure 266—One type of arthroplasty of the knee. The arms of the metal hinge are impacted or cemented into the shafts of the femur and tibia.

TUBERCULOUS ARTHRITIS OF THE KNEE

(General description of tuberculous arthritis, p. 51).

After the hip, the knee is the joint most commonly affected by tuberculosis, usually in children or young adults. The knee is painful, diffusely swollen from thickening of the synovial membrane, and warm. Movements are limited, the thigh muscles are wasted, and an abscess or sinus is sometimes apparent. *Radiographic examination :* The earliest change is diffuse rarefaction throughout the area of the knee (Fig. 267). Later, unless the disease is arrested, there are narrowing of the cartilage space and erosion of the underlying bone.

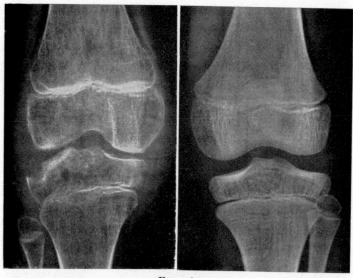

Fig. 267

Tuberculous arthritis of right knee in a child. The normal left knee is shown for comparison. Note the rarefaction, the diminution of cartilage space, and the small area of erosion near the lateral margin of the tibial joint surface.

Treatment. *Constitutional treatment* is the same as that for other tuberculous joints (p. 54). *Local treatment* is at first by rest in a splint or plaster, generally for three to six months depending on severity and progress. Subsequent management depends upon the response to treatment and the state of the joint at the end of this period of immobilisation. If the articular cartilage and bone are still intact, if the general health is good and the local signs have subsided, and if the erythrocyte sedimentation rate has steadily improved, it is likely that the disease has been aborted. In that event active joint movements are encouraged and walking is gradually resumed.

On the other hand, if the review at the end of the initial period of immobilisation shows that the disease is still active and that articular cartilage or bone has been destroyed, sound bony fusion becomes the ultimate aim. Immobilisation is therefore continued until the disease becomes quiescent. Arthrodesis is then undertaken if the patient is over 12 years old. In children under that age the joint is protected in a walking caliper or splint until the age of 12 is reached.

OSTEOARTHRITIS OF THE KNEE
(General description of osteoarthritis, p. 55.)

The knee is affected by osteoarthritis more often than any other joint. The condition is particularly common in fat women.
Cause. It is caused by wear and tear : but nearly always some factor is present that has caused the joint to wear out sooner than usual. Overweight is the commonest factor : for some reason it seems to impose a harmful stress upon the knee whereas it does not adversely affect the hip or ankle. Other important predisposing factors are : previous fracture causing irregularity of the joint surfaces ; previous disease with damage to the joint surfaces (especially old rheumatoid arthritis) ; and mal-alignment of the femur on the tibia (as in long-established bow leg).
Pathology. The articular cartilage is worn away and the underlying bone becomes eburnated. There is hypertrophy of bone at the joint margins, with the formation of osteophytes. The changes may affect predominantly the femoro-tibial joint or the patello-femoral joint ; but usually the whole joint is affected.
Clinical features. The patient is commonly an elderly fat woman. Often both knees are affected. There is slowly increasing pain in the joint, worse after unusual activity. The symptoms are often exacerbated by a slight strain or twist. There is usually evidence

of one of the predisposing factors mentioned above. *On examination* the knee is slightly thickened from hypertrophy of

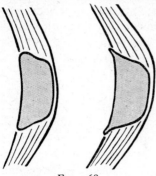

bone at the joint margins, where a rim of osteophytes may be palpable. Effusion of fluid into the joint is a common but not a constant feature. Movement is moderately restricted and is accompanied by coarse crepitation. The quadriceps muscle is wasted. In severe cases there is a tendency to fixed flexion deformity. *Radiographic examination :* Narrowing of the cartilage space, which is the first sign of osteoarthritis in most joints, is often not discernible until a later stage in the case of the knee. The first clear sign of osteoarthritis in the knee is sharpening

FIG. 268

Spiking of the articular margins of the patella, as seen in the lateral radiograph, is an early sign of osteoarthritis. The normal (*left*) is shown for comparison.

or 'spiking' of the joint margins, especially of the patella (Fig. 268) and tibia. Later, narrowing of the cartilage space is obvious, osteophytes form at the joint margins, and the subchondral bone may become sclerotic (Fig. 269). Opacities that appear to be loose bodies are often seen, but most are not in fact loose but are attached to the synovial membrane.

Treatment. Conservative treatment is usually effective in relieving the symptoms, although the structural changes in the joint are clearly irreversible. The most effective treatment is by physiotherapy. Intensive active exercises are carried out to strengthen the wasted quadriceps muscle. Local heat therapy is often also given, but it is less important than the exercises. The knee is largely dependent upon the quadriceps for its stability, and if a powerful muscle can be developed there may be no symptoms despite marked osteoarthritis. This is evidenced by the fact that many footballers with osteoarthritis of the knees have been able to continue in first-class football.

Intra-articular injections of hydrocortisone have been tried, but the results are uncertain. Repeated injections sometimes seem to accelerate the degenerative process.

Operative treatment. In the worst cases, with severe persistent

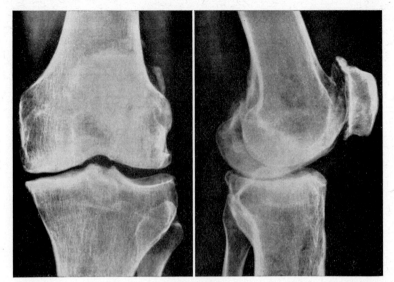

FIG. 269

Advanced osteoarthritis of the knee. Note the narrowing of the cartilage space,
sclerosis of the articulating bone surfaces, and osteophytes at the joint margins.

pain especially when associated with deformity, operation may be
advisable. Its nature will depend upon the circumstances of each
case. The following are the operations most used : 1) removal of
loose bodies ; 2) upper tibial osteotomy ; 3) excision of patella ;
4) arthroplasty ; 5) arthrodesis. *Removal of loose bodies :* When
loose bodies cause recurrent locking of the joint they should be
removed. This is a simple operation that gives good results.
Upper tibial osteotomy : This is valuable if uneven wear of articular
cartilage has caused bow-leg or knock-knee deformity. The main
points were discussed in relation to rheumatoid arthritis (p. 366).
Excision of patella : This is appropriate only when the arthritic
process is largely confined to the patello-femoral joint, the
femoro-tibial joint being relatively healthy. *Arthroplasty :* This
is undertaken less often for osteoarthritis than for rheumatoid
arthritis. Its limitations were discussed on page 367.
Arthrodesis may be appropriate in a severe case, especially
when other operations have failed and when the other knee is
healthy.

HAEMOPHILIC ARTHRITIS OF THE KNEE

(General description of haemophilic arthritis, p. 60.)

Haemophilic arthritis affects the knee more often than any other joint.

Pathology. Initially there is simply a haemorrhage into the joint (haemarthrosis). With rest, this is slowly absorbed. But further bleeding usually occurs, and it leads eventually to degenerative changes in the articular cartilage and to fibrous thickening of the synovial membrane.

Clinical features. The findings on examination vary according to the phase and duration of the disease. After each fresh episode of bleeding the knee is swollen, partly from contained blood and partly from synovial thickening caused by interstitial extravasation of blood. The overlying skin is abnormally warm. Joint movements are restricted, and painful if forced. In a quiescent phase between attacks of haemarthrosis there is some thickening of the joint from synovial fibrosis, movements are slightly impaired, and often there is moderate flexion deformity. *Investigations :* The clotting time of the blood is usually increased.

Diagnosis. Because of the synovial thickening, increased warmth of the skin and restriction of knee movements, haemophilic arthritis is easily mistaken for chronic inflammatory arthritis. A history of previous bleeding incidents and the increased clotting time of the blood are the important distinguishing features. Biopsy should be avoided because it may cause further bleeding.

Treatment. In centres where the necessary haematological facilities are available the ideal treatment is to aspirate the knee under the temporary cover of antihaemophilic factor (cryoprecipitate) as if it were an ordinary traumatic haemarthrosis. Such treatment might well prevent or delay chronic joint changes. If cryoprecipitate is not available aspiration should usually be avoided. The knee should be firmly bandaged and immobilised on a Thomas's splint or in a plaster. After four to eight weeks the residual blood is absorbed and cautious activity may be resumed.

The chronic degenerative arthritis that results from multiple repeated haemarthroses may have to be controlled by the permanent use of a polythene knee splint. Operation should be avoided.

NEUROPATHIC ARTHRITIS OF THE KNEE

(General description of neuropathic arthritis, p. 62.)

The knee is one of the joints most commonly affected by neuropathic arthritis (Charcot's osteoarthropathy). The commonest underlying cause is tabes dorsalis.

Pathology. The changes may be regarded as a much exaggerated form of osteoarthritis. The articular cartilage and parts of the underlying bone are worn away, but at the same time there is often considerable hypertrophy of bone at the joint margins. The ligaments become lax and the joint is unstable.

Clinical features. The knee is greatly thickened, mostly from irregular hypertrophy of the bone ends. There is slight or moderate restriction of movement, and there is marked lateral laxity, often giving a severe bow-leg deformity. Pain is slight or absent. Further examination will reveal evidence of the underlying disease—usually tabes dorsalis. *Radiographs* show marked destructive changes, usually with some new bone formation at the joint margins (Fig. 270).

Treatment. In many cases function is adequate despite the marked disorganisation of the knee, and treatment is not required. In other cases marked deformity — usually lateral bowing — may demand some form of protective appliance, such as a moulded plastic splint or a caliper. Arthrodesis of the joint is practicable but fusion is often slow. Because of this and the absence of severe pain operation is seldom advised.

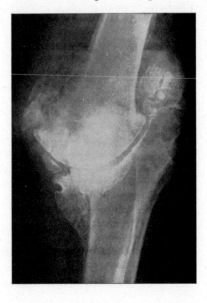

FIG. 270

Neuropathic arthritis of the knee. Degenerative destruction is accompanied by massive new bone formation.

SYPHILITIC HYDRARTHROSIS

Symmetrical hydrarthrosis of the knees (Clutton's joints) occurs in children as a manifestation of congenital syphilis. It is now rare. Clinically, there is an effusion of clear fluid into the joints, but there is little or no pain and good function is preserved. Other signs of syphilis are usually present, and the Wassermann reaction is positive. *Treatment* is by general antisyphilitic remedies and firm bandaging.

CHONDROMALACIA OF THE PATELLA

This is an uncommon affection of adolescents or young adults, in which the cartilage of the articular surface of the patella is roughened and 'fibrillated.' It is distinct from patello-femoral osteoarthritis, a condition occurring in older patients. Nevertheless chondromalacia predisposes to the later development of osteoarthritis. The cause is uncertain : repeated friction of the patella against an abnormally prominent ridge on the medial femoral condyle is at least partly responsible.

Clinical features. There is aching pain deep in the knee, behind the patella. Pain is exacerbated by climbing or descending stairs. There is often an effusion of fluid, and tenderness may be found on palpating the deep surface of the patella after displacing it to one side. There may also be a point of marked tenderness over the front of the medial femoral condyle. Movements may be accompanied by a fine crepitation transmitted to the examiner's hand upon the patella. *Radiographs* are normal.

Treatment. At first this should be expectant. A firm elastic bandage is applied and strenuous activities are curtailed. These precautions will often allow spontaneous improvement. If troublesome symptoms persist for many months operation may be required. Often it is sufficient to chisel away the abnormal ridge on the front of the medial femoral condyle, but in some cases it is necessary to remove the patella.

TEARS OF THE MENISCI

Injuries of the menisci [semilunar cartilages] are common in men under the age of 45. A tear is usually caused by a twisting force with the knee semi-flexed or flexed. It is usually a football

injury, but it is also common among men who work in a squatting
position, such as coal miners.   The medial meniscus is torn much
more often than the lateral.

Pathology.   There are three types of meniscus tear (Figs. 273-
275).   All begin as a longitudinal split (Fig. 271).   If this extends
throughout the length of the meniscus it becomes a *bucket-handle
tear*, in which the fragments remain attached at both ends

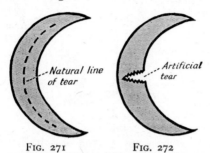

FIG. 271   FIG. 272

Figure 271—Direction of tear in a meniscus.
Figure 272—Transverse tears do not occur
in nature ; a tear such as this is always an
artefact.

(Fig. 273).   This is much the commonest type.   The ' bucket
handle ' (that is, the central fragment) is displaced towards the
middle of the joint, so that the condyle of the femur rolls upon the
tibia through the rent in the meniscus (Fig. 273).   Since the
femoral condyle is so shaped that it requires most space when
the knee is straight the chief effect of a displaced ' bucket handle '
fragment is that it limits full extension (= locking).

If the initial longitudinal tear emerges at the concave border
of the meniscus a pedunculated tag is formed.   In *posterior horn
tear* the fragment remains attached at its posterior horn (Fig. 274) ;
in *anterior horn tear* it remains attached at its anterior horn
(Fig. 275).   A transverse tear through the meniscus is always an
artefact, produced at the time of operation (Fig. 272).

The menisci are almost avascular : consequently when they
are torn there is not an effusion of blood into the joint.   But
there is an effusion of synovial fluid, secreted in response to
the injury.   Torn menisci do not heal spontaneously.

Clinical features of torn medial meniscus.   The patient is 18
to 45 years old.   The history is characteristic, especially with

' bucket-handle ' tears. In consequence of a twisting injury the patient falls and has pain at the antero-medial aspect of the joint. He is unable to continue what he was doing, or does so

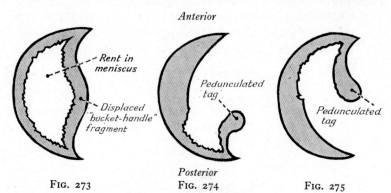

Anterior

Rent in meniscus

Displaced "bucket-handle" fragment

Pedunculated tag

Pedunculated tag

Posterior

FIG. 273   FIG. 274   FIG. 275

The three types of meniscus tear. Figure 273—Bucket-handle tear, the commonest type. Figure 274—Posterior horn tear. Figure 275—Anterior horn tear.

only with difficulty. He is unable to straighten the knee fully. The next day he notices swelling of the whole knee. He rests the knee. After about two weeks the swelling lessens, the knee seems to go straight, and he resumes his activities. Within weeks or months the knee suddenly gives way again during a twisting movement ; there are pain and subsequent swelling as before. Similar incidents occur repeatedly.

Locking : By ' locking ' is meant inability to extend the knee fully. It is not a true jamming of the joint because there is a free range of flexion. Locking is a common feature of torn medial meniscus, but the limitation of extension is often so slight that it is not noticed by the patient. Persistent locking can occur only in ' bucket-handle ' tears : tag tears cause momentary catching but not true locking in the accepted sense.

On examination in the recent stage the typical features are effusion of fluid, wasting of the quadriceps, local tenderness at the level of the joint antero-medially, and (characteristically in ' bucket-handle ' tears) limitation of the *last few degrees* of extension by a springy resistance, with sharp antero-medial pain if passive extension is forced.

In the ' silent ' phase between attacks there are often no signs other than wasting of the quadriceps.

Clinical features of torn lateral meniscus. The features are broadly similar, but the clinical picture is often less clearly defined. The history may be vague. Pain is at the lateral rather than the medial side of the joint, but it is often poorly localised.

Radiographs are normal, whether the tear be of the medial or lateral meniscus.

Diagnosis. In the ' silent ' phase diagnosis often depends largely upon the history. The surgeon should be very cautious in diagnosing a torn meniscus unless there is a clear history of injury and unless there have been recurrent incidents, each followed by synovial effusion. Often a period of observation is required before the diagnosis becomes reasonably certain.

Late effects. Long-continued internal derangement from a torn meniscus predisposes to the later development of osteo-arthritis.

Treatment. Once the diagnosis is established the correct treatment is to excise the whole meniscus.

Treatment of the locked knee. Manipulation under anaesthesia is the standard practice when there is a marked block to extension. But it cannot be expected that manipulation will restore the displaced ' bucket handle ' to its normal position : it merely extends the tear longitudinally and thereby allows the ' bucket-handle ' fragment to move farther towards the middle of the joint—that is, to the intercondylar region. In this position the displaced fragment presents less impediment to joint movement, but completely full extension is seldom restored. Manipulation is therefore worth while only in so far as it increases the patient's comfort while he is awaiting admission for operation.

CYSTS OF THE MENISCI

A cyst of a meniscus [semilunar cartilage] forms a tense, almost solid swelling at the level of the joint, usually on the lateral side.

Cause. Cysts arise spontaneously, but there is often a previous history of direct injury at the site of the cyst.

Pathology. The swelling is formed by a proliferation of fibrous

13

tissue, which is honeycombed with small cystic cavities containing clear gelatinous fluid.

Clinical features. The lateral meniscus is affected much more often than the medial. There is visible swelling, most obvious when the knee is held slightly flexed, at the level of the joint and usually anterior to the lateral (or medial) ligament (Fig. 276).

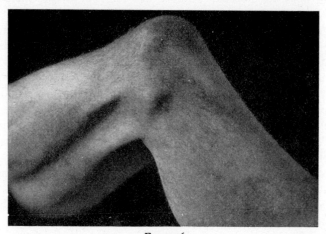

Fig. 276
Cyst of lateral meniscus.

The swelling tends to be painful at night and it is usually tender on firm pressure. The swelling is so tense that fluctuation can seldom be elicited (indeed it is sometimes mistaken for bone). *Radiographs* may show an indentation of the side of the tibial condyle where the cyst has been in contact with it.

Treatment. If the disability justifies operation the cyst should be excised together with the meniscus from which it arises.

DISCOID LATERAL MENISCUS

Rarely the lateral meniscus [semilunar cartilage] fails to assume its normal crescentic form during development, but persists in its embryonic form as a thick disc-like mass intervening between the lateral condyles of the femur and tibia.

A discoid meniscus may cause recurrent discomfort in the knee, with a tendency to giving way. Usually a loud ' clonk ' can be demonstrated on flexion-extension movements. These symptoms often become prominent during adolescence. If the disability becomes troublesome the meniscus should be removed.

OSTEOCHONDRITIS DISSECANS OF THE KNEE

(General description of osteochondritis dissecans, p. 67).

Osteochondritis dissecans is characterised by local necrosis of a segment of the articular surface of a bone and of the overlying articular cartilage, with eventual separation of the fragment to form an intra-articular loose body. The knee is affected much more often than any other joint.

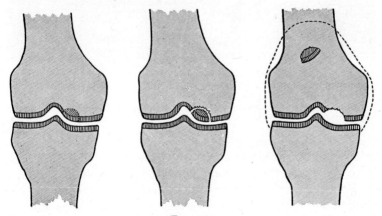

FIG. 277

The evolution of osteochondritis dissecans. *Left*—A segment of the articular surface dies. *Middle*—A line of demarcation forms around it. *Right*—The fragment breaks away and lies loose in the joint, leaving a cavity in the femoral condyle.

Cause. This is unknown. Impairment of the blood supply to the affected segment of bone by thrombosis of an end-artery has been suggested. Injury is possibly a predisposing factor. There is also a constitutional predisposition to the disease, because it may affect several members of a family or several joints in the same patient.

Pathology. The lesion nearly always affects the articular surface of the medial condyle of the femur (Fig. 277). The size of

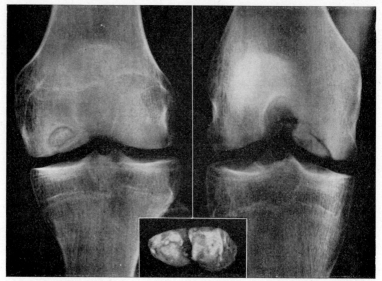

FIG. 278   FIG. 279

Osteochondritis dissecans.   Figure 278—Routine antero-posterior radiograph.
Figure 279—Tangential postero-anterior projection with knee semiflexed. This
shows clearly the large crescentic cavity in the medial femoral condyle, with
the separating fragment *in situ*.   Inset shows the loose fragment after removal.

the affected segment varies—it is often about two centimetres
in diameter. Within the area of the lesion the subchondral bone
is avascular and the overlying cartilage softens. A clear line of
demarcation forms between the avascular segment and the
surrounding normal bone and cartilage. After many months the
fragment separates as a loose body (sometimes two or three),
leaving a shallow cavity in the articular surface which is ultimately
filled with fibro-cartilage. The damage to the joint surface
predisposes to the later development of osteoarthritis.

Clinical features. The patient is an adolescent or a young adult.
He complains of discomfort or pain in the knee after exercise, a
feeling of insecurity, and intermittent swelling. When a loose
body has already separated within the joint the predominant
symptom is recurrent sudden locking. *On examination* there is
a fluid effusion. The quadriceps muscle is wasted. Movements
are not usually impaired. *Radiographs* show a clear-cut defect
of the bone at the articular surface of the medial femoral condyle
(Fig. 278). At first the cavity is occupied by the separating

fragment of bone ; later the cavity may be empty, and a loose body will then be seen elsewhere in the joint. The lesion is shown best in tangential postero-anterior projections with the knee semi-flexed (Fig. 279).

Treatment. In the developing stage treatment should be expectant : the knee is supported with a crepe bandage and strenuous activities are curtailed. Sometimes in these early cases the lesion will heal spontaneously, especially in children. When the lesion is ' ripe '—that is, when a clear line of demarcation has formed between the separating fragment and the surrounding normal bone—the loose piece should usually be removed, especially if it is small. A shallow cavity is left in the femoral condyle, but this gradually fills with fibrocartilage and adequate function is usually restored.

Because of the risk of the later development of osteoarthritis if a large part of the femoral condyle has been excavated, some surgeons recommend that the loose fragment be replaced in position and fixed with a pin. It has been shown that the fragment may unite again with its bed, but it is by no means certain yet that the incidence of late osteoarthritis will be reduced by this method of treatment. Probably it should be reserved for cases in which the separated fragment is large.

LOOSE BODIES IN THE KNEE

The knee is the joint most commonly affected by the formation of loose bodies.[1] There are four main causes : 1) osteochondritis dissecans (1 to 3 loose bodies) ; 2) osteoarthritis (1 to 10 loose bodies) ; 3) chip fracture of a joint surface (1 to 3 loose bodies) ; 4) synovial chondromatosis (50 to 500 loose bodies).

Pathology. *Osteochondritis dissecans* was described on page 379. The loose body or bodies are formed by spontaneous separation of a fragment of bone and cartilage from the articular surface of the medial femoral condyle. A shallow cavity remains in the condyle.

Osteoarthritis was described on page 369. Some of the loose bodies that may be found in osteoarthritis are probably formed

---

[1] A clear distinction must be made between *loose* bodies (*i.e.*, fragments of the joint tissues that have separated off to lie free in the joint) and *foreign* bodies (*i.e.*, pieces of extraneous matter introduced into the body from outside). Students often confuse the two terms.

by detachment of marginal osteophytes. Most separated osteo-phytes, however, retain a synovial attachment and cause no trouble : though they appear loose in radiographs they should not be regarded as such unless symptoms of locking indicate that they are moving freely within the joint. True loose bodies may possibly form from flakes of articular cartilage shed into the joint.

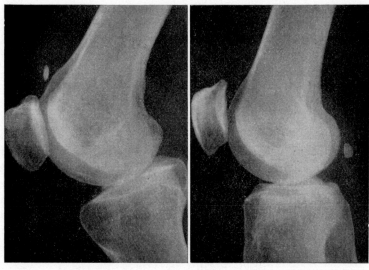

FIG. 280   FIG. 281

Figure 280—Loose body in the knee. As in this case, loose bodies often lie in the suprapatellar pouch. Figure 281—The fabella, a sesamoid bone in the lateral head of the gastrocnemius, present in many normal persons. It is sometimes mistaken for a loose body in the joint.

Chip fractures of the joint surfaces are an infrequent cause of intra-articular loose bodies. There is a clear history of the causative injury.

Synovial chondromatosis (osteochondromatosis) is a rare disease of the synovial membrane. It is characterised by the formation of numerous small villous processes, which become pedunculated. Later their bulbous extremities become cartilaginous and they are detached to lie free in the joint. Finally, some or all of the numerous loose bodies become calcified.

Whatever the cause of a loose body, its repeated jamming

between the joint surfaces will predispose to osteoarthritis or will aggravate existing osteoarthritis.

Clinical features. The characteristic symptom of a loose body in the knee is recurrent locking of the joint from interposition of the loose piece between the joint surfaces. Suddenly, without warning, the knee becomes jammed during movement. Locking is accompanied by severe pain. After a variable interval the patient is usually able, by manœuvring the limb, to disengage the loose body and free the joint. The next day the knee is found to be swollen with fluid. In many cases the patient is able to feel the mobile body through the soft tissues when it lies in a superficial part of the joint. *On examination* the findings are often slight, for a patient is seldom seen when the knee is locked. If he is seen soon afterwards a fluid effusion is present. Between attacks the only constant sign is wasting of the quadriceps. Sometimes the loose body can be palpated. The features of an underlying condition such as osteoarthritis may be present. *Radiographic examination :* With few exceptions, loose bodies are shown radiographically. They often lie in the suprapatellar pouch (Fig. 280). Care should be taken not to mistake the fabella (a sesamoid bone in the lateral head of the gastrocnemius) (Fig. 281) for a loose body. The position of the fabella is constant—it lies slightly above the level of the joint well behind the femur and towards the lateral side—and it is always oval in shape with its long axis vertical.

Treatment. In general the treatment for an intra-articular loose body is to remove it. Removal should always be advised if the body is causing recurrent locking. If there are no symptoms of locking operation is not essential. In such cases the fragment, though appearing loose in the radiographs, is often attached to the synovial membrane and is kept out of harm's way. This applies particularly to detached osteophytes in cases of osteoarthritis.

RECURRENT DISLOCATION OF THE PATELLA

The patello-femoral joint is one of the three joints that are most liable to recurrent displacement, the others being the shoulder and the ankle. In the case of the patello-femoral joint, unlike the other two, the instability is often caused by congenital factors rather than by an initial violent injury.

Pathological anatomy. In dislocations of the patella the displacement is always lateral, the patella slipping over the lateral condyle of the femur while the knee is flexed. Four factors predispose to recurrent dislocation : 1) general ligamentous laxity (' double-jointedness '), which may be an inherited defect ; 2) under-development of the lateral femoral condyle, with a shallow intercondylar groove ; 3) an abnormally high position of the patella, which consequently does not lie so deeply as usual in the intercondylar groove ; and 4) genu valgum, which causes the line of pull of the quadriceps to lie too far to the lateral side ; this last factor is seldom an important one.

Clinical features. Recurrent dislocation of the patella is more common in girls than in boys. Often both knees are affected. Trouble usually begins during adolescence or in early adult life. The dislocations occur while the patient is engaged in some activity that entails flexing the knees—not necessarily a violent exertion. Suddenly, while the knee is flexed or semi-flexed, there is severe pain in the front of the knee, and the patient is unable to straighten it. Often the displacement of the patella is recognised and reduced on the spot, either by the patient herself or by an onlooker.

On examination in the dislocated state the knee is swollen, and the patella is seen and felt upon the lateral side of the lateral femoral condyle. After reduction the main signs are an effusion (usually of blood-stained fluid), and tenderness over the medial part of the quadriceps expansion, which is usually strained or torn. One of the minor anatomical anomalies mentioned above may be observed. In particular, generalised ligamentous laxity is often found, as evidenced by the patient's ability to hyperextend the knee (genu recurvatum) or other joints such as the wrists or the joints of the fingers : this double-jointedness may be present also in parents or other relatives. *Radiographs* are seldom obtained in the state of dislocation. After reduction the knee may appear normal radiographically, but commonly the patella is seen at a slightly higher level than usual—often in both knees.

Course. Dislocation of the patella does not always become recurrent : some patients have no further trouble after one or two dislocations. But in many cases dislocations recur with ever-increasing ease and frequency, so that the patient may become seriously handicapped. Oft-repeated dislocations predispose to the later development of osteoarthritis.

Treatment. Treatment should be expectant at first. After a dislocation the patient should receive a course of physiotherapy designed to strengthen the quadriceps muscle, and especially the vastus medialis.

If the dislocations recur with such frequency that the patient is seriously disabled, operation should be advised. The method recommended is to detach the bony insertion of the patellar tendon and transpose it to a new bed in the tibia, medial and distal to the original insertion. In this way the patella is drawn lower into the intercondylar groove of the femur, and the line of pull of the quadriceps mechanism is transferred more to the medial side.

An alternative but usually less satisfactory operation is to excise the patella. It has been claimed that this gives better long-term results because the liability to osteoarthritis is reduced, but the claim is not yet proved.

HABITUAL DISLOCATION

It is important to distinguish between recurrent dislocation of the patella and habitual dislocation. Whereas in recurrent dislocation the knee may seem normal for weeks or months between dislocations, in habitual dislocation the patella dislocates laterally each time the knee is flexed beyond a certain range. This condition becomes apparent at an earlier age than recurrent dislocation—usually in early childhood. The underlying pathology is also distinct : there is shortening of the quadriceps muscle and in particular of the vastus lateralis, which may show a fibrous contracture. It is this shortened vastus lateralis that pulls the patella laterally every time the knee is markedly flexed. In the absence of treatment the patella may eventually become permanently dislocated. *Treatment* is directed entirely to releasing the tight vastus lateralis muscle by dividing as much of it as is necessary to permit full flexion of the knee without displacement of the patella.

EXTRA-ARTICULAR DISORDERS IN THE REGION OF THE KNEE

GENU VARUM AND GENU VALGUM

Genu varum (bow leg) and genu valgum (knock knee) occur commonly in childhood. In the vast majority of instances there is no underlying disease, and the deformity need not cause anxiety because it is gradually corrected spontaneously.

13*

Genu varum or valgum may also occur, either in children or in adults, in consequence of injury or disease. The commonest causes are : 1) fracture of the lower part of the femur or the upper part of the tibia with mal-union (for example, depressed fracture of the lateral tibial condyle causing genu valgum) ; 2) rarefying diseases of the bones, such as rickets or osteomalacia ;

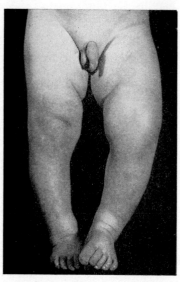

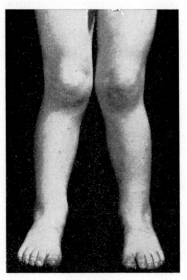

FIG. 282

Genu varum. Slight bowing is common in infants but it is usually corrected spontaneously as the child grows.

FIG. 283

Genu valgum. Deformity of this degree in young children is usually corrected spontaneously during growth.

3) other bone-softening diseases such as osteitis deformans (Paget's disease) (Fig. 80, p. 111) ; 4) in children, uneven growth of the epiphysial plates, such as may occur after injury or osteomyelitis or in dyschondroplasia (p. 106).

In assessing a case of genu varum or genu valgum the surgeon must always be careful to exclude such underlying organic disorders by full clinical examination, and if necessary by radiography, before diagnosing the benign childhood affections described below.

BENIGN GENU VARUM OF TODDLERS

The knee and leg are bowed outwards (Fig. 282). A mild degree of this deformity is so common as to be almost normal in children of 1 to 3 years. It does not require treatment unless it persists into later childhood. Care should be taken to exclude the possibility of rickets or other underlying disease.

BENIGN GENU VALGUM OF CHILDHOOD

The knee is angled inwards, the tibia being abducted in relation to the femur. With the knees straight, the medial malleoli cannot be brought into contact (Fig. 283). The deformity is common in children of 3 to 5 years. In the absence of underlying bone disease it usually corrects itself spontaneously in the course of years.

Treatment. In early childhood treatment is unnecessary, but it is common practice to fit a wedge, base medially and 3 to 5 millimetres deep, to the heel of the shoe to shift the line of weight-bearing medially (Fig. 304, p. 419).

Severe genu valgum persisting after the age of 10 requires active treatment. In growing children two methods of correction are available. One is to retard the growth at the medial side of the epiphysial cartilage of femur or tibia by bridging the epiphysis to the diaphysis with metal staples (epiphysiodesis). The other and more certain method is by supracondylar osteotomy of the femur, with excision of a suitable wedge from the medial side. After the cessation of epiphysial growth genu valgum can be corrected only by osteotomy.

RUPTURE OF THE QUADRICEPS APPARATUS

The quadriceps muscle gains insertion into the tibia through the medium of the patella (enclosed within the quadriceps expansion) and the patellar tendon. Complete rupture may occur at three points (Fig. 284) : 1) at the point of attachment of the quadriceps tendon to the upper pole of the patella ; 2) through the patella and the surrounding quadriceps expansion (fractured patella) ; or 3) at the attachment of the patellar tendon to the tibial tubercle. In all cases the injury is caused by an unexpected flexion force, resisted automatically by a sudden contraction of the quadriceps.

AVULSION FROM PATELLA

Avulsion of the quadriceps tendon from the upper pole of the patella occurs mainly in elderly men, in whom the quadriceps tendon is often degenerate. The tendon should be re-attached to the bone by sutures of stainless steel wire.

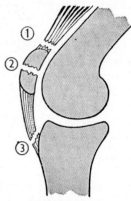

FIG 284

The three points at which the quadriceps apparatus may rupture. 1. At insertion of quadriceps into patella. 2. Through the patella. 3. At insertion of patellar tendon into tibial tubercle.

DISRUPTION THROUGH PATELLA

This is the usual site of rupture, and it forms a common variety of fractured patella. The injury occurs mainly in adults of middle age. If the patella is cleanly broken into two pieces and the patient is under 40 the fragments should be fixed together by a screw. Otherwise the patellar fragments should be excised and the quadriceps expansion sutured.

AVULSION AT TIBIAL TUBERCLE

This is the least common injury, occurring mainly in children or young adults. A fragment of bone may be pulled off with the tendon. The torn tendon should be re-attached by sutures.

APOPHYSITIS OF THE TIBIAL TUBERCLE
(Osgood-Schlatter's disease)

Apophysitis of the tibial tubercle is a childhood affection in which the tibial tubercle becomes enlarged and temporarily painful. The precise nature of the condition is unknown. Often known as Osgood-Schlatter's disease, it has been widely accepted as an example of osteochondritis juvenilis (p. 97), but most surgeons are now agreed that it is nothing more than a strain of the developing tibial tubercle, from the pull of the patellar tendon. **Clinical features.** The patient is a child of 10 to 14 years, usually a boy. The complaint is of pain in front of and below the knee, worse on strenuous activity. *On examination* the tibial tubercle is unduly prominent, and tender on palpation. Pain is increased when the quadriceps is tensed, as in straight leg raising

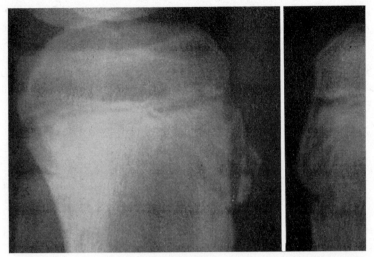

FIG. 285

Apophysitis of the tibial tubercle (Osgood-Schlatter's disease). The tibial tubercle appears enlarged and fragmented. The normal tubercle of the other tibia is shown for comparison.

against resistance. The symptoms and signs are confined to the region of the tibial tubercle, and the knee joint itself is normal. *Radiographs* show enlargement and sometimes fragmentation of the tibial tubercle (Fig. 285).

Course. The disorder is self-limiting, and normal function is always restored.

Treatment. In many cases treatment is not required. If local pain and tenderness are severe the knee should be rested for two months in a plaster cylinder extending from groin to malleoli.

PREPATELLAR BURSITIS

The bursa that lies in front of the lower half of the patella and the upper part of the patellar tendon is prone to inflammation.

Types. There are two types of prepatellar bursitis : 1) irritative ; and 2) infective or suppurative.

IRRITATIVE PREPATELLAR BURSITIS

This is caused by repeated friction ; it occurs especially in those who do much kneeling. There is fibrous thickening of the wall of the bursa, which is distended with fluid.

Clinical features. There is a softly fluctuant swelling in front of the lower part of the patella ('house-maid's knee'). The swelling is clearly demarcated. It is manifestly confined to a plane in front of the joint, and the joint itself is unaffected.

Treatment. A trial may be made of aspiration under local anaesthesia, but the effusion tends to recur unless further friction can be avoided. The risk of recurrence may possibly be reduced if hydrocortisone is injected into the emptied sac. Operative excision of the bursa affords a more certain permanent cure.

Suppurative Prepatellar Bursitis

This is caused by infection of the bursa with pyogenic organisms, which reach the bursa directly through a puncture wound, or through the lymphatics from an infected lesion on the leg. The wall of the bursa is acutely inflamed and the sac is distended with pus.

Clinical features. There are pain and swelling in front of the knee, often with pyrexia. The swelling is confined to the site of the prepatellar bursa. It is acutely tender on palpation, and the overlying skin is hot and reddened. The inguinal lymphatic glands are often enlarged and tender. The knee joint itself is unaffected, but the patient is unwilling to bend it fully because flexion increases the pain by tensing the skin over the bursa.

Treatment. Appropriate chemotherapy should be instituted and the bursal abscess should be drained by incision.

POPLITEAL CYSTS

Cystic swellings are not infrequently found in the popliteal fossa. Most are examples of irritative bursitis, usually of the semimembranosus bursa. A few are caused by herniation of the synovial cavity of the knee (Baker's cyst). Care must be taken to distinguish popliteal cysts from other swellings in this region, such as aneurysm and synovial sarcoma.

Semimembranosus Bursitis

The semimembranosus bursa lies between the medial head of the gastrocnemius and the semimembranosus. The bursa may become distended with fluid to form an elongated sac that bulges backwards between the muscle planes. *Clinically*, there is a soft cystic swelling at the back of the knee, close to the medial condyle of the femur.

Treatment is not always required. If the swelling becomes uncomfortably large the sac should be excised.

Baker's Cyst

A Baker's cyst is simply a herniation of the synovial cavity of the knee, with the formation of a fluid-filled sac extending backwards and downwards (Fig. 286). It is not a primary condition but is always secondary to a disorder of the knee with persistent synovial effusion, such as osteoarthritis. In long-standing cases the hernial sac is much elongated, and may extend a considerable distance down the calf. *Clinically* there is a soft cystic bulge near the midline behind the knee or in the upper calf. The underlying abnormality of the knee, with synovial effusion, will usually be obvious.

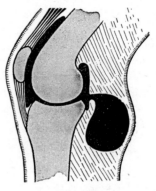

Fig. 286

To show how a Baker's cyst is formed as a herniation of the synovial membrane.

Treatment. In most cases treatment should be directed towards the underlying condition of the knee rather than to the cyst itself. Nevertheless if the cyst is extensive it is sometimes advisable to excise it.

PELLEGRINI-STIEDA'S DISEASE

Pellegrini-Stieda's disease is the name sometimes used to describe ossification in the subligamentous haematoma after partial avulsion of the medial ligament from the medial condyle of the femur. *Clinically* there is persistent discomfort at the medial side of the knee after an injury to the medial ligament. There are thickening and slight tenderness over the site of attachment of the ligament to the medial femoral condyle. *Radiographs* show a thin plaque of new bone close to the medial condyle.

Treatment is by active mobilising and muscle-strengthening exercises.

Calcified Deposit in Medial Ligament

It is probable that many supposed cases of Pellegrini-Stieda's disease are in fact examples of calcified deposit within the medial ligament. A similar deposit may occur in the lateral ligament. These lesions are homologous with the calcified deposit that occurs more commonly in the supraspinatus tendon (p. 236). If the symptoms are acute the calcified material should be removed by aspiration or by operation.

EXTRINSIC DISORDERS WITH REFERRED SYMPTOMS IN THE KNEE

From time to time patients are seen whose main complaint is of pain in the knee, but local examination reveals no satisfactory explanation for it. In such cases the possibility that the pain is referred from a disorder distant from the knee should always be considered. The commonest source of such referred pain is a disorder of the hip. Much less often a disorder of the spine is responsible.

DISORDERS OF THE HIP

The conditions of the hip in which the pain may be felt predominantly in the knee are the various types of arthritis, of which osteoarthritis is the most common. Pain in the knee may also be the main complaint in cases of slipped upper femoral epiphysis—a fact that should be well remembered. The pain is referred along the course of one of the nerves—especially the obturator nerve, which takes a large share in the innervation of the hip.

Differential diagnosis. There should be little difficulty in determining the true source of the pain if the possibility of a hip lesion is borne in mind. Whenever knee symptoms cannot be adequately explained after a local examination of the knee the hip should be investigated and, if necessary, radiographed.

DISORDERS OF THE SPINE

The only disorders of the spine that may cause symptoms predominantly in the region of the knee are those that cause pressure on the roots of the lumbar or sacral plexus, especially prolapsed intervertebral disc. It is only rarely that such referred symptoms are unassociated with other symptoms in the back, buttock, or thigh.

References and bibliography, page 445.

CHAPTER TEN

The Leg, Ankle, and Foot

IN the orthopaedic out-patient clinic disorders of the foot
are second in frequency only to disorders of the back. Their
prevalence may have several causes. *Hereditary factors* : The
foot is probably in a state of relatively rapid evolution consequent
upon man's assumption of the upright posture, and perhaps for
that reason it is prone to variations in structure and form which
may impair its efficiency. *Postural stresses* : Overweight throws
an increased burden on the feet, and they may be unable to with-
stand the stress without ill-effect, especially if the intrinsic muscles
are poorly developed. *Footwear* : The wearing of shoes is a potent
cause of foot disorders. Many types of shoe interfere seriously
with the mechanics of the foot, and the ladies' shoe with high heel
and pointed toe is particularly to blame.

SPECIAL POINTS IN THE INVESTIGATION OF LEG, ANKLE, AND FOOT COMPLAINTS

In nearly all cases symptoms in the leg, ankle, or foot can be
explained by a local abnormality. Only rarely are they referred from
a distant lesion. In this respect the lower limb differs markedly from
the upper, for in many cases symptoms in the hand have no local
cause but are referred from a proximal lesion.

History
The precise distribution of pain should be ascertained. The occupation
and habits of the patient, or a history of previous injury, may be
significant. Specific inquiry should be made into the effect upon the
symptoms of standing and walking.

Exposure
It is essential that socks or stockings be removed and that the whole
leg be exposed up to the knee. Both limbs must always be examined
so that the two may be compared. The first part of the examination
is conducted with the patient sitting, the heel being supported on a

stool ; or, better still, the patient may recline on a couch.   Later, the
foot is examined while the patient stands.

Steps in Clinical Examination

A suggested plan for the routine clinical examination of the leg,
ankle, and foot is summarised in Table XII.

Assessing the State of the Peripheral Circulation

An essential part of the examination of the foot that is often
forgotten is to study the efficiency of the arterial circulation.   A
reasonably accurate assessment may be made on clinical evidence alone,
but if surgical treatment is contemplated for vascular insufficiency it is
necessary to have more precise information which can be provided only
by certain special investigations.

Clinical assessment.   This is based on a study of the texture of the
skin and nails, colour changes, skin temperature, the arterial pulses,
auscultation, and exercise tolerance.   *Texture of skin and nails :* The
skin of an ischaemic foot loses its hair and becomes thin and inelastic.
The nails are coarse, thickened and irregular.   *Colour changes :* A
brick-red rubor or cyanosis when the foot is dependent, with rapid
blanching on elevation, denotes serious impairment of the arterial
circulation.   *Temperature :* A foot with impaired arterial supply is colder
than normal, but little reliance can be placed on this test as applied
clinically at the bedside.   *Arterial pulses :* The pulses to be felt for are
the dorsalis pedis, the posterior tibial, the popliteal and the femoral.
Pulsation of the dorsalis pedis artery is best felt at the dorsum of the
foot between the bases of the first and second metatarsals.   The posterior
tibial artery is felt about two centimetres behind and below the tip
of the medial malleolus.   Absence or impairment of arterial pulsation is
an important sign of defective circulation.   It should be remembered,
however, that a normal pulse is easily masked by thickening or oedema
of the soft tissues.   *Auscultation :* A bruit over one of the major limb
vessels may denote partial obstruction or an arterio-venous communication.   *Exercise tolerance :* The patient is instructed to walk at a controlled
speed (timed by a metronome) on level ground to test whether symptoms
of claudication arise and, if so, at what distance.

Special investigations.   These include arteriography to determine
the state of the major arteries, and skin temperature recordings and
plethysmography to show the state of the peripheral and collateral
circulation.   *Arteriography :* The arterial tree is outlined by radiography
after injection of opaque fluid into the main vessel.   Any narrowing
or occlusion of a vessel is clearly revealed.   *Skin temperature recordings :*
Accurate measurement, by thermocouples, of the skin temperature of
the foot at the basic room temperature (usually maintained at 20 degrees
Centigrade to promote vasoconstriction) and after inhibition or
temporary paralysis of the vasoconstrictor fibres (by heating the other

limbs in water at 44 degrees Centigrade or by procaine nerve block or spinal anaesthesia) gives a valuable indication of the peripheral blood flow. With healthy vessels the rise of temperature on vasodilation

TABLE XII

ROUTINE CLINICAL EXAMINATION IN SUSPECTED DISORDERS
OF THE LEG, ANKLE, AND FOOT

---

1. LOCAL EXAMINATION OF THE LEG, ANKLE, AND FOOT

Inspection

Bone contours and alignment
Soft-tissue contours
Colour and texture of skin
Scars or sinuses

Palpation

Skin temperature
Bone contours
Soft-tissue contours
Local tenderness

State of peripheral circulation

Dorsalis pedis pulse
Posterior tibial pulse
Popliteal pulse
Femoral pulse
? Cyanosis of foot when dependent

Movements (active and passive, compared with normal side)

At the ankle :
Plantarflexion
Extension (dorsiflexion)
At the subtalar joint :
Inversion-adduction
Eversion-abduction
At the midtarsal joint :
Inversion-adduction
Eversion-abduction

At the toes :
Flexion
Extension

Power (tested against resistance of examiner)

Each muscle group to be tested in turn. (*N.B.*—Power of calf muscles is best tested with the patient standing)

Stability

Integrity of ligaments—particularly the lateral ligament of the ankle

Appearance of foot on standing

Shape of longitudinal arch
Shape of forefoot
Efficiency of toes
Efficiency of calf muscles (? ability to raise heel from ground while standing on affected leg)

Gait

Condition of footwear

Sites of greatest wear

---

2. GENERAL EXAMINATION

General survey of other parts of the body. The local symptoms may be only one manifestation of a widespread disease.

---

should be to a maximum of 34 degrees Centigrade, whereas in severe arterial disease there may be little or no rise of temperature. The speed of the vascular response is also significant. *Plethysmography :* The plethysmograph records changes in the volume of a limb or digit enclosed within a special rigid cylinder. Plethysmography gives an accurate indication of the pulse pressure and peripheral blood flow. Like temperature recordings, it may be used to measure the increase in peripheral blood flow that is brought about by vasodilation, and thus to predict the likely effect of sympathectomy.

Movements at the Ankle and Tarsal Joints

Since the joints are close together, movement at the tarsal joints is easily mistaken for movement at the ankle, and vice versa. Careful examination is required to determine the range at each individual joint.

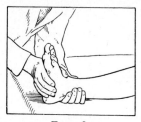

FIG. 287

Examining ankle movement.

Ankle movement. The ankle is strictly a hinge joint. The only movements are extension (dorsiflexion) and plantarflexion. The range should be judged from the excursion of the hindfoot rather than the forefoot, so that any contribution from the tarsal joints is disregarded. Similarly, in testing the passive range, the foot should be controlled from the heel (Fig. 287). The normal range of ankle movement varies in different subjects; so the normal ankle must be used as a control. An average range is about 25 degrees of extension and 35 degrees of plantarflexion.

Subtalar and midtarsal movement. In normal use the subtalar and midtarsal joints work together as a single unit. The movements permitted are: 1) combined inversion and adduction (supination), and 2) combined eversion and abduction (pronation).

In clinical examination the range of movement contributed by each component can be determined separately. To test *subtalar movement* support the lower leg by a hand gripping the ankle. With the other hand lightly grasp the calcaneus from below (Fig. 288). Instruct the

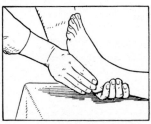

FIG. 288

Examining subtalar movement.

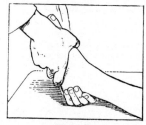

FIG. 289

Examining midtarsal movement.

patient alternately to invert and evert the foot, observing the range through which the heel rocks from side to side. Compare with the sound foot. The normal range is about 20 degrees on each side of the vertical.

To test *midtarsal movement* grasp the calcaneus firmly so that subtalar movement is eliminated. With the other hand lightly grasp the midfoot near the bases of the metatarsals (Fig. 289). Instruct the patient alternately to twist the foot inwards and outwards into inversion and eversion, and compare the range with that on the sound side. The normal is a rotation of about 20 degrees on each side of the neutral.

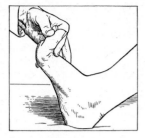

FIG. 290

The normal range of dorsiflexion at the metatarsophalangeal joint of the great toe is nearly 90 degrees.

Toe movements. Determine the active and passive range at the metatarso-phalangeal and interphalangeal joints. It should be remembered that the normal range of dorsiflexion of the great toe at the metatarsophalangeal joint is nearly 90 degrees (Fig. 290). Limitation to less than 60 degrees of dorsiflexion is certainly abnormal.

Examination of the Feet under Weight-bearing Stress

Instruct the patient to stand evenly on both feet. Observe the general shape of the ankle, foot, and toes. Study the shape of the longitudinal arch. Is it of normal shape? Is it flattened so that the navicular region is in contact with the ground (pes planus or valgus)? Or is it higher than normal (pes cavus)? Next study the forefoot. Is it splayed and broader than normal? Assess the function of the toes. Normally they can be pressed upon the ground by the action of the intrinsic muscles so that the metatarsal heads are lifted up and relieved of weight-bearing pressure. Finally, examine the efficiency of the calf muscles. The crucial test is to ask the patient to stand on the affected leg and to raise the heel from the ground.

Gait

Look especially for abnormal posture of the feet such as turning in (intoeing) or turning out, or drop foot. Observe whether weight is borne correctly on the sole of the foot or whether it is taken too much on the medial or lateral border. Observe also whether the heel is raised normally from the ground at the beginning of each step.

Footwear

The examination of the foot is not complete until the patient's shoes have been inspected and compared on the two sides. Note the position of greatest wear. When the foot is normal the greatest wear in the sole occurs beneath the ball of the foot and slightly to the medial side. In the heel it is at the posterior border slightly to the lateral side. The state of the uppers is also important: excessive bulging on the medial side suggests a valgus foot and excessive bulging on the lateral side an inverted foot.

Radiographic Examination

The ankle. Routine radiographs of the ankle comprise an antero-posterior and a lateral projection centred at the level of the joint. The films should include a reasonable length of the shafts of the tibia and fibula, and the whole of the talus.

When laxity of the lateral ligament is suspected a special inversion film is required. This is an antero-posterior projection taken while the heel is held in fullest inversion by an assistant. If the lateral ligament is torn or lax the talus will be shown tilted in the ankle mortise (p. 407).

The foot. Routine radiographs of the foot comprise an antero-posterior (strictly a supero-inferior) projection and a lateral projection. Special techniques are used to show the calcaneus (axial view) and the subtalar joint (oblique projection).

CLASSIFICATION OF DISORDERS OF THE LEG, ANKLE, AND FOOT

DISORDERS OF THE LEG

INJURIES
> Rupture of the tendo calcaneus

INFECTIONS
> Acute osteomyelitis
> Chronic osteomyelitis
> Syphilitic infection

TUMOURS
> Benign tumours of bone
> Malignant tumours of bone

CIRCULATORY DISORDERS
> Intermittent claudication

DISORDERS OF THE ANKLE

ARTHRITIS
> Pyogenic arthritis
> Rheumatoid arthritis
> Tuberculous arthritis
> Osteoarthritis
> Gouty arthritis
> Haemophilic arthritis
> Neuropathic arthritis

POST-**TRAUMATIC** MECHANICAL DERANGEMENTS
> Recurrent subluxation

DISORDERS OF THE FOOT

DEFORMITIES

Congenital club foot (talipes equino-varus)
Talipes calcaneo-valgus
Accessory bones in the foot
Pes cavus
Pes planus (flat foot)

POSTURAL DISORDERS

Foot strain

ARTHRITIS

Osteoarthritis of the tarsal joints
Other forms of tarsal arthritis

OSTEOCHONDRITIS

Osteochondritis of the navicular bone

MISCELLANEOUS

Painful heel
Pain in the forefoot
Plantar wart
Callosities
Ganglion

DISORDERS OF THE TOES

DEFORMITIES

Hallux valgus
Hammer toe
Under-riding toe

ARTHRITIS

Osteoarthritis
Gouty arthritis

OSTEOCHONDRITIS

Osteochondritis of a metatarsal head

MISCELLANEOUS

Ingrowing toe nail
Subungual exostosis
Onychogryposis

DISORDERS OF THE LEG

RUPTURE OF THE TENDO CALCANEUS

Surprising as it may seem, a ruptured tendo calcaneus [tendo Achillis] is often overlooked, the symptoms being wrongly ascribed to a strain or to a ruptured plantaris muscle.

Pathology. The rupture is always complete. It occurs about five centimetres above the insertion of the tendon. If it is left untreated the tendon unites spontaneously, but with lengthening.

Clinical features. While running or jumping the patient feels a sudden agonising pain at the back of the ankle. He may believe that something has struck him. He is able to walk, but with a limp. *On examination* there is tenderness at the site of rupture. There is general thickening from effusion of blood and from oedema of the paratenon, but a gap can usually be felt in the course of the tendon. The power of plantarflexion at the ankle is greatly weakened, though some power remains through the action of the tibialis posterior, the peronei, and the toe flexors.

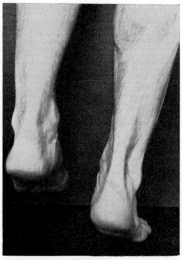

Fig. 291

The crucial test of intact calf function is to raise the heel from the ground while standing only on the affected leg. Inability to do this after an injury to the calcaneal tendon is diagnostic of complete rupture.

Diagnosis. The retention of some power of plantarflexion may deflect the unwary from the correct diagnosis. The crucial test is to ask the patient to lift the heel from the ground while standing only upon the affected leg (Fig. 291). This is impossible if the tendon is ruptured.

Treatment. In the case of a recent rupture operative repair is to be recommended. The tendon should be sutured with stainless steel wire, tension on the suture line being relaxed by immobilising the limb with right-angled knee flexion and moderate ankle plantarflexion for two weeks. For the next four weeks a below-knee plaster with the ankle at 90 degrees is worn. The plaster is then discarded, and increasingly vigorous exercises for the calf muscles are practised until full strength is restored.

If the rupture has been overlooked or neglected for more than two months it is doubtful whether operation is worth while : probably as good a result will be gained from conservative treatment by intensive exercise as from delayed operation. In such a case the shoe-heels may be raised by one or two centimetres to relieve the strain on the healing tendon.

ACUTE OSTEOMYELITIS
(General description of acute osteomyelitis, p. 69.)

The tibia is one of the commonest sites of haematogenous osteomyelitis. Because of its liability to open (compound) fracture it is also the commonest site of osteomyelitis from direct contamination. The fibula is less often affected.

The pathological and clinical features and treatment conform to the general description on p. 69.

CHRONIC OSTEOMYELITIS
(General description of chronic osteomyelitis, p. 74).

Chronic osteomyelitis in the lower leg, as elsewhere, is nearly always a sequel of acute osteomyelitis. It may follow either the haematogenous type of infection or an infected open fracture.

BRODIE'S ABSCESS

This rather uncommon lesion was described on page 75. It is a special form of chronic osteomyelitis which arises insidiously, without a recognised acute infection preceding it. The tibia is the commonest site.

SYPHILITIC INFECTION OF THE TIBIA
(General description of syphilitic osteitis, p. 79.)

Although skeletal syphilis is now rare in Western countries, when it does occur the tibia is often the bone affected. The infection may take the form of a localised gumma or diffuse osteoperiostitis (Fig. 51). There is a gradually enlarging swelling, with moderate pain. It is important to bear the possibility of syphilis in mind, because the swelling is easily mistaken for a tumour.

TUMOURS OF BONE
BENIGN TUMOURS

(General description of benign bone tumours, p. 81.)

Of the four main types of benign tumours of bone—osteoma, chondroma, osteochondroma, and giant-cell tumour—only the chondroma and giant-cell tumour require further mention here.

CHONDROMA

In the tibia or fibula this is seldom found except in multiple form in the condition of dyschondroplasia (p. 106). The individual tumours in this condition resemble enchondromata. They arise from the growing epiphysial cartilage plate, and they interfere with the normal growth of the bone. An important effect is that the growth of the tibia and fibula may be unequal, with the consequence that the bones may become curved or the plane of the ankle joint may be tilted away from the horizontal (Fig. 19, p. 41 ; Fig. 75, p. 106).

GIANT-CELL TUMOUR (Osteoclastoma)

The upper end of the tibia or fibula, like the lower end of the femur, is a favourite site for this tumour. It usually arises in a young adult, expanding the bone and extending to within a short distance of the articular surface.

Treatment. If the tumour is in the fibula the whole of the affected end of the bone should be excised together with an adequate margin of healthy bone. If the tumour is in the upper end of the tibia, the problem of treatment is much more difficult. The discussion relating to this tumour when it affects the lower end of the femur (p. 363) applies here also. As in the femur, to ensure full eradication of the tumour it is probably wise to excise the upper end of the tibia entire, to sacrifice the knee joint, to bridge the gap with bone grafts, and to provide stability by means of a long intramedullary nail.

MALIGNANT TUMOURS

(General description of malignant bone tumours, p. 86.)

The tibia, like the femur, is a common site for primary malignant bone tumours, especially osteosarcoma and Ewing's tumour.

OSTEOSARCOMA (Osteogenic sarcoma)

This tumour usually affects the upper metaphysis of the tibia : the lower end of the tibia and the fibula are affected much less often. The tumour metastasises rapidly through the blood stream, especially to the lungs.

Treatment. Amputation is the usual method if pulmonary metastases are not already demonstrable. The place of radiotherapy was discussed on p. 90.

EWING'S TUMOUR

This usually affects the shaft of a long bone, again in childhood or early adult life. The tibia is one of the commonest sites.

Treatment. Although it is ultimately fatal from metastases, Ewing's tumour is radio-sensitive, and treatment by radiotherapy is probably as effective as amputation.

INTERMITTENT CLAUDICATION

Intermittent claudication is a symptom of arterial insufficiency in the lower limb. In its typical form it is characterised by cramp-like pain in the calf, induced by walking.

Cause. The usual underlying cause is arteriosclerosis with local thrombosis of the main limb vessel. Thrombo-angiitis obliterans and arterial embolism are less common causes.

Pathology. The basic disturbance is ischaemia of muscle, in consequence of which metabolites cannot be removed speedily enough when the muscle is exercised. The accumulation of metabolites is believed to be responsible for the pain, which subsides when the muscle is rested. The muscles usually affected are those of the calf, but in some instances other muscle groups are involved. The vascular lesion is usually a complete occlusion of the femoral or the popliteal artery. In claudication affecting the buttock the aortic bifurcation or the iliac artery may be occluded.

Clinical features. Intermittent claudication is much more common in men than in women. In the usual arteriosclerotic type the patient is past middle life, but in cases due to thrombo-angiitis obliterans or embolism the symptoms may develop in early adult life.

With gradual arterial occlusion the onset is insidious and the symptoms are slowly progressive ; but in cases precipitated by thrombosis or embolism the onset may be sudden. In a typical case the patient complains that after walking a certain distance—perhaps a hundred yards or so—he is forced to stop by severe cramp-like pain in the calf, or occasionally in another muscle group, such as the buttock. After a few minutes' rest the pain disappears and he is able to walk on again for a similar distance.

On examination there is objective evidence of impaired arterial circulation in the lower limb (p. 394). The posterior tibial, dorsalis pedis, and popliteal pulses are absent. There may be ischaemic changes in the skin of the foot. Evidence of widespread arterial or cardiac disease is nearly always found on general examination. *Radiographic examination :* Plain radiographs often show patches of calcification in the walls of several arteries. Arteriographs demonstrate the site and extent of the arterial occlusion.

Diagnosis. Intermittent claudication is frequently misdiagnosed. Unless a detailed history is obtained, the patient's complaint of pain in the calf may suggest to the unwary doctor the likelihood of foot strain or flat foot. Moreover, such a diagnosis may seem to be supported by the finding of flattened arches or deformed feet, common in the elderly. The clues to the correct diagnosis are the typical history and the impairment of the arterial pulses.

Prognosis. The outlook is serious. In progressive cases increasing ischaemia may lead eventually to gangrene of the foot, if the patient does not die first from cardiac disease.

Treatment. Except in rare instances, treatment is rather unsatisfactory. If the nutrition of the limb as a whole is not in danger it is doubtful whether any treatment is worth while. The exceptional cases are those in which there is a localised occlusion, the general state of the arteries being reasonably good. In these circumstances the channel may often be restored by thrombo-endarterectomy or by replacement or by-passing of the occluded section by a prosthetic (Dacron) tube or vein graft. In cases of severe pain tenotomy of the tendo calcaneus has been tried. It affords relief by reducing the activity of the calf muscles.

If the nutrition of the foot is threatened lumbar ganglion-ectomy is often worth a trial as a means of improving the circulation in the skin, but it cannot be expected to have a significant effect on the symptoms of claudication.

DISORDERS OF THE ANKLE

PYOGENIC ARTHRITIS OF THE ANKLE

(General description of pyogenic arthritis, p. 43.)

Pyogenic arthritis of the ankle is uncommon. The organisms reach the joint through the blood stream or through a penetrating wound ; local spread from a focus of osteomyelitis of the tibia or fibula is rare because the bony metaphyses are entirely extra-capsular (Fig. 37, p. 71).

RHEUMATOID ARTHRITIS OF THE ANKLE

(General description of rheumatoid arthritis, p. 46.)

One or both ankles are often affected by rheumatoid arthritis in common with other joints.

Treatment. General treatment is along the lines suggested for the disease as a whole (p. 49). *Local treatment :* In the active phase rest in bed or in a plaster is sometimes required. But in most cases the patient should be encouraged to remain active so far as possible, with such help as may be gained from short-wave diathermy, active exercises, and hot paraffin-wax baths. Operation is advised mainly when destruction of articular cartilage has led to intractable pain with marked impairment of capacity for walking. Arthrodesis is then the operation of choice. If the subtalar and midtarsal joints are also severely affected they should be included in the fusion.

TUBERCULOUS ARTHRITIS OF THE ANKLE

(General description of tuberculous arthritis, p. 51.)

Tuberculosis is much less common in the ankle than it is in the hip and knee. In Britain it is now seen very seldom.

The clinical features correspond to those of tuberculous arthritis of other superficial joints, with pain, swelling, increased warmth of the overlying skin, restriction of movement, and limp.

Treatment. Early conservative treatment (p. 54) may restore a mobile ankle, but if in a resistant case articular cartilage is badly eroded or destroyed arthrodesis may have to be undertaken.

OSTEOARTHRITIS OF THE ANKLE
(General description of osteoarthritis, p. 55.)

Degenerative destruction of the articular cartilage is less common in the ankle than in the knee. There is nearly always a known predisposing factor which causes the joint to wear out prematurely. The commonest is irregularity or mal-alignment of the joint surfaces after a fracture. Sometimes articular disease such as ' burnt out ' rheumatoid arthritis is the primary factor.

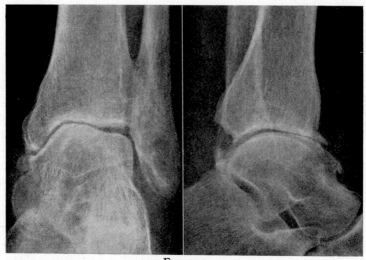

FIG. 292

Osteoarthritis of the ankle complicating injury ten years before. Note the marked narrowing of the cartilage space and the prominent osteophytes.

Clinical features. The symptoms are pain which slowly increases over months and years, and limp. *On examination* the joint is a little thickened from the marginal bony hypertrophy. Movements are limited slightly or severely according to the degree of arthritis. *Radiographs* show the usual features of osteoarthritis—narrowing of the cartilage space, a tendency to sclerosis of the bone adjacent to the joint, and hypertrophy (osteophyte formation) at the joint margins (Fig. 292).

Treatment. In mild cases treatment is often unnecessary, because the patient may be willing to accept the disability when the nature of the trouble has been explained. When treatment is called for, conservative measures should be tried first if the disability is only moderate. Physiotherapy by short-wave diathermy, hot baths, and active exercises is usually advised. Such treatment, however, is only palliative, and if the disability increases to the extent of becoming a serious handicap operation should be undertaken. The only satisfactory operation is arthrodesis.

GOUTY ARTHRITIS OF THE ANKLE

Although gout is commonest in the joints of the great toe it should be remembered that it can occur in the ankle and in other peripheral joints. The general features of gouty arthritis were described in Chapter II (p. 58).

HAEMOPHILIC ARTHRITIS OF THE ANKLE
(General description of haemophilic arthritis, p. 60.)

Haemophilic arthritis is much less common in the ankle than in the knee or elbow, but it should be remembered as an occasional cause of a warm, swollen ankle in boys. Treatment is by rest in plaster for several weeks until the irritative reaction settles down.

NEUROPATHIC ARTHRITIS OF THE ANKLE
(General description of neuropathic arthritis, p. 62.)

Neuropathic arthritis is uncommon but nevertheless well recognised in the ankle. The underlying neurological disease is tabes dorsalis, diabetic neuropathy, syringomyelia, cauda equina lesion or, in some countries, leprosy.

Treatment. In many cases protection by a firm surgical boot, reinforced if necessary by a below-knee brace, is all that is required. Occasionally arthrodesis of the ankle may have to be considered. Appropriate treatment must be given for the underlying neurological disorder.

RECURRENT SUBLUXATION OF THE ANKLE

When the lateral ligament of the ankle is torn and fails to heal there may be persistent instability with recurrent attacks of giving way in which the talus tilts medially in the ankle mortise. The causative injury is always a severe inversion force.

Clinical features. The patient complains that the ankle goes over at frequent intervals, often causing him to fall. Each incident is accompanied by pain at the lateral side of the ankle. There is always a history of previous severe injury, followed by much swelling and extensive bruising at the lateral side of the joint. *On examination* there is often some oedema about the ankle. There is tenderness over the site of the lateral ligament. The normal ankle movements—dorsiflexion and plantarflexion— are unchanged, but abnormal mobility is present as shown by the fact that the heel can be inverted passively beyond the normal range permitted by the subtalar joint. Moreover, when the heel is fully inverted a dimple or depression of the skin may be visible in front of the lateral malleolus, where the soft tissues have been ' sucked ' into the gap created between tibia and talus. *Radiographic examination :* Routine radiographs do not show any abnormality. Antero-posterior films must be taken while the heel is held fully inverted. If the lateral ligament is torn or lax the talus will be shown tilted away from the tibio-fibular mortise at the lateral side through 20 or 30 degrees or more (Fig. 293).

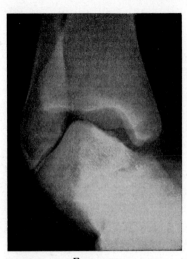

FIG. 293

Tilting of the talus in the ankle mortise under adduction stress, an indication of torn lateral ligament.

Diagnosis. Chronic strain of the lateral ligament may cause similar symptoms, but in that condition radiographs will not show the talus tilted on forced inversion.

Treatment. If the disability is slight it may be sufficient to strengthen the evertor muscles (mainly the peronei) by exercises, to enable them to control the ankle more efficiently. But if the disability is severe operation is required. A new lateral ligament is constructed from the peroneus brevis tendon.

DISORDERS OF THE FOOT

CONGENITAL CLUB FOOT
(Talipes equino-varus)

The rather vague term ' club foot ' has come to be synonymous in the minds of most surgeons with the most important congenital deformity of the foot—talipes equino-varus. The less serious form of club foot, talipes calcaneo-valgus, will be considered later under that title.

Cause. In most cases a defect of foetal development is responsible. Minor degrees of the deformity may possibly be explained by prolonged mal-position of the foetal foot in the uterus, but this cannot be accepted as the usual cause.

Pathology. The soft tissues at the medial side of the foot are under-developed and shorter than normal. The foot is adducted and inverted at the subtalar, midtarsal, and anterior tarsal joints, and is held in equinus (plantarflexion) at the ankle. In many cases the calf and peroneal muscles are under-developed. In the absence of early effective treatment the developing tarsal bones become misshapen, perpetuating the deformity.

Clinical features. The deformity is much commoner in boys than in girls. (Contrast congenital dislocation of the hip, which is much commoner in girls.) One or both feet may be affected. When the infant is born it is noticed that the foot is turned inwards so that the sole is directed medially (Fig. 294). The deformity, to be more precise, consists of three elements : 1) inversion (twisting inwards) of the foot ; 2) adduction (inward deviation) of the forefoot relative to the hindfoot ; and 3) equinus (plantarflexion). The foot cannot be pushed passively through the normal range of eversion and dorsiflexion. In an older child there may be obvious under-development of the muscles of the lower leg.

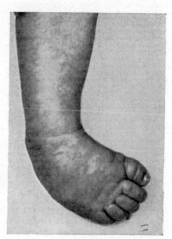

FIG. 294
Congenital club foot. The typical deformity.

14

Diagnosis. Newborn infants should be examined routinely for evidence of club foot. It is not sufficient, for purposes of diagnosis, that the foot be found to rest in the position described, for often the feet of normal infants tend to lie naturally in a somewhat

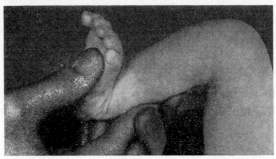

FIG. 295

Correcting a club-foot deformity by manual pressure without anaesthesia.

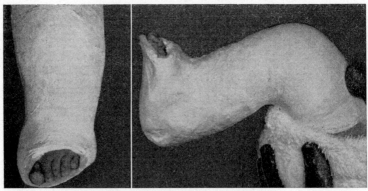

FIG. 296

Plaster for maintaining correction in congenital club foot. It is essential to include the thigh, with the knee flexed to a right angle.

inverted position. The criterion for the diagnosis of club foot is that the deformity cannot readily be corrected and over-corrected to bring the foot into eversion and dorsiflexion. It should be remembered that in normal infants under one year old it is possible to evert and dorsiflex the foot far enough to bring the little toe into contact with the shin.

Prognosis. The prognosis depends largely upon the age at which primary treatment is begun, and upon the efficiency with which it is carried out. The longer the delay before treatment, the smaller is the prospect of complete cure. Yet even with prompt treatment the outcome is uncertain. In a proportion of cases, despite the greatest care from the time of birth, there is a tendency to relapse when treatment is discontinued. These are usually the cases that present well marked hypoplasia of the muscles of the lower leg, especially of the peroneal group.

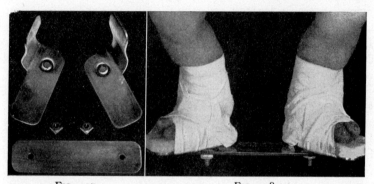

Fig. 297   Fig. 298

Metal splints for congenital club foot (Denis Browne pattern). The feet are held to the sole plates by adhesive strapping, as shown in Figure 298.

Treatment in fresh cases. Although it is seemingly a simple deformity talipes equino-varus presents difficult problems in treatment, and there is no unanimity about the best method to adopt. Hitherto the most widely accepted practice has been to rely upon conservative treatment by correction and splintage during the first year of life and often well beyond that. But it has to be admitted that in many cases the results have been disappointing. All too often operation has been needed later to correct recurrent deformity, and even then the foot has been far from normal. Because of this there has recently been a trend towards operative correction in early infancy if full and lasting correction is not obtained quickly by the traditional methods of conservative treatment. The idea behind early operation is to set the tarsal bones in normal relationship to one another and to remove deforming stresses, thus allowing the bones to develop in their normal shape from an early age. This plan of treatment may be summarised as follows.

Primary conservative treatment. Ideally treatment should be begun immediately after birth—certainly not more than one week later. The principles of treatment are : 1) to correct and over-correct the deformity by repeated firm manual pressure ; and 2) to hold the foot in the over-corrected position until there is no longer a tendency for the deformity to recur.

Correction of deformity. The deformity is corrected by firm manual pressure without anaesthesia (Fig. 295). The adduction and inversion are corrected first, and finally the equinus. Depending on the severity of the deformity, it may be possible to correct it fully by two or three manipulations, or as many as six or eight manipulations (at weekly intervals) may be required.

Maintenance of correction. Two methods are available for holding the foot in the corrected position between manipulations : 1) a plaster of Paris case ; and 2) metal splints as advocated by Denis Browne. Retention in a plaster is preferred, because it holds the foot in the over-corrected position more efficiently and for a longer period than metal splints. The plaster must extend to the upper thigh, with the knee flexed 90 degrees (Fig. 296) ; otherwise the infant is able to draw the foot up inside the plaster. The plaster must be changed every week at first, but the interval may be extended to two and then three weeks as the child grows larger. In the Denis Browne method both feet are fixed to the metal splints by strips of adhesive strapping, and the splints are then clamped rigidly to a cross bar with the feet rotated outwards (Figs. 297 and 298). To remain effective, the splints must be reapplied every day or at least on alternate days.

Operative treatment. If at the end of four months the feet are not normal clinically and radiologically operation is undertaken. All taut ligaments at the medial side of the ankle and foot are divided and any tendon that is too tight to allow full correction is lengthened—including the calcaneal tendon. Finally, under direct vision the tarsal bones are restored to their normal relationships, particular attention being paid to the talus and the navicular bone. After operation a plaster is worn for two or three months.

Treatment in neglected or relapsed cases. Repeated manipulation and retention in plaster can produce worth-while improvement in children of up to 2 years of age. If significant deformity is still present after the age of 2, operative treatment is required. It should be appreciated that in these late cases no method of treatment—whether conservative or operative—is capable of restoring the foot to normal. The most that can be done is to restore a plantigrade [1] foot.

Types of operation : In children of from 2 to 12 years four operations are to be considered : 1) division of the short soft tissues at the medial side of the foot, the foot thereafter being forced into a plantigrade position and immobilised in plaster for three months ; 2) transfer of the tendon of the tibialis posterior through the interosseous membrane to the lateral side of the foot to supplement the action of the evertor muscles ; 3) lengthening of a short calcaneal tendon ; and 4) when inversion of the heel is a prominent feature, osteotomy of the calcaneus with insertion of a bone wedge in the medial side to correct the line of weight-bearing (Dwyer, 1963).

In children over the age of 12 resort must be had to operation upon the bones : a wedge of bone of appropriate size (with base dorso-laterally) is removed from the tarsus so that when the resulting gap is closed the foot is plantigrade. This operation is not recommended for children under 12 because it may impair the growth of the foot.

CONGENITAL TALIPES CALCANEO-VALGUS

This is the opposite deformity to talipes equino-varus. The foot is everted and dorsiflexed. It is a much less serious deformity than talipes equino-varus because it responds more readily to treatment.

Cause. The cause is unknown. In some cases it may simply be a postural deformity, from folding of the foot against the shin for a long time in intra-uterine life.

Clinical features. One or both feet may be affected. The foot rests in a position of eversion and dorsiflexion, so that its dorsum lies almost in contact with the shin (Fig. 299). Tightness of the

---

[1] Plantigrade = sole-walking ; with the sole on the ground.

dorso-lateral soft tissues prevents the foot from being brought down easily into inversion and equinus, though with steady pressure a fair degree of correction can usually be obtained.

Treatment. In most cases the deformity will respond readily to repeated manual stretching by the parents, who should be carefully instructed how to coax the foot into the over-corrected position of inversion and equinus by steady pressure upon the dorsum of the foot. The manipulations should be begun immediately after birth and should be carried out several times a day.

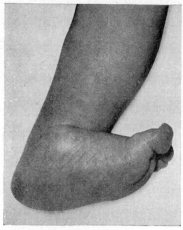

FIG. 299

Congenital talipes calcaneo-valgus.
The typical deformity.

If calcaneo-valgus deformity still persists when the child is a month old more intensive supervision is required. The surgeon should gently over-correct the deformity as far as possible by manipulation without anaesthesia, thereafter applying a plaster with the foot in the over-corrected position. The plaster is changed weekly until a full range of inversion and equinus is gained. At that stage the plaster may be discarded without fear of relapse.

ACCESSORY BONES IN THE FOOT

Many accessory bones have been described in the foot, but most are of little or no practical importance. The commonest is the **os trigonum,** which lies immediately behind the talus, on the upper surface of the tuberosity of the calcaneus (Fig. 300). It does not cause symptoms. It may be confused with a fracture of the talus. The only tarsal accessory bone that is frequently responsible for symptoms is the **os tibiale externum** (accessory navicular bone) (Fig. 301). This lies medial to the navicular bone, and forms a well marked prominence at the inner border of the foot which may become painful and tender from the

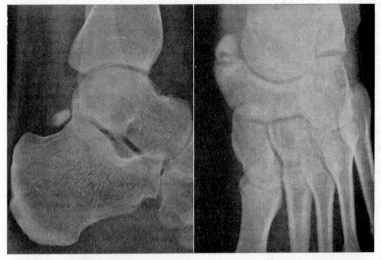

FIG. 300   FIG. 301
Os trigonum.   Os tibiale externum.

pressure of the shoe. If the symptoms justify operation the accessory bone should be removed.

PES CAVUS

In pes cavus or ' hollow foot ' the longitudinal arch of the foot is accentuated.

Cause. In many cases the deformity has a congenital basis. It is sometimes familial. In other cases there is an underlying neurological disorder causing muscle imbalance. For instance, it is sometimes associated with spina bifida, or it may follow poliomyelitis.

Pathology. The metatarsal heads are lowered in relation to the hind part of the foot, with consequent exaggeration of the longitudinal arch. The soft tissues in the sole are abnormally short, and eventually the bones themselves alter shape, perpetuating the deformity. There is always associated clawing of the toes, which are hyperextended at the metatarso-phalangeal joints and flexed at the proximal and distal interphalangeal joints (Fig. 302). This clawing seems to result from defective action of the intrinsic muscles—lumbricals and interossei. The effect is that the toes are almost functionless, and unable to take their normal share in weight-bearing. Consequently excessive weight falls upon the metatarsal heads on walking or standing, and hard callosities form in the underlying skin. The mal-alignment of the tarsal joints predisposes to the later development of osteoarthritis.

Clinical features. The deformity often becomes evident in childhood. It may affect one foot or both. In some cases the symptoms are negligible. When symptoms do arise they may take three forms: 1) painful callosities beneath the metatarsal heads; 2) tenderness over the deformed toes from pressure

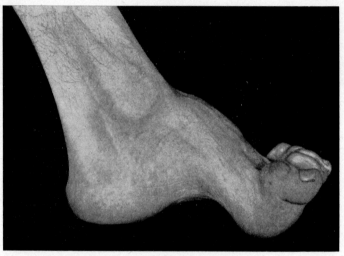

Fig. 302

Pes cavus. Typical deformity with high arch, clawed toes, and prominence of the metatarsal heads in the sole.

against the shoe; and 3) pain in the tarsal region from osteo-arthritis of the tarsal joints. *On examination* the deformity is characteristic and easily recognised (Fig. 302). The longitudinal arch is high; the forefoot is thick and splayed; the toes are clawed; the metatarsal heads are prominent in the sole. Callosities beneath the metatarsal heads indicate that they take excessive weight. The toes cannot be straightened at will by the patient, nor can they be pressed firmly upon the ground to take a share in weight-bearing. There may also be tender callosities where the tops of the toes have rubbed against the shoes.

The base of the spine should be examined for a congenital anomaly such as spina bifida.

Treatment. In many cases treatment is not required. Mild symptoms can often be relieved by regular chiropody and by the provision of a sponge-rubber pad beneath the metatarsal heads to distribute the weight more widely. It is often helpful to prescribe surgical shoes, made to fit the altered shape of the feet.

If the symptoms are severe operation may be required. The nature of the operation should depend upon the cause of the main symptoms.

Operations on the toes. When local pressure upon the toes or beneath the metatarsal heads is the main complaint, adequate relief can often be afforded simply by straightening the clawed toes. This may be done by arthrodesing all the interphalangeal joints or, if the toes are still mobile, by transplanting the long flexor tendon into the extensor expansion to supplement the action of the intrinsic muscles.

Operations on the soft tissues of the sole. In appropriate cases arthrodesis of the toes may be supplemented by the Steindler muscle-slide operation, in which the taut ligamentous tissues in the sole of the foot are detached from the calcaneus and allowed to slide forwards as the height of the arch is reduced by strong manual force. After operation the correction is maintained by immobilising the foot in plaster for two months

Operations on the tarsal joints. When osteoarthritis of the tarsal joints is the main cause of the symptoms arthrodesis of the affected joints (usually the subtalar, calcaneo-cuboid, talo-navicular, and naviculo-cuneiform) is required. At the same time the deformity is corrected by excising a wedge of bone, base upwards, from the metatarsal region. When necessary, this operation may be combined with operations to straighten the toes.

PES PLANUS
(Flat foot ; valgus foot)

In this common condition the longitudinal arch of the foot is reduced so that, on standing, its medial border is close to, or in contact with, the ground (Fig. 303). It is usually associated with some degree of twisting outwards of the foot on its longitudinal axis (eversion or valgus deformity).

Cause. In many cases it probably has a congenital basis, but it may be caused by selective muscle weakness or paralysis.

Pathology. All infants have flat feet for a year or two after they begin to stand. When the deformity persists into adult life it becomes a permanent structural defect, the tarsal bones being so shaped that when articulated they tend to form a straight line rather than an arch.

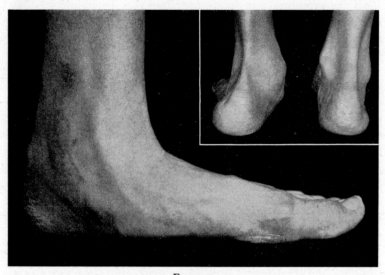

FIG. 303

Pes planus. Marked flattening of the longitudinal arch, with valgus deformity seen well from behind (inset).

Clinical features. In children, flat feet are usually symptomless, but the parents commonly complain that the uppers of the shoes persistently bulge inwards and that the heels wear down quickly at the inner sides.

In adults, too, flat feet are often free from symptoms, but they are more liable than are normal feet to suffer foot strain (p. 419), and when pain is complained of it is usually from that cause.

In later life pain may also arise from osteoarthritis of the tarsal joints consequent upon their mal-alignment.

Treatment. In children under 3 years old treatment is not required. In children over 3 the accepted method of treatment is to tilt the shoe slightly to the lateral side by inserting a wedge, base medially, between the layers of the heel (not the sole) (Fig. 304). This helps to overcome the valgus twist and reduces the bulging-over of the uppers at the medial side. In older children this treatment is supplemented by a course of supervised exercises to strengthen the intrinsic muscles of the foot.

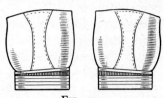

FIG. 304

Shoes drawn from behind, to illustrate medial heel wedges.

In cases of severe valgus deformity, —especially when it is a consequence of selective muscle paralysis, as after poliomyelitis—operation to restore the correct relationship between the talus and the calcaneus, and to fuse the two bones together (talo-calcaneal arthrodesis), may be considered. In children this operation is best done by placing bone grafts extra-articularly in the sinus tarsi, from the lateral side (Grice, 1952).

In adults treatment is not needed unless symptoms are present. If symptoms are due to superimposed foot strain, as is usually the case, treatment appropriate to that condition is advised. At first reliance is placed upon a course of exercises and electrical (faradic) stimulation, under the supervision of a physiotherapist, to strengthen the intrinsic muscles of the foot and the calf muscles. If these measures fail to give relief the advisability of fitting an arch support should be considered. Supports are seldom of benefit when the foot is completely flat, but they often afford relief when the longitudinal arch is diminished but not lost. They should be made from a plaster model of the foot. In persistently troublesome cases manipulation of the feet under an anaesthetic is worth a trial.

If the symptoms in a case of long-established flat foot are ascribed to superimposed osteoarthritis of the tarsal joints, treatment should be directed against the arthritis (p. 421).

FOOT STRAIN

The term ' foot strain ' implies a subacute or chronic strain of the tarsal ligaments, not an acute injury from sudden violence.
Cause. In feet previously normal foot strain is caused by excessive standing by a person unaccustomed to it. In feet whose intrinsic

structure is already impaired (for example, by flattened arches) strain often arises from the ordinary amount of standing demanded in everyday life.

Pathology. In the normal foot the tarsal ligaments are protected from strain by the action of muscles. Thus a force tending to deform the longitudinal arch is resisted by the muscles responsible for maintaining the arch, and not by the tarsal ligaments. When the muscles are unequal to their task the stress falls upon the ligaments, which become strained. The mechanical irritation of recurrent strains leads to chronic inflammatory changes in and around the ligaments. This inflammation is responsible for the characteristic aching after activity.

Clinical features. During and after prolonged walking or standing there is aching pain either in the foot alone or in the foot and calf. Pain in the foot is felt mainly in the midtarsal region : commonly it extends along the under side of the medial border of the foot and along the dorsum of the foot. Calf pain is usually posterior, but it may be felt in the anterior leg muscles. *On examination* the foot may be of normal shape and appearance, but often there is flat foot or other deformity. In severe cases there is tenderness over the tarsal ligaments in the sole.

Diagnosis. Foot strain is easily confused with intermittent claudication (p. 403) from occlusive vascular disease, the symptoms of which are in some respects similar. With careful inquiry and clinical examination there should be no difficulty in making the distinction. The history of intermittent claudication is highly characteristic, and the absence of palpable pulses at the foot (and usually also at the knee) is important confirmatory evidence.

Treatment. The methods of treatment have already been outlined in the section on pes planus in adults (p. 417), the symptoms of which are in fact usually the consequence of superimposed foot strain. In mild cases it is sufficient to curtail the amount of standing and walking, and to arrange a course of supervised exercises and electrical (faradic) stimulation to strengthen the muscles of the leg and foot

When these measures are unsuccessful recourse may be had to manipulation of the feet under anaesthesia, and perhaps to arch supports. In severe cases it may be necessary for the patient to change to a sedentary occupation.

OSTEOARTHRITIS OF THE TARSAL JOINTS

Osteoarthritis may affect any of the tarsal joints, but in practice it is seen most often in the subtalar and midtarsal joints. It seldom arises primarily : there is nearly always a predisposing cause such as previous fracture or disease involving the joint surfaces (especially fractures of the calcaneus), or mal-alignment of the tarsal bones (as in severe flat foot or severe pes cavus).

Clinical features. The main symptom is pain, which gradually increases over months or years and finally leads to a limp and impaired capacity for walking. Pain is localised fairly accurately to the particular joint or joints affected. A history will usually be obtained of previous injury, disease, or deformity of the foot. *On examination* movements of the affected joint are impaired, and painful if forced. *Radiographs* confirm the diagnosis and may give an indication of the primary underlying cause.

Treatment. In mild cases treatment is not required, especially if the patient can curtail his activities. When the disability is troublesome more active measures are needed. Conservative treatment is only palliative, but it is usually worth a trial. It should take the form of short-wave diathermy or hot paraffin-wax baths, muscle exercises, and support from an elastic bandage.

If conservative treatment fails to give adequate relief operation must be considered. The only effective method is by arthrodesis of the affected joint or joints.

OTHER FORMS OF ARTHRITIS OF THE TARSAL JOINTS

Like all true synovial joints, the tarsal joints are liable to any of the recognised forms of arthritis, including pyogenic arthritis, rheumatoid arthritis, tuberculous arthritis, gouty arthritis, and neuropathic arthritis. Of these, the only one that is at all common is rheumatoid arthritis.

OSTEOCHONDRITIS OF THE NAVICULAR BONE
(Köhler's disease)

The general subject of osteochondritis was discussed in Chapter II (p. 97). The growing navicular bone is one of its best recognised sites. The developing nucleus of the bone is temporarily softened and usually becomes compressed by the mechanical forces entailed in walking. A disturbance of blood supply is possibly a causative factor.

Pathology. The pathology is believed to be like that of osteo-chondritis of other growing bony nuclei (Fig. 70, p. 99). The bone loses its normal trabecular structure and may become fragmented. After about two years the normal bone structure is restored. Slight deformation of the bone may remain, but the growing foot seems to adapt itself to the altered shape and little or no disability persists.

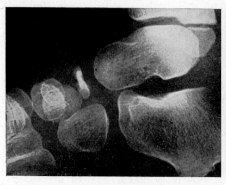 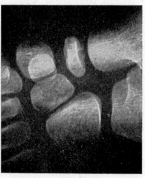

Fig. 305   Fig. 306

Köhler's osteochondritis of the navicular bone. Figure 305—Early stage. Bony nucleus dense and flattened antero-posteriorly. Figure 306—Two years later. Bone texture restored ; slight residual flattening.

Clinical features. Köhler's disease is confined to children of about 3 to 5 years. The child complains of pain in the midtarsal part of the foot and is noticed to limp. *On examination* there may be slight swelling in the midtarsal region, and tenderness on firm palpation over the navicular bone. There may be some restriction of midtarsal movements with pain on forcing, but these signs are slight and sometimes absent. *Radiographs* are diagnostic. The bony nucleus of the navicular bone appears squashed from before backwards (Fig. 305) ; it is denser than normal, and some-times has a fragmented appearance. Serial radiographs during the two-year span of the disease show the gradual evolution of the bone changes. After a stage of maximal density and deformation a few months after the onset there is gradual improvement until the normal bone texture is restored (Fig. 306).

Treatment. Despite the slow evolution of the bone changes prolonged treatment is not required. Good results follow symptomatic treatment, and usually all that is necessary is to rest the foot for two or three months in a walking plaster.

PAINFUL HEEL

The causes of painful heel are conveniently classified according to the site of the pain (Fig. 307).

PAIN WITHIN THE HEEL
> Disease of the calcaneus
> > (osteomyelitis ; tumour ; Paget's disease)
> Arthritis of the subtalar joint

PAIN BEHIND THE HEEL
> Rupture of the tendo calcaneus (p. 400)
> Calcaneal paratendinitis
> Post-calcaneal bursitis
> Calcaneal apophysitis

PAIN BENEATH THE HEEL
> Tender heel pad
> Plantar fasciitis

DISEASE OF THE CALCANEUS

The calcaneus is subject, although rarely, to all types of infection of bone, the commonest being pyogenic infection (osteomyelitis). Occasionally it is the seat of a benign or malignant tumour. It may also be affected by other disorders of bone, such as Paget's disease.

ARTHRITIS OF THE SUBTALAR JOINT

The commonest type of arthritis in the subtalar joint is osteo-arthritis secondary to fracture of the calcaneus (p. 421). The joint is occasionally subject to other forms of arthritis, such as pyogenic arthritis, rheumatoid arthritis, tuberculous arthritis, and gout.

CALCANEAL PARATENDINITIS
(Calcaneal tenosynovitis)

The calcaneal tendon is surrounded by loose connective tissue, or paratenon, which allows gliding movements. Rarely, this becomes inflamed from excessive friction. The condition should be termed paratendinitis rather than tenosynovitis, for there is no true synovial sheath.

Clinical features. The patient is usually an active young adult. There is pain in the region of the calcaneal tendon, made worse by activities such as running or dancing. *On examination* there is tenderness on palpation between finger and thumb deep to the tendon (Fig. 307), and there is slight local thickening in this region. The tendon itself is of normal size and consistency.

Treatment. In many cases relief is afforded by local injection of hydrocortisone deep to the tendon. If this fails, the ankle should be rested in a below-knee walking paster for four weeks. In an exceptionally resistant case operation may be required : it consists in excising the loose connective tissue surrounding and deep to the tendon.

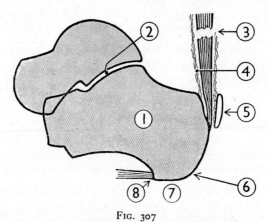

FIG. 307

Eight causes of painful heel, with site of pain. 1. Disease of the calcaneus. 2. Arthritis of the subtalar joint. 3. Ruptured calcaneal tendon. 4. Calcaneal paratendinitis. 5. Post-calcaneal bursitis. 6. Calcaneal apophysitis. 7. Tender heel pad. 8. Plantar fasciitis.

POST-CALCANEAL BURSITIS

This is the commonest cause of pain behind the heel. It is often a cause of troublesome disability in young women.

Pathology. An adventitious bursa forms at the back of the heel, between the tuberosity of the calcaneus and the skin. Repeated friction against the back of the shoe leads to chronic inflammation and thickening of the walls of the bursa, and the sac may be distended with fluid.

Clinical features. There is troublesome tenderness where the swelling is in contact with the shoe (Fig. 307). The symptoms are aggravated by walking, and they tend to be worse in winter than in summer ; hence the term ' winter heel.' *On examination* there is an obvious gristly prominence at the back of the heel ; the overlying skin is thickened and may be red.

Treatment. In mild or recent cases the symptoms can be controlled by protecting the back of the heel with a double layer of elastic adhesive strapping and by wearing shoes with soft backs. If these measures fail the bursa should be excised : its recurrence must be prevented by excising the prominent upper posterior corner of the calcaneal tuberosity, immediately above the attachment of the calcaneal tendon.

CALCANEAL APOPHYSITIS
(Sever's disease)

This harmless condition occurs only in children, during the period of active growth of the calcaneal apophysis. It was formerly believed to be an example of osteochondritis (p. 97), but most authorities now agree that it is nothing more than a chronic strain at the attachment of the posterior apophysis of the calcaneus to the main body of the bone, possibly from the pull of the calcaneal tendon. It may thus be regarded as analogous to Osgood-Schlatter's disease of the tibial tubercle, and totally unrelated to osteochondritis.

Clinical features. The child is usually between 8 and 13 years old. He complains of pain behind the heel, and a slight limp may be noticed. *On examination* there is tenderness over the lower posterior part of the tuberosity of the calcaneus (Fig. 307). *Radiographs* usually fail to show any alteration from the normal. Importance has sometimes been attached to an appearance of fragmentation of the calcaneal apophysis, but this is a normal state, often seen in children without pain in the heel.

Treatment. In most cases treatment is not required, because the symptoms will gradually subside spontaneously. If the pain is severe, rest for a few weeks in a below-knee walking plaster will afford adequate relief.

TENDER HEEL PAD

This is a distinct clinical condition characterised by pain beneath the hind part of the heel on standing or walking.

Pathology. The site of the tenderness is the tough fibro-fatty tissue beneath the prominent weight-bearing part of the calcaneus. In some cases the lesion is probably no more than a simple contusion ; but in most cases injury seems to play no part and it must be assumed that there is mild inflammation, of uncertain origin.

Clinical features. Pain beneath the heel on standing or walking is the only symptom. *On examination* there is well marked local tenderness on firm palpation over the heel pad (Fig. 307).

Treatment. There is a tendency to slow spontaneous improvement. Recovery may be hastened by providing a sponge-rubber heel cushion on an insole, and by a course of short-wave diathermy to the tender area.

PLANTAR FASCIITIS

In this condition, which is believed to be inflammatory, there is pain beneath the anterior part of the calcaneus.

Pathology. The lesion affects the soft tissues at the site of attachment of the plantar aponeurosis to the inferior aspect of the tuberosity of the calcaneus. The precise cause of the inflammation is uncertain.

Clinical features. The complaint is of pain beneath the heel on standing or walking ; the pain may extend forwards into the sole. The disability is sometimes severe. *On examination* there is marked tenderness over the site of attachment of the plantar fascia to the calcaneus. The site of tenderness is farther forward than it is in tender heel pad (Fig. 307). *Radiographs* usually do not show any abnormality. A sharp spur projecting forwards from the tuberosity of the calcaneus is sometimes found, but its significance is doubtful because such spurs may be present in patients without heel symptoms.

Treatment. Conservative treatment usually suffices if continued for long enough, though recovery may be slow. The heel should be protected by a sponge-rubber cushion on an insole, and a course of short-wave diathermy to the tender area should be arranged. If these measures fail, local injection of hydrocortisone into the tender area may be tried. Only in exceptionally severe and resistant cases—if at all—should resort be had to operation. Spurred bone may be removed and the plantar fascia stripped from its posterior attachment.

PAIN IN THE FOREFOOT
(Metatarsalgia)

Pain in the forefoot is one of the commonest orthopaedic complaints. There are three main causes, of which the first is the most frequent: 1) anterior flat foot (dropped transverse arch); 2) stress fracture of a metatarsal bone (march fracture); 3) plantar digital neuritis (Morton's metatarsalgia).

ANTERIOR FLAT FOOT
(Dropped transverse arch)

Permanent flattening of the transverse arch of the foot, with excessive weight-bearing pressure beneath the metatarsal heads, is the commonest cause of metatarsalgia. In most cases the primary cause is inefficiency of the intrinsic muscles of the foot.
Pathology. Even in normal feet the transverse arch is only a potential arch, not a constant one. But in the normal state the

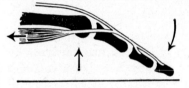 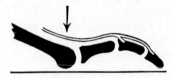

FIG. 308   FIG. 309

Figure 308—Diagram to show the normal action of the toes in raising the metatarsal heads from the ground, whereby they share the weight with the metatarsal heads. This action is controlled mainly by the intrinsic muscles. Figure 309—If the intrinsic muscles are inefficient all the weight must be borne by the metatarsal heads.

metatarsal heads can be raised from the ground at will by the action of the toes, held straight at the interphalangeal joints by the intrinsic muscles and flexed strongly at the metatarso-phalangeal joints by the intrinsic muscles in conjunction with the long and short flexors (Fig. 308). Thus the weight is shared between the metatarsal heads and the toes. If the intrinsic muscles are inefficient the toes are unable to fulfil their important weight-sharing function and all the pressure falls upon the metatarsal heads (Fig. 309). The excessive pressure leads to the formation of callosities.

Clinical features. The main complaint is of pain beneath the forefoot. There may be secondary symptoms from pressure of the shoes upon deformed toes. *On examination* the forefoot is often splayed, appearing broader than normal. There are callosities beneath some or all of the metatarsal heads. The toes are often curled or otherwise deformed. The patient is unable to raise the metatarsal heads from the ground by pressing downwards with the toes—an indication that the intrinsic muscles are inefficient.

Treatment. In patients under 50 worth-while improvement can usually be gained by a prolonged course of physiotherapy, designed to strengthen the intrinsic muscles by special exercises aided by faradic stimulation. In older patients this treatment is seldom effective, and resort must usually be had to a sponge-rubber support to distribute the weight-bearing pressure over a wide area of the metatarsus.

STRESS FRACTURE OF A METATARSAL BONE
(March fracture ; fatigue fracture)

Stress or fatigue fractures are unusual in that there is no history of violence. The possibility of fracture may therefore be overlooked. A stress fracture of a metatarsal is not a common cause of pain in the forefoot but the possibility of its occurrence should be remembered.

Cause. The fracture is ascribed to long-continued or oft-repeated stress ; it has been likened to the fatigue fractures that sometimes occur in metals.

Pathology. The fracture usually affects the shaft of the second or third metatarsal bone. It is no more than a hairline crack, and there is no displacement of the fragments. In the process of healing a large mass of callus may form around the bone at the site of fracture.

Clinical features. The complaint is of severe pain in the forefoot on walking. The onset is rapid but the patient is usually unable to ascribe it to an obvious cause. Inquiry may reveal, however,

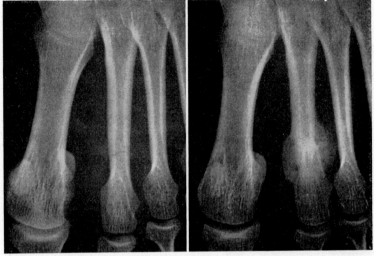

FIG. 310   FIG. 311

Stress fracture of second metatarsal. Figure 310 shows the initial radiograph, taken a week after the onset of pain. The fracture is seen as a fine crack across the bone. Figure 311 shows the condition three weeks later, in the stage of healing. Abundant callus has formed about the site of fracture.

that he has done an unusual amount of walking a day or two before the onset. *On examination* there is swelling at the dorsum of the forefoot, with marked and well localised tenderness over the affected metatarsal bone. *Radiographs* at first show only a faint hairline crack which is easily overlooked (Fig. 310), but after two or three weeks the callus surrounding the fracture is clearly visible (Fig. 311).

Treatment. The fracture heals spontaneously; so treatment is purely symptomatic. Indeed in some cases treatment is not needed; but if pain is severe immobilisation in a below-knee walking plaster for three or four weeks is advised.

PLANTAR DIGITAL NEURITIS
(Morton's metatarsalgia; interdigital neuroma)

This condition, which is primarily an affection of a digital nerve, is characterised typically by metatarsal pain combined with a radiating pain in the third and fourth toes.

Pathology. The underlying lesion is a fibrous thickening or ' neuroma ' of the digital nerve of the 3-4 cleft just proximal to its point of division into terminal branches. It takes the form of a fusiform swelling one and a half to two centimetres long, surrounding the nerve as it lies in the space between the heads of the third and fourth metatarsals (Fig. 312). Occasionally the nerve to the 2-3 cleft is the one affected. The cause of the fibrous thickening is uncertain.

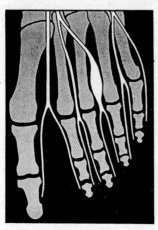

Fig. 312

Fibrous thickening of an inter-digital nerve, as found in plantar digital neuritis (Morton's meta-tarsalgia). The ' neuroma ' is usually in the 3-4 cleft.

Clinical features. The patient is often a woman of middle age. She complains of pain in the forefoot on standing or walking. A characteristic feature is that the pain, arising in the metatarsal region, radiates forwards into the contiguous sides of the third and fourth toes, or to the fourth toe alone. Rarely, the cleft between the second and third toes is affected. Patients often state that they can relieve the pain by taking the shoe off and squeezing or manipulating the forefoot. *On examination* the forefoot is often splayed, as in anterior flat foot. Sometimes a painful click can be elicited by compressing the metatarsal heads from side to side, and upward pressure on the sole between the third and fourth metatarsal heads is painful ; but the significance of these signs is doubtful.

Diagnosis. This depends mainly upon the typical history.

Treatment. The patient should try first the effect of wearing a sponge-rubber metatarsal pad to support the anterior arch. If this fails to relieve the symptoms operative excision of the thickened segment of the nerve is recommended.

PLANTAR WART
(Verruca plantaris)

Plantar warts may occur in any part of the sole of the foot, including the under surface of the heel. They are like warts elsewhere, except that they do not project beyond the skin surface.

They are distinct from plantar callosities, which are simply localised thickenings of the skin at points of excessive pressure.

Cause. The exact cause is unknown. A virus infection has been thought responsible.

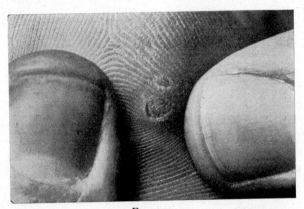

FIG. 313

Plantar wart. Note the clearly circumscribed outline and the slight cleft when the skin is stretched away from the wart.

Pathology. A wart is a simple papilloma, growing outwards from the basal layers of the skin. It is prevented by the pressure of weight-bearing from projecting much beyond the skin surface, but the surrounding skin is thickened, so the wart may have a total depth of up to half a centimetre (Fig. 314). It slowly enlarges, but seldom reaches a diameter of more than a centimetre.

Clinical features. The chief complaint is of severe localised pain on walking. *On examination* the skin surrounding the wart is thickened and therefore raised. The wart, a little darker in colour and with a mosaic surface, is seen in the centre of the raised area (Fig. 313). Its edge is clearly demarcated from the surrounding skin : this can be discerned easily if the skin is stretched away from the wart, when a tiny cleft becomes apparent between wart and skin. There is always marked local tenderness on pressure over the wart.

Diagnosis. The main difficulty is to distinguish warts from callosities. Warts occur anywhere on the sole, callosities only over points of pressure. Warts are also much more tender than callosities. But the most reliable distinguishing feature is that a wart has a mosaic surface and a clearly defined margin with a potential cleft between it and the skin (Fig. 314), whereas a callosity blends imperceptibly with the surrounding normal skin (Fig. 315).

Treatment. The wart should be curetted out and the base lightly cauterised.

CALLOSITIES

A callosity is simply a localised thickening of the skin in response to abnormal pressure. It is nearly always secondary to a pre-existing disorder of the foot.

Plantar callosities are callosities on the sole of the foot. They occur under a prominent bone. They are commonest beneath the metatarsal heads when deficient intrinsic muscles prevent the toes from taking their proper share in weight-bearing (anterior flat foot, p. 427). They are also common beneath the base of the fifth metatarsal in patients who for any reason walk with the foot inverted.

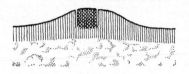

FIG. 314

Diagrammatic section of a plantar wart. It is clearly demarcated from the surrounding skin.

Callosities on the toes often take the form of localised thickenings, when they are termed corns. They are caused by pressure against the shoe, and they are especially common when the dorsum of a toe is made unduly prominent by a fixed flexion deformity, as in hammer toe (Fig. 322, p. 437).

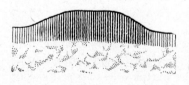

FIG. 315

Diagrammatic section of a callosity. It blends imperceptibly with the surrounding normal skin.

Treatment. The treatment is mainly that of the underlying condition. Palliative measures include paring of excess epidermis (preferably by a chiropodist), and sponge-rubber padding to distribute the weight-bearing pressure over a wider area.

GANGLION

Ganglia are common on the dorsum of the foot and around the ankle. They are similar in all respects to the ganglia that occur at the back of the wrist and hand. They consist of thin-walled sacs filled with glairy viscous fluid, and the fibrous wall is usually connected deeply with a ligament, tendon sheath, or joint capsule. Clinically, a ganglion appears as a fluctuant subcutaneous swelling, which may be either soft or tense. If it causes trouble it should be excised.

DISORDERS OF THE TOES

HALLUX VALGUS

In hallux valgus the great toe is deviated laterally at the metatarso-phalangeal joint. It is common in women past middle age.

Cause. In a few cases congenital factors are responsible. But in most the deformity is caused by the toe's being persistently forced laterally by enclosure in tight stockings and narrow pointed shoes. The wearing of high heels favours the development of hallux valgus because the forefoot is forced into the narrow pointed part of the shoe.

Pathology. Outward deviation of the big toe is the most obvious feature of the deformity, but a further, almost constant feature is that the first metatarsal is deviated medially, so that the gap between the heads of the first and second metatarsals is unduly wide (metatarsus primus varus). Indeed this may often be the primary defect. After several years two secondary changes occur. One is the formation of a thick-walled bursa (bunion) over the medial prominence of the joint ; this may become inflamed, occasionally

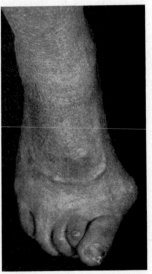

Fig. 316

Hallux valgus. A typical example. There is also fixed flexion deformity of the adjacent toe.

with suppuration. The second, a later development, is osteo-arthritis of the metatarso-phalangeal joint consequent upon its mal-alignment (Fig. 317).

Clinical features. The patient is nearly always a woman, who is often at or past middle age when she seeks advice. The early symptoms arise from tenderness over the bunion from pressure against the shoe. There is also difficulty in getting comfortable footwear. Later, additional symptoms arise from osteoarthritis of the metatarso-phalangeal joint, and from flattening of the transverse arch (anterior flat foot, p. 427), which is a common associated deformity. *On examination* the deformity is obvious at a glance (Fig. 316). The skin over the prominent joint is hard, reddened, and tender. Often a thick-walled bursa can be felt, and occasionally it is distended with fluid. In relatively early cases metatarso-phalangeal joint movements are free and painless, but in severe cases of many years' duration the secondary osteoarthritis makes movement limited and painful. In late cases the forefoot is often flat and splayed, and the toes may be severely curled.

Treatment. In mild cases treatment is not required, but footwear must be selected with care to obtain adequate width.

In moderate cases sufficient relief is often afforded by regular chiropody, protection of the bunion with pads of felt, and some-times by wearing a rubber wedge between the great and second toes to reduce the deformity.

In severe cases operation is often advisable. Mention will be made here of only five of the many methods that are available. *Trimming of ' exostosis.'* When the deviation of the toe is slight, but troublesome symptoms arise from localised prominence or ' exostosis ' of the first metatarsal head at the medial side of the foot, it may sometimes be sufficient to excise the bursa and chisel away the medial prominence of the metatarsal head without disturbing the joint itself. There is a tendency for the symptoms to recur after this operation, and in general the results are rather disappointing.

Excision arthroplasty of the metatarso-phalangeal joint by Keller's method is widely used. The object is to create a flail, freely movable false joint between the first metatarsal and the proximal phalanx, with correction of the mal-alignment. This is done by excising the proximal half or two-thirds of the proximal phalanx so that a centimetre gap is left between the two bones; at the same time the bursa is excised and the medial prominence of the metatarsal head is smoothed off with a chisel (Fig. 318).

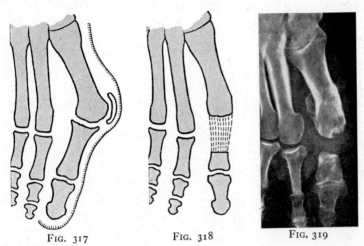

FIG. 317   FIG. 318   FIG. 319

Hallux valgus. Figure 317—Diagram showing the prominent metatarsal head with overlying bunion, and osteoarthritis from mal-alignment of the joint. Figure 318—Excision arthroplasty (Keller's operation): removal of the promixal two-thirds of the proximal phalanx. The resulting gap fills with flexible fibrous tissue. The bursa and the underlying prominence of the metatarsal head have also been removed. Figure 319—Radiograph ten years after Keller's operation for hallux valgus.

The space created by excision of the base of the phalanx fills with rubbery fibrous tissue, and a false joint forms which allows a reasonable range of movement (Fig. 319). This operation leaves the big toe slightly shorter than normal and rather floppy, with poor active control over toe movements. Nevertheless the main symptoms are relieved and the result is usually satisfactory in patients beyond middle age who do not wish to walk long distances or to indulge in athletic pursuits.

Mayo's operation is similar in principle, and is in fact another form of excision arthroplasty: the head of the first metatarsal is excised instead of the base of the proximal phalanx. The operation is open to the criticism that the weight-bearing end of the metatarsal and the bearing surfaces for the sesamoid bones are sacrificed.

Arthrodesis of the metatarso-phalangeal joint of the hallux in a position of slight extension allows full and permanent correction of the valgus deformity, and is preferred by some surgeons. Its chief disadvantage is that the joint must be immobilised in plaster for about eight weeks, to ensure sound bony fusion.

Displacement osteotomy of the neck of the first metatarsal bone is illustrated in Figures 320-321. After division of the neck of the metatarsal the head fragment is displaced markedly laterally (Fig. 321). (A spike of lateral cortex is left on the shaft fragment to impale the head in its new position.) The outward shift of the metatarsal head eliminates the prominence of the 'exostosis' without the need for its removal. The soft tissues between the heads of the first and second metatarsals are also relaxed, allowing permanent reduction of the subluxation at the first metatarso-phalangeal joint. By a process of remodelling (Fig. 321), the alignment of the first metatarsal is gradually altered after operation so that it lies closer to the second metatarsal. In this operation the joint itself is left undisturbed, indeed unopened. After

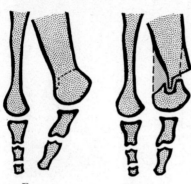

FIG. 320   FIG. 321

Displacement osteotomy of neck of first metatarsal. Figure 320—Before operation. Note wide gap between first and second metatarsals. The line of osteotomy is indicated. Figure 321—After division of the bone the head fragment is displaced markedly laterally, so that its medial prominence (the ' exostosis ') disappears. The metatarso-phalangeal subluxation is automatically reduced. Remodelling (interrupted line) alters the shape of the metatarsal and the intermetatarsal gap is narrowed.

operation the toe is immobilised in plaster for eight weeks to ensure union at the site of osteotomy without loss of position.

This operation gives good results in patients with relatively slight deformity : it does not shorten the toe appreciably or impair active movement, and it is therefore particularly suitable for young patients who wish to lead an energetic life.

COMMENT

There is much variation of opinion among different surgeons on the choice of treatment. The author's preference is to advise Keller's excision arthroplasty for the usual middle-aged or elderly patient, and displacement osteotomy of the neck of the metatarsal for the younger and more active patients.

When severe hallux valgus is associated with flattening of the transverse arch and marked clawing of the toes, operation of any type may be disappointing and it may be wiser to rely upon well made surgical shoes.

HAMMER TOE

The term hammer toe denotes a fixed flexion deformity of an interphalangeal joint.

Cause. Presumably an imbalance of the delicate arrangement of flexor and extensor tendons is responsible ; but the precise explanation of its occurrence is unknown.

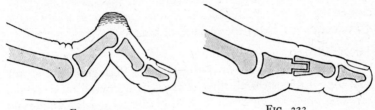

FIG. 322   FIG. 323

Figure 322—Hammer toe: the typical deformity, with callosity over the prominent proximal joint. Figure 323—Peg arthrodesis, for correction of hammer toe.

Pathology. The affected joint is sharply angled into flexion. Secondary contracture of the plantar aspect of the joint capsule fixes the deformity, and a callosity usually forms over the dorsum of the flexed joint, from pressure against the shoe.

Clinical features. Typically the deformity affects only one toe— usually the second. In the characteristic deformity the proximal interphalangeal joint is in fixed flexion, and the distal interphalangeal joint, though still mobile, rests in compensatory hyperextension (Fig. 322). The symptoms, if any, are caused by the overlying callosity.

Treatment. If symptoms are slight the deformity may be accepted, or conservative treatment by protective felt pads may be sufficient. In severe cases operation gives gratifying results. The joint surfaces are excised and the joint is arthrodesed in the straight position by the pegging technique shown in Figure 323.

UNDER-RIDING TOE
(Congenital curled toe)

Children are often brought in for advice because one of the smaller toes, often the fourth, is curled inwards and lies beneath the adjacent toe. The condition does not cause any symptoms during childhood, and it should be left alone until adolescence or early adult life, when the toe can easily be straightened if it begins to cause symptoms. Similar principles apply to the management of over-riding toe.

OSTEOARTHRITIS OF THE TOE JOINTS

In practice, osteoarthritis in the toes is seen commonly only in the metatarso-phalangeal joint of the great toe. This has been termed *hallux rigidus*. Occasionally the metatarso-phalangeal joint of one of the smaller toes is affected, usually as a late result of Freiberg's disease of the metatarsal head.

HALLUX RIGIDUS

This is osteoarthritis of the metatarso-phalangeal joint of the great toe. Like osteoarthritis elsewhere, it is caused by wear and tear, but previous injury or disease of the joint is an important predisposing factor.

Pathology. The changes are like those of osteoarthritis in other joints. The articular cartilage is gradually worn away from both surfaces of the joint until eventually the subchondral bone is exposed. The exposed bone becomes hard and glossy (eburnation). The marginal bone hypertrophies to form osteophytes, which often cause obvious thickening, especially at the dorsum of the toe.

Clinical features. The complaint is of pain in the base of the great toe on walking. *On examination* the metatarso-phalangeal joint is palpably thickened from osteophyte formation. If an osteophyte is especially prominent on the dorsal or medial aspect of the joint a thick-walled bursa (bunion) may form over it; occasionally the bursa is distended with fluid. Flexion and extension of the toe at the metatarso-phalangeal joint are restricted —usually markedly so by the time the patient seeks advice (Fig. 324). Forced dorsiflexion of the painful joint on walking is the main source of the disability.[1] *Radiographs* confirm the presence of osteoarthritis. The cartilage space is narrowed, the

---

[1] It should be remembered that the normal range of dorsiflexion at the metatarso-phalangeal joint of the great toe is nearly 90 degrees.

subchondral bone tends to be sclerotic, and there is osteophytic spurring of the joint margins (Fig. 325).

Treatment. In mild cases treatment is not required. When treatment is called for, conservative measures are usually worth a trial first. A metatarsal bar should be fitted beneath the sole of the foot at the metatarso-phalangeal level. This acts as a rocker in walking, and so reduces the dorsiflexion required of the toes when weight is brought onto the forefoot from the heel. A course of short-wave diathermy to the joint may also be helpful.

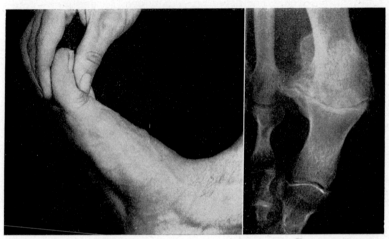

FIG. 324   FIG. 325

Hallux rigidus. Figure 324 shows the marked impairment of dorsiflexion. Figure 325 shows the radiographic changes typical of osteoarthritis, namely narrowing of the cartilage space, subchondral sclerosis, and the formation of osteophytes.

When the disability is severe operation should be advised. One method is to create a flail joint by excision of the base of the proximal phalanx (Keller's arthroplasty), as for hallux valgus. Many surgeons find, however, that arthrodesis of the metatarso-phalangeal joint in a position of slight extension gives better results, with complete relief of pain.

OSTEOARTHRITIS OF OTHER TOE JOINTS

Osteoarthritis of the other metatarso-phalangeal joints is uncommon except as a sequel to Freiberg's disease of a metatarsal head (p. 441).

GOUTY ARTHRITIS OF THE GREAT TOE JOINTS

(General description of gouty arthritis, p. 58.)

The joints of the great toe are those most often affected in gout, especially in the first attack.

Cause. The precise cause of gout is unknown. A predisposition to the disease may be inherited. An attack of gout occurs when uric acid is deposited as sodium biurate crystals in the cartilage of the joint.

Clinical features. The patient is usually over 40, and more often a man than a woman. There is a sudden onset (often during the night) of severe pain in the great toe. *On examination* the toe is swollen, red, and extremely tender. Joint movements are impossible because of pain. There is sometimes slight pyrexia. The patient will usually recall previous similar attacks lasting a few days, with freedom from pain in the intervals. *Radiographs* are normal in the early stages. *Investigations :* There is sometimes a mild leucocytosis. The blood uric acid level is usually raised. Aspiration of the joint may yield sterile fluid containing urate crystals. *Chronic gout.* In this form deposits of sodium biurate in and around the joints of the great toe lead to persistent nodular thickening. *Radiographs* show rounded areas of transradiance in the bone ends ; these represent deposits of sodium biurate (which is transradiant) in the subchondral bone.

Diagnosis. Acute gout is easily mistaken for acute infective arthritis. Features suggestive of gout are : a raised blood uric acid level ; a history of previous attacks, with symptom-free intervals ; the presence of tophi in the ears or elsewhere ; mild rather than severe leucocytosis ; the characteristic features of aspirated synovial fluid ; and a good response to phenylbutazone.

Course. Gout usually occurs in recurrent attacks. In the early years, an acute attack subsides within a few days, leaving the joint clinically normal. In chronic gout the joint is gradually disorganised, causing permanent disability.

Treatment. Acute attacks respond to phenylbutazone, begun in high dosage which is reduced after two or three days, or to colchicum. Meanwhile the foot should be rested, and the toe should be protected from pressure by a bulky wool dressing. The treatment of recurrent and chronic gout was detailed on p. 60.

FREIBERG'S DISEASE OF A METATARSAL HEAD
(Metatarsal osteochondritis)

Freiberg's disease of a metatarsal head is regarded by some as an example of osteochondritis juvenilis (p. 97) and by others as osteochondritis dissecans (p. 67). It may therefore be well to use the non-committal eponymous title for the present. The essential feature of Freiberg's disease is partial necrosis and fragmentation of a metatarsal head, which may become deformed under the pressure of weight-bearing.

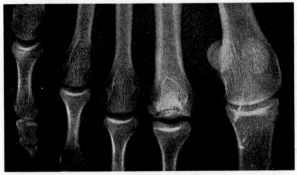

Fig. 326

Freiberg's disease of the second metatarsal head. Note the fragmentation and the square-shaped deformity of the articular surface.

Pathology. The epiphysis of one of the metatarsal heads— nearly always the second or third—is the part affected. The bony nucleus becomes necrotic and granular. Part of the articular surface separates, usually remaining attached only by a hinge of articular cartilage. While it is in this crumbly state the metatarsal head is crushed by the pressure against it of the base of the proximal phalanx of the toe. The articular surface of the metatarsal head thus loses its normal dome-shaped contour and becomes flat (Fig. 326). After about two years the texture of the bone returns to normal, but flattening of the articular surface remains. Later, the distortion of the joint surface often leads to osteoarthritis.

Clinical features. At the time of onset the patient is 14 to 18

15

years old. There is pain in the affected metatarso-phalangeal joint, worse on standing or walking. *On examination* there is slight thickening in the region of the head of the metatarsal, which is tender on pressure. Movements of the metatarso-phalangeal joint are slightly restricted and painful. *Radiographs* reveal the nature of the trouble, though at first the changes are very slight and may be overlooked. Later the head of the metatarsal appears fragmented, with patches of increased density. Finally, the articular surface is flattened, so that the end of the bone appears square-cut instead of round (Fig. 326).

Treatment. When the diagnosis can be made in the early stage—before marked radiographic changes are apparent—operation offers a hope of preventing permanent distortion of the joint surface. Through a window cut in the dorsal surface of the metatarsal neck the necrotic bone of the head is curetted out and replaced by cancellous chip bone grafts, packed firmly enough to restore the normal dome-shaped contour of the articular surface. Thereafter the toe is supported in a plaster cuff for two months.

When deformity of the metatarsal head is already well established at the time of diagnosis attempted restoration of the articular surface is of no avail. Expectant treatment is then recommended. If pain is troublesome rest in a walking plaster for two months may afford relief. But if disabling osteoarthritis develops later the head of the metatarsal should be excised.

INGROWING TOE NAIL
(Embedded toe nail)

Ingrowing toe nail is common only in the big toe.

Cause. Some persons have toes that are prone to develop ingrowing toe nail. But the main causative factors are incorrect cutting of the nail, pressure on the nail-wall (lateral skin fold) by the shoe or by the adjacent second toe, and accumulation of dirt and sweat. When the nail is cut its sides should be left long enough to project beyond the terminal pulp (Fig. 327) : if it is cut too short a sharp corner of nail lies in contact with the lateral skin fold (Fig. 328), and this corner may tend to embed itself in the skin, especially if there is local pressure at the side of the toe. In the presence of dirt and sweat, infection is then liable to arise.

Clinical features. The lesion may be at the medial or (more commonly) the lateral border of the nail, or both. There is pain at the affected anterior corner of the nail. *On examination* the skin fold is inflamed, and there may be local suppuration where the corner of the nail digs into the skin.

Treatment. In mild cases conservative treatment may suffice. Pledgets of gauze soaked in alcohol (surgical spirit) are tucked beneath the corner of the nail twice a day, and the nail is allowed to grow until its edges project beyond the skin folds (Fig. 327).

In long-standing cases operation is advisable. If only one side of the nail is involved it is sufficient to avulse a strip of nail at the

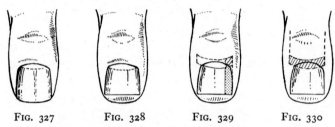

Fig. 327   Fig. 328   Fig. 329   Fig. 330

Figure 327—Nail cut correctly. Figure 328—Nail cut too short : corners dig into pulp. Figure 329—Operation for ingrowing toe nail. A strip of nail is avulsed and its re-growth is prevented by excision of a segment of the germinal matrix. Figure 330— Operation for permanent ablation of the whole nail. After avulsion of the nail, only the germinal matrix need be excised to prevent re-growth. The raw area is covered by advancing a proximal skin flap.

affected side and then to prevent re-growth of this part. Since the nail is formed only from the germinal matrix—the proximal curved segment of the nail bed that corresponds to the lunula—and not from the nail bed as a whole, it is necessary to remove only an appropriate piece of the germinal matrix to prevent re-growth (Fig. 329).

In the worst cases, with infection at both sides of the nail, permanent ablation of the entire nail by excision of the whole of the germinal matrix is more satisfactory (Fig 330). It is not necessary to shorten the toe to obtain adequate skin cover : the small raw area can be covered simply by advancing a dorsal skin flap, based proximally and with its free edge at the nail fold.

15*

SUBUNGUAL EXOSTOSIS

A subungual exostosis is a bony outgrowth from the dorsal surface of the distal phalanx of a toe—usually the great toe. It projects upwards and forwards between the tip of the nail and the terminal pulp. The nail is raised and deformed, and the skin of the pulp overlying the outgrowth is thickened and hard. There is sharp pain when pressure is applied over the nail or terminal pulp. *Radiographs* show the exostosis, which is seen best in the lateral projection.

Treatment. The exostosis should be excised through a terminal incision just beyond the tip of the nail.

ONYCHOGRYPOSIS

Translated from the Greek, this means 'hooked nail.' The term is descriptive. The nail—usually of the big toe—is enormously thickened and curved, eventually resembling a miniature ox-horn (Fig. 331).

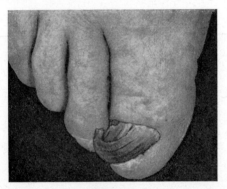

Fig. 331
Onychogryposis.

Treatment. Simple removal of the nail is an adequate temporary measure ; but the new nail will become similarly deformed. For permanent cure the nail bed must be ablated permanently by excision of the germinal matrix, as described in the section on ingrowing toe-nail (p. 443).

References and bibliography, page 445.

References and Bibliography

THIS list is not intended as a comprehensive guide even to the more recent literature on orthopaedic surgery : space does not permit the inclusion of more than a limited selection. The aim has been to choose books and papers that will be of the greatest service to those seeking detailed information on a given subject, and a paper has generally been selected for one or more of the following reasons : 1) it reports recent work ; 2) it reports authoritative opinion ; 3) it is of special intrinsic interest ; 4) it contains a comprehensive list of references. An original description or a classic paper has not always been listed when reference to it is made in more recent works, because it can thereby be easily traced. In the main the references are to works in the English language which will be readily accessible to most readers.

The list is arranged in two parts, ' general ' and ' specific.' The general list cites comprehensive works of reference on orthopaedic surgery as a whole or on branches of it. The specific list refers to papers or chapters on a particular topic.

Titles printed in italics refer to books or monographs ; those in roman type refer to papers in journals.

GENERAL WORKS

ADAMS, R. D., DENNY-BROWN, D. & PEARSON, C. M. (1962) : *Diseases of Muscle*, 2nd ed. London : Henry Kimpton.

APLEY, A. G. (1968) : *A System of Orthopaedics and Fractures*. London: Butterworth.

APLEY, A. G. (ed.) (1969) : *Recent Advances in Orthopaedics*. London : Churchill.

BOURNE, G. H. (ed.) (1956) : *The Biochemistry and Physiology of Bone*. New York : Academic Press.

CAMPBELL, W. C. (1971) : *Operative Orthopaedics*, 5th ed., ed. Crenshaw. London : Henry Kimpton.

COPEMAN, W. S. C. (ed.) (1969) : *Textbook of the Rheumatic Diseases*, 4th ed. Edinburgh : Livingstone.

EASTCOTT, H. H. G. (1969) : *Arterial Surgery*. London : Pitman.

FAIRBANK, H. A. T. (1951) : *An Atlas of General Affections of the Skeleton*. Edinburgh : Livingstone.

GRAHAM, W. D. (ed.) (1967) : *Modern Trends in Orthopaedics* (5). London : Butterworth.

JAMES, J. I. P. (1970) : The Orthopaedic Surgeon and Research. Journal of Bone and Joint Surgery, **52B,** 14.

LLOYD-ROBERTS, G. C. (ed.) (1967) : Orthopaedics. Vol. 13 of *Clinical Surgery*, ed. Rob and Smith. London : Butterworth.

McKUSICK, V. A. (1966): *Heritable Disorders of Connective Tissue*. London: Henry Kimpton.

445

MERCER, W. & DUTHIE, R. B. (1964): *Orthopaedic Surgery.* London : Arnold.
NANGLE, E. J. (1951): *Instruments and Apparatus in Orthopaedic Surgery.* Oxford : Blackwell Scientific Publications.
PERKINS, G. (1961): *Orthopaedics.* London : London University, Athlone Press.
RANG, M. (ed.) (1969): *The Growth Plate and its Disorders.* Edinburgh : Livingstone.
TAYLOR, G. W. & WILKINSON, J. F. (1967): Vascular Surgery. Vol. 14 of *Clinical Surgery*, ed. Rob & Smith. London : Butterworth.
VAUGHAN, J. (1970): *The Physiology of Bone.* Oxford : Oxford University Press.
WILES, P. & SWEETNAM, R. (1965) : *Essentials of Orthopaedics,* 4th ed. London : Churchill.

SPECIFIC WORKS

INTRODUCTION

ANDRY, N. (1743, reprod. 1961): *Orthopaedia.* Philadelphia : Lippincott.
BIGELOW, H. J. (1846): Insensibility during Surgical Operations produced by Inhalation. Boston Medical and Surgical Journal, **35,** 309.
COOPER, A. (1823) : *Treatise on Dislocations and Fractures of the Joints,* 2nd ed., London : Longmans [etc.].
DUBOS, R. J. (1951) : *Louis Pasteur: Freelance of Science.* London : Gollancz.
HOLDSWORTH, F. W. (1964): Surgical Training. Journal of Bone and Joint Surgery, **46B,** 3.
JONES, A. ROCYN (1956) : A Review of Orthopaedic Surgery in Britain. Journal of Bone and Joint Surgery, **38B,** 27.
JONES, A. ROCYN (1948): Hugh Owen Thomas. Journal of Bone and Joint Surgery, **30B,** 547.
JONES, A. ROCYN (1948): Lister. Journal of Bone and Joint Surgery, **30B,** 196.
JONES, A. ROCYN (1948): John Hunter. Journal of Bone and Joint Surgery, **30B,** 357.
LISTER, J. (1867): On the Antiseptic Principle in the Practice of Surgery. Lancet, **2,** 353.
LONG, C. W. (1849): An Account of the First Use of Sulphuric Ether by Inhalation as an Anaesthetic in Surgical Operations. Southern Medical and Surgical Journal, **5,** 705.
MAYER, L. (1950): Orthopaedic Surgery in the United States of America. Journal of Bone and Joint Surgery, **32B,** 461.
MORTON, W. T. G. (Quoted by Bigelow ; see above).
MORTON, W. T. G. Letheon [a circular]. Boston : Dutton & Wentworth.
OSMOND-CLARKE, H. (1950): Half a Century of Orthopaedic Progress in Great Britain. Journal of Bone and Joint Surgery, **32B,** 620.
PLATT, H. (1950): The Evolution and Scope of Modern Orthopaedics. In *Modern Trends in Orthopaedics* (1). London : Butterworth.
PLATT, H. (1950): Orthopaedics in Continental Europe, 1900-50. Journal of Bone and Joint Surgery, **32B,** 570.
RÖNTGEN, W. C. (1896): On a New Kind of Rays. Nature, **53,** 274, 377.

CHAPTER ONE

Clinical Methods

Joint Movement : Method of Recording

AMERICAN ACADEMY OF ORTHOPAEDIC SURGEONS (1960): *Joint Motion : Method of Measuring and Recording.* Edinburgh: Livingstone.

Radiographic Examination

BRAILSFORD, J. F. (1953): *The Radiology of Bones and Joints*. London: Churchill.

CAFFEY, J. (1961): *Pediatric X-Ray Diagnosis*. Chicago: Year Book Medical Publishers.

FREIBERGER, R. H. & HALPERN, M. (1967): Orthopaedic Radiology. In *Modern Trends in Orthopaedics* (5) (ed. Graham). London: Butterworth.

SHANKS, S. C. & KERLEY, P. (eds.) (1970): *A Text-book of X-Ray Diagnosis*, 4th ed. *Vol. VI, Bones, Joints and Soft Tissues*. London: Lewis.

SUTTON, D. (1962): *Arteriography*. Edinburgh: Livingstone.

Pathology

CANTAROW, A. & TRUMPER, M. (1962): *Clinical Biochemistry*, 6th ed. Philadelphia: Saunders.

DYKE, S. C. (ed.) (1968): *Recent Advances in Clinical Pathology* (Series 5). London: Churchill.

GRAY, J. D. A., & DISCOMBE, G. (1966): *Clinical Pathology*. Oxford: Blackwell Scientific Publications.

SOLOMON, L. (1967): Laboratory Investigations in Connective Tissue Disease. In *Modern Trends in Orthopaedics* (5) (ed. Graham). London: Butterworth.

WOODS, C. G. (1971): *Diagnostic Orthopaedic Pathology*. Oxford: Blackwell Scientific Publications.

Electrodiagnosis

PARRY, C. B. WYNN (1961): Electrodiagnosis. Journal of Bone and Joint Surgery, **43B**, 222.

Treatment of Orthopaedic Disorders

ANDERSON, W. V. (1967): Lengthening of the Lower Limb. In *Modern Trends in Orthopaedics* (5) (ed. Graham). London: Butterworth.

BAADSGAARD, K. (1969): Kiel Bone in the Treatment of Pseudarthrosis. Acta Orthopaedica Scandinavica, **40**, 696.

BURROWS, H. J. & COLTART, W. D. (1951): *Treatment by Manipulation*. London: Eyre & Spottiswoode.

BURWELL, G. (1969): The Fate of Bone Grafts. In *Recent Advances in Orthopaedics* (ed. Apley). London: Churchill.

CAMPBELL, W. C. (1971): *Operative Orthopaedics*, 5th ed., ed. Crenshaw. London: Henry Kimpton.

CHARNLEY, J. (1953): *Compression Arthrodesis*. Edinburgh: Livingstone.

COZEN, L. (1966): *An Atlas of Orthopaedic Surgery*. London: Henry Kimpton.

CYRIAX, J. (1965): *Text-book of Orthopaedic Medicine, Vol. 2*. London: Cassell.

HALLEN, L. G. (1966): Heterologous Transplantation with Kiel Bone. Acta Orthopaedica Scandinavica, **37**, 1.

HENRY, A. K. (1957): *Extensile Exposure*, 2nd ed. Edinburgh: Livingstone.

HØSTRUP, H. & PILGAARD, S. (1969): Epiphysiodesis and Epiphysial Stapling in the Lower Limbs. Acta Orthopaedica Scandinavica, **40**, 130.

McGREGOR, I. A. (1968): *Fundamental Techniques of Plastic Surgery and their Surgical Application*, 4th ed. Edinburgh: Livingstone.

PARRY, C. B. WYNN (1966): *Rehabilitation of the Hand*, 2nd ed. London: Butterworth.

PERKINS, G. (1953): Rest and Movement. Journal of Bone and Joint Surgery, **35B**, 521.

PLEWES, L. W. (1963): Rehabilitation. In *Recent Advances in Surgery of Trauma*. London: Churchill.

POIRIER, H. (1968): Epiphysial Stapling and Leg Equalisation. Journal of Bone and Joint Surgery, **50B**, 61.
THOMAS, H. O. (1875, reprod. 1962): *Diseases of the Hip, Knee and Ankle Joints.* Boston : Little, Brown.

CHAPTER TWO

General Survey of Orthopaedic Disorders

Injuries

ADAMS, J. C. (1968): *Outline of Fractures,* 5th ed. Edinburgh : Livingstone.
WATSON-JONES, R. (1952-55): *Fractures and Joint Injuries.* Edinburgh : Livingstone.

Deformities and Malformations

DUTHIE, R. B. & TOWNES, P. L. (1967): The Genetics of Orthopaedic Conditions. Journal of Bone and Joint Surgery, **49B**, 229.
HENKEL, L. & WILLERT, H-G (1969): Dysmelia. Journal of Bone and Joint Surgery, **51B**, 399.
JAMES, J. I. P. & WYNNE-DAVIES, R. (1969) : Genetic Factors in Orthopaedics. In *Recent Advances in Orthopaedics* (ed. Apley). London : Churchill.
McKENZIE, D. S. (1957): The Prosthetic Management of Congenital Deformities of the Extremities. Journal of Bone and Joint Surgery, **39B**, 233.
NANCE, W. E., ELMORE, S. M. & HILLMAN, J. W. (1965): Genetics and Orthopaedics. (Instructional Course Lecture, American Academy of Orthopaedic Surgeons.) Journal of Bone and Joint Surgery, **47A**, 1260.
NORMAN, A. P. (ed.) (1963) : *Congenital Abnormalities in Infancy.* Oxford : Blackwell Scientific Publications.

Arthritis

ADAM, A., MACDONALD, A. & MACKENZIE, I. G. (1967): Monarticular Brucellar Arthritis in Children. Journal of Bone and Joint Surgery, **49B**, 652.
BAUM, D. (1963) : Rheumatic Fever. Pediatric Clinics of North America, **10**, 899.
BIGGS, R. & MacFARLANE, R. G. (1970) : *Human Blood Coagulation and its Disorders,* 4th ed. Oxford : Blackwell Scientific Publications.
COPEMAN, W. S. C. (1968) : Some Thoughts on the Surgical Treatment of Rheumatic Diseases. Annals of the Royal College of Surgeons of England, **43**, 274.
CURREY, H. L. F. & MASON, R. M. (1969) : Gout and Chondrocalcinosis (Pseudogout). In *Recent Advances in Orthopaedics* (ed. Apley). London : Churchill.
FISK, G. R. (1952) : Hyperplasia and Metaplasia in Synovial Membrane. Annals of the Royal College of Surgeons of England, **2**, 157.
FRANCE, W. G. & WOLF, P. (1965) : Treatment and Prevention of Chronic Haemorrhagic Arthropathy and Contractures in Haemophilia. Journal of Bone and Joint Surgery, **47B**, 247.
HILL, A. G. S. (ed.) (1966) : *Modern Trends in Rheumatology.* London : Butterworth.
KELLGREN, J. H. (1964) : The Epidemiology of Rheumatic Diseases. Annals of the Rheumatic Diseases, **23**, 109.
LIPSCOMB, P. R. (1968) : Surgery for Rheumatoid Arthritis. Journal of Bone and Joint Surgery, **50A**, 575.
LLOYD-ROBERTS, G. C. (1960) : Suppurative Arthritis of Infancy. Journal of Bone and Joint Surgery, **42B**, 706.

McEWEN, C. (1968): Early Synovectomy in the Treatment of Rheumatoid Arthritis. New England Journal of Medicine, **279**, 420.

NUKI, G. & DICK, W. C. (1969): Rheumatoid Arthritis: Drug Therapy. Hospital Medicine, **2**, 1962.

NUKI, G., FREEMAN, P. & JACKSON, I. (1969): Rheumatoid Arthritis: Surgical Management. Hospital Medicine, **2**, 1951.

PATERSON, D. C. (1970): Acute Suppurative Arthritis in Infancy and Childhood. Journal of Bone and Joint Surgery, **52B**, 424.

ROAF, R., KIRKALDY-WILLIS, W. H. & CATHRO, A. J. M. (1959): *Surgical Treatment of Bone and Joint Tuberculosis.* Edinburgh: Livingstone.

SCHWARZ, G. S., BERENYI, M. R. & SIEGEL, M. W. (1969): Atrophic Arthropathy and Diabetic Neuritis. American Journal of Roentgenology, **106**, 523.

SWEETNAM, R. (1969): Corticosteroid Arthropathy and Tendon Rupture. Journal of Bone and Joint Surgery, **51B**, 397.

WHALEY, K. & DICK, W. C. (1969): Rheumatoid Arthritis: Aetiological and Pathogenic Considerations. Hospital Medicine, **2**, 1916.

Osteochondritis Dissecans; Loose Bodies

JEFFREYS, T. E. (1967): Synovial Chondromatosis. Journal of Bone and Joint Surgery, **49B**, 530.

MURPHY, F. P., DAHLIN, D. C. & SULLIVAN, C. R. (1962): Articular Synovial Chondromatosis. Journal of Bone and Joint Surgery, **44A**, 77.

ROBERTS, N. W. (1957): Osteochondritis Dissecans. Journal of Bone and Joint Surgery, **39B**, 219.

SMILLIE, I. S. (1960): *Osteochondritis Dissecans.* Edinburgh: Livingstone.

Infections of Bone

BLOCKEY, N. J. & WATSON, J. T. (1970): Acute Osteomyelitis in Children. Journal of Bone and Joint Surgery, **52B**, 77.

CLAWSON, D. K. & DUNN, A. W. (1967): Management of Common Bacterial Infections of Bones and Joints. (Instructional Course Lecture: American Academy of Orthopaedic Surgeons.) Journal of Bone and Joint Surgery, **49A**, 164.

CLAWSON, D. K. & STEVENSON, J. K. (1965): Treatment of Chronic Osteomyelitis. Surgery, Gynecology and Obstetrics, **120**, 59.

EVANS, E. M. & DAVIES, D. M. (1969): Treatment of Chronic Osteomyelitis by Saucerisation and Secondary Skin Grafting. Journal of Bone and Joint Surgery, **51B**, 454.

ROWE, R. C. (1962): Management of Osteomyelitis following Fractures of the Extremities. New York Journal of Medicine, **62**, 1200.

TRONZO, R. G. & DOWLING, J. J. (1962): Acute Haematogenous Osteomyelitis of Children in the Era of Broad-spectrum Antibiotics. Clinical Orthopaedics, **22**, 108.

WILKINSON, M. C. (1965): The Treatment of Bone and Joint Tuberculosis. Annals of the Royal College of Surgeons of England, **37**, 19.

Tumours of Bone

BARNES, R. & CATTO, M. (1966): Chondrosarcoma of Bone. Journal of Bone and Joint Surgery, **48B**, 729.

DAHLIN, D. C., COVENTRY, M. B. & SCANLON, P. (1961): Ewing's Sarcoma. Journal of Bone and Joint Surgery, **43A**, 185.

DAHLIN, D. C. & COVENTRY, M.B. (1967). Osteogenic Sarcoma. Journal of Bone and Joint Surgery, **49A**, 101.

DAHLIN, D. C. & IVINS, J. C. (1969): Fibrosarcoma of Bone. Cancer, **23**, 35.

EYRE-BROOK, A. L. & PRICE, C. H. G. (1969): Fibrosarcoma of Bone. Journal of Bone and Joint Surgery, **51B**, 20.

GOLDENBERG, R. R., CAMPBELL, C. J. & BONFIGLIO, M. (1970): Giant-Cell Tumour of Bone: Analysis of 218 Cases. Journal of Bone and Joint Surgery, 52A, 619.

GRIFFITHS, D. LL. (1966): Orthopaedic Aspects of Myelomatosis. Journal of Bone and Joint Surgery, 48B, 703.

JAFFE, H. L. (1958): Tumors and Tumorous Conditions of the Bones and Joints. London: Henry Kimpton.

LEE, E. S. & MACKENZIE, D. H. (1964): Osteosarcoma. British Journal of Surgery, 51, 252.

LICHTENSTEIN, L. (1965): Bone Tumours. St. Louis: The C. V. Mosby Co.

MARCOVE, R. C., MIKE, M., HAJEK, J. V., LEVIN, A. G. & HUTTER, R. V. P. (1970): Osteogenic Sarcoma under the Age of Twenty-one. Journal of Bone and Joint Surgery, 52A, 411.

MOORE, M. (1971): Tumour-specific Antigens: Their Possible Significance in the Etiology and Treatment of Malignant Disease. Journal of Bone and Joint Surgery, 53B, 13.

PRICE, C. H. G. & GOLDIE, W. (1969): Paget's Sarcoma of Bone. Journal of Bone and Joint Surgery, 51B, 205.

SCHAJOWICZ, F. (1961): Giant Cell Tumours of Bone. Journal of Bone and Joint Surgery, 43A, 1.

SWEETNAM, R. (1969): Osteosarcoma. Annals of the Royal College of Surgeons of England, 44, 38.

WANG, C. C. & FLEISCHLI, D. J. (1968): Primary Reticulum Cell Sarcoma of Bone with Emphasis on Radiation Therapy. Cancer, 22, 994.

WATT, J. (1968): The Use of Cytotoxic Drugs in the Surgery of Malignant Disease. Journal of Bone and Joint Surgery, 50B, 511.

WOODRUFF, M. (1969): The Challenge of Osteosarcoma. Annals of the Royal College of Surgeons of England, 44, 299.

Other Local Affections of Bone

BOSEKER, E. H., BICKEL, W. H. & DAHLIN, D. C. (1968): Clinico-pathologic Study of Simple Unicameral Bone Cysts. Surgery, Gynecology and Obstetrics, 127, 550.

CLOUGH, J. R. & PRICE, C. H. G. (1968): Aneurysmal Bone Cysts. Journal of Bone and Joint Surgery, 50B, 116.

DABSKA, M. & BURACZEWSKI, J. (1969): Aneurysmal Bone Cyst. Cancer, 23, 371.

FOWLES, J. V. & BOBECHKO, W. P. (1970): Solitary Eosinophilic Granuloma in Bone. Journal of Bone and Joint Surgery, 52B, 238.

HENRY, A. (1969): Monostotic Fibrous Dysplasia. Journal of Bone and Joint Surgery, 51B, 300.

NEER, C. S., FRANCIS, K. C., MARCOVE, R. C., TERZ, J. & CARBONARA, P. N. (1966): Treatment of Unicameral Bone Cyst. Journal of Bone and Joint Surgery, 48A, 731.

POULSEN, J. O. (1969): Osteoid Osteoma. Acta Orthopaedica Scandinavica, 40, 198.

General Affections of the Skeleton

BAILEY, J. A. (1970): Orthopaedic Aspects of Achondroplasia. Journal of Bone and Joint Surgery, 52A, 1285.

BURNETT, C. H., DENT, C. E., HARPER, C. & WARLAND, B. J. (1964): Vitamin D-Resistant Rickets. American Journal of Medicine, 36, 222.

BURROWS, H. J. (1950): The Bone Dystrophies. In Modern Trends in Ortho-paedics (2). London: Butterworth.

CHALMERS, J., CONACHER, W. D. H., GARDNER, D. L. & SCOTT, P. J. (1967): Osteomalacia: A Common Disease in Elderly Women. Journal of Bone and Joint Surgery, 49B, 403.

DENT, C. E. & HARRIS, H. (1956) : Hereditary Forms of Rickets and Osteo-malacia. Journal of Bone and Joint Surgery, 38B, 204.
DENT, C. E. & SMITH, R. (1969) : Nutritional Osteomalacia. Quarterly Journal of Medicine, 38, 195.
FAIRBANK, H. A. T. (1951) : *An Atlas of General Affections of the Skeleton.* Edinburgh : Livingstone.
FIRAT, D. & STUTZMAN, L. (1968) : Fibrous Dysplasia of Bone. American Journal of Medicine, 44, 421.
FLYNN, J. E. & GRAHAM, J. H. (1964) : Myositis Ossificans. Surgery, Gyne-cology and Obstetrics, 118, 1001.
HARRIS, W. H., DUDLEY, H. R. & BARRY, R. J. (1962) : Natural History of Fibrous Dysplasia. Journal of Bone and Joint Surgery, 44A, 207.
HUNT, J. C. & PUGH, D. G. (1961) : Skeletal Lesions in Neurofibromatosis. Radiology, 76, 1.
JACKSON, W. P. U. (1967) : *Calcium Metabolism and Bone Disease.* London : Edward Arnold.
KING, J. D. & BOBECHKO, W. P. (1971) : Osteogenesis Imperfecta. Journal of Bone and Joint Surgery, 53B, 72.
MURRAY, R. O. (1961) : Steroids and the Skeleton. Radiology, 77, 729.
PIERCE, D. S., WALLACE, W. M. & HERNDON, C. H. (1964) : Long-term Treat-ment of Vitamin-D Resistant Rickets. Journal of Bone and Joint Surgery, 46A, 978.
PYRAH, L. N., HODGKINSON, A. & ANDERSON, C. K. (1966) : Primary Hyper-parathyroidism. British Journal of Surgery, 53, 245.
SIFFERT, R. S. (1966) : The Growth Plate and its Affections. (Instructional Course Lecture, American Academy of Orthopaedic Surgeons.) Journal of Bone and Joint Surgery, 48A, 546.
SISSONS, H. A., ROSE, G. A., JASANI, C., NORDIN, B. E. C., SMITH, D. A. & SWANSON, I. (1966) : Osteoporosis (Symposium). Proceedings of the Royal Society of Medicine, 58, 435.
SOFIELD, H. A. (1959) : Fragmentation, Realignment and Intramedullary Rod Fixation of Deformities of the Long Bones in Children. Journal of Bone and Joint Surgery, 41A, 1371.
URIST, M. R. (1964) : Recent Advances in the Physiology of Calcification. (Instructional Course Lecture, American Academy of Orthopaedic Surgeons.) Journal of Bone and Joint Surgery, 46A, 889.

Tumours of Soft Tissue

HAMPOLE, M. K. & JACKSON, B. A. (1968) : Analysis of Twenty-four Cases of Malignant Synovioma. Canadian Medical Association Journal, 99, 1025.
PACK, G. T. & ANGLEM, T. J. (1939) : Tumours of the Soft Somatic Tissues in Infancy and Childhood. Journal of Pediatrics, 15, 372.
TILLOTSON, J. F., McDONALD, J. R. & JANES, J. M. (1951) : Synovial Sarcomata. Journal of Bone and Joint Surgery, 33A, 459.

Poliomyelitis

CLARK, J. M. P. (1956) : Muscle and Tendon Transposition in Poliomyelitis. In *Modern Trends in Orthopaedics* (2). London : Butterworth.
European Association against Poliomyelitis (1959) : Symposium. Journal of Bone and Joint Surgery, 41B, 883.
SHARRARD, W. J. W. (1967) : Paralytic Deformity of the Lower Limb. Journal of Bone and Joint Surgery, 49B, 731.
STUART-HARRIS, C. H. (1964) : Poliovirus Vaccines and the Control of Polio-myelitis. Proceedings of the Royal Society of Medicine, 57, 459.

Cerebral Palsy

CRAIG, J. J. (1967) : Cerebral Palsy. In *Modern Trends in Orthopaedics* (5) (ed. Graham). London : Butterworth.

MORTENS, J. (1965) : Surgery of the Hand in Cerebral Palsy. Acta Orthopaedica Scandinavica, **36,** 411.

POLLOCK, G. A. & ENGLISH, T. A. (1967) : Transplantation of the Hamstring Muscles in Cerebral Palsy. Journal of Bone and Joint Surgery, **49B,** 80.

SHARRARD, W. J. W. (1969) : The Orthopaedic Surgery of Cerebral Palsy and Spina Bifida. In *Recent Advances in Orthopaedics* (ed. Apley). London : Churchill.

Spina Bifida

MENELAUS, M. B. (1969) : Dislocation and Deformity of the Hip in Children with Spina Bifida Cystica. Journal of Bone and Joint Surgery, **51B, 205.**

SHARRARD, W. J. W. & GROSFIELD, I. (1968): The Management of Deformity and Paralysis of the Foot in Myelomeningocele. Journal of Bone and Joint Surgery, **50B,** 456.

WALKER, G. F. (1968) : The Orthopaedics of Myelomeningocele in Infancy. Hospital Medicine, **2,** 900.

Peripheral Nerve Injuries

BARNES, R. (1956) : Peripheral Nerve Injuries. In *Modern Trends in Orthopaedics* (2). London : Butterworth.

GUPTA, S. K., HELAL, B. H. & KIELY, P. (1969): The Prognosis in Zoster Paralysis. Journal of Bone and Joint Surgery, **51B,** 593.

KOPELL, H. P. & THOMPSON, W. A. L. (1963) : *Peripheral Entrapment Neuropathies.* Baltimore : Williams & Wilkins.

Medical Research Council (1943) : Aids to the Investigation of Peripheral Nerve Injuries. War Memorandum No. 7. London : H.M.S.O.

SEDDON, H. J. (1942) : Classification of Nerve Injuries. British Medical Journal, **2,** 237.

SEDDON, H. J. (1954) : Clinical Manifestations of Nerve Injury. In *Peripheral Nerve Injuries.* Medical Research Council Special Report Series, No. 282. London : H.M.S.O.

SEDDON, H. J. (1963) : Nerve Grafting. Journal of Bone and Joint Surgery, **45B,** 447.

SUNDERLAND, S. (1968): *Nerves and Nerve Injuries.* Edinburgh: Livingstone.

YEOMAN, P. M. (1963) : Peripheral Nerve Injuries. In *Recent Advances in the Surgery of Trauma.* London : Churchill.

YEOMAN, P. M. (1968): Cervical Myelography in Traction Injuries of the Brachial Plexus. Journal of Bone and Joint Surgery, **50B,** 253.

CHAPTER THREE

Neck and Cervical Spine

Deformities

BONOLA, A. (1956) :   Surgical Treatment of the Klippel-Feil Syndrome. Journal of Bone and Joint Surgery, **38B,** 440.

GARBER, N. (1964) : Abnormalities of the Atlas and Axis Vertebrae. (Instructional Course Lecture, American Academy of Orthopaedic Surgeons.) Journal of Bone and Joint Surgery, **46A,** 1782.

GRAY, S. W., ROMAINE, C. B. & SKANDALAKIS, J. E. (1964) : Congenital Fusion of the Cervical Vertebrae. Surgery, Gynecology and Obstetrics, **118,** 373.

JONES, P. G. (1968) : *Torticollis in Infancy and Childhood.* Springfield, Illinois : Charles C. Thomas.

MACDONALD, D. (1969): Sternomastoid Tumour and Muscular Torticollis. Journal of Bone and Joint Surgery, 51B, 432.
WOODWARD, J. W. (1961): Congenital Elevation of the Scapula. Journal of Bone and Joint Surgery, 43A, 219.

Infections

GARCIA, A. & GRANTHAM, S. A. (1960): Haematogenous Pyogenic Vertebral Osteomyelitis. Journal of Bone and Joint Surgery, 42A, 429.
HODGSON, A. R., STOCK, F. E., FANG, H. S. Y. & ONG, G. B. (1960): Anterior Spinal Fusion [for tuberculosis]. British Journal of Surgery, 48, 172.

Arthritis and Disc Lesions

CRELLIN, R. Q., MACCABE, J. J. & HAMILTON, E. B. D. (1970): Severe Subluxation of the Cervical Spine in Rheumatoid Arthritis. Journal of Bone and Joint Surgery, 52B, 244.
HARRIS, P. (1963): The Anterior Approach to Excision of Cervical Discs. Proceedings of the Royal Society of Medicine, 56, 807.
HIRSCH, C. (1960): Cervical Disc Rupture. Acta Orthopaedica Scandinavica, 30, 172.
LIVERSEDGE, L. A. (1959): Cervical Spondylosis. Postgraduate Medical Journal, 35, 380.
LOGUE, V. (1959): Cervical Spondylosis. In *Modern Trends in Diseases of the Vertebral Column*. London: Butterworth.
ROBINSON, A. R. et al. (1962): The Results of Anterior Interbody Fusion of the Cervical Spine. Journal of Bone and Joint Surgery, 44A, 1569.
ROGERS, L. (1961): The Surgical Treatment of Cervical Spondylotic Myelopathy. Journal of Bone and Joint Surgery, 43B, 3.
WILKINSON, M., BONNEY, G., BREWERTON, D. A. & KNIGHT, G. (1964): Symposium on Cervical Spondylosis. Proceedings of the Royal Society of Medicine, 57, 159.

Cervical Rib

BONNEY, G. (1965): The Scalenus Medius Band. Journal of Bone and Joint Surgery, 47B, 268.
BRANNON, E. W. (1963): Cervical Rib Syndrome. Journal of Bone and Joint Surgery, 45A, 977.
EASTCOTT, H. H. G. (1962): Reconstruction of the Subclavian Artery for Complications of Cervical-rib and Thoracic-outlet Syndrome. Lancet, 2, 1243.
GRIFFITHS, D. LL. (1952): The Thoracic Inlet. Journal of Bone and Joint Surgery, 34B, 167.

Spondylolisthesis

DUNBAR, H. S. & RAY, B. S. (1961): Chronic Atlanto-axial Dislocation with Late Neurologic Manifestations. Surgery, Gynecology and Obstetrics, 113, 757.
SOUTHWICK, W. O. & ROBINSON, R. A. (1961): Recent Advances in Surgery of the Cervical Spine. Surgical Clinics of North America, 41, 1661.

CHAPTER FOUR

Trunk and Spine

General

BIANCO, A. J. (1968): Low Back Pain and Sciatica: Diagnois and Indications for Treatment. Journal of Bone and Joint Surgery, 50A, 170.

HOOVER, N. W. (1968): Methods of Lumbar Fusion. Journal of Bone and Joint Surgery, 50A, 194.

Deformities and Anomalies

BLUMEL, J., EVANS, E. B., HADNOTT, J. L. & EGGERS, G. W. N. (1962): Congenital Skeletal Anomalies of the Spine. American Surgeon, 28, 501.

COLLIS, D. K. & PONSETI, I. V. (1969): Long-term Follow-up of Patients with Idiopathic Scoliosis not Treated Surgically. Journal of Bone and Joint Surgery, 51A, 425.

GOLDSTEIN, L. A. (1966): Surgical Management of Scoliosis. (Instructional Course Lecture, American Academy of Orthopaedic Surgeons.) Journal of Bone and Joint Surgery, 48A, 167.

HARRINGTON, P. R. (1967): Instrumentation in Structural Scoliosis. In *Modern Trends in Orthopaedics* (5) (ed. Graham). London : Butterworth.

HARRIS, R. I. (1959): Congenital Anomalies. In *Modern Trends in Diseases of the Vertebral Column.* London : Butterworth.

JAMES, E. S. & LASSMAN, L. P. (1962): Spinal Dysraphism. Journal of Bone and Joint Surgery, 44B, 828.

JAMES, J. I. P. (1967): *Scoliosis.* Edinburgh : Livingstone.

JAMES, J. I. P. (1970): The Etiology of Scoliosis. Journal of Bone and Joint Surgery, 52B, 410.

MOE, J. H. (1966): Evaluation of the Surgical Treatment of Idiopathic Scoliosis (Symposium at Dixième Congrès International de Chirurgie Orthopédique et de Traumatologie). Brussels : Acta Medica Belgica.

RISSER, J. C. (1964): Scoliosis: Past and Present. (Instructional Course Lecture, American Academy of Orthopaedic Surgeons.) Journal of Bone and Joint Surgery, 46A, 167.

ROAF, R. (1966): *Scoliosis.* Edinburgh : Livingstone.

SCOTT, J. C. (1965): Scoliosis and Neurofibromatosis. Journal of Bone and Joint Surgery, 47B, 240.

TAMBORNINO, J. M., ARMBRUST, E. N. & MOE, J. H. (1964): Harrington Instrumentation in Correction of Scoliosis. Journal of Bone and Joint Surgery, 46A, 313.

TILL, K. (1969): Spinal Dysraphism. Journal of Bone and Joint Surgery, 51B, 415.

Infections

AHN, B. H. (1968): Treatment of Pott's Paraplegia. Acta Orthopaedica Scandinavica, 39, 145.

BAKALIM, G. (1960): Tuberculous Spondylitis. Acta Orthopaedica Scandinavica, Supplement 47.

GARCIA, A. & GRANTHAM, S. A. (1960): Haematogenous Pyogenic Vertebral Osteomyelitis. Journal of Bone and Joint Surgery, 42A, 429.

GRIFFITHS, D. LL., SEDDON, H. J. & ROAF, R. (1956): *Pott's Paraplegia.* Oxford : Oxford University Press.

HODGSON, A. R. & STOCK, F. E. (1960): Anterior Spine Fusion for Treatment of Tuberculosis of Spine. Journal of Bone and Joint Surgery, 42A, 295.

KIRKALDY-WILLIS, W. H. & THOMAS, T. G. (1965): Anterior Approaches in the Diagnosis and Treatment of Infections of the Vertebral Bodies. Journal of Bone and Joint Surgery, 47A, 87.

KONSTAM, P. G. & BLESOVSKY, A. (1962): The Ambulant Treatment of Spinal Tuberculosis. British Journal of Surgery, 50, 26.

MARTIN, N. S. (1970): Tuberculosis of the Spine. Journal of Bone and Joint Surgery, 52B, 613.

MENELAUS, M. B. (1964): Discitis. Journal of Bone and Joint Surgery, 46B, 16.

Osteoarthritis and Disc Lesions

ADKINS, E. W. O. (1955): Lumbo-sacral Arthrodesis after Laminectomy. Journal of Bone and Joint Surgery, **37B**, 208.

ARMSTRONG, J. R. (1965): *Lumbar Disc Lesions*, 3rd ed. Edinburgh: Livingstone.

PENNYBACKER, J. (1968): Lumbar Disc Protrusions. Hospital Medicine, **2**, 1088.

ROBINSON, R. G. (1965): Massive Protrusions of Lumbar Disks. British Journal of Surgery, **52**, 858.

SACKS, S. (1965): Anterior Interbody Fusion of the Lumbar Spine. Journal of Bone and Joint Surgery, **47B**, 211.

WILTBERGER, B. R. (1963): Surgical Treatment of Degenerative Disease of the Back. (Instructional Course Lecture, American Academy of Orthopaedic Surgeons.) Journal of Bone and Joint Surgery, **45A**, 1509.

Ankylosing Spondylitis

ADAMS, J. C. (1952): Technique, Dangers and Safeguards in Osteotomy of the Spine. Journal of Bone and Joint Surgery, **34B**, 226.

GRAHAM, D. C. (1960): Leukaemia Following X-ray Therapy for Ankylosing Spondylitis. American Medical Association Archives of Internal Medicine, **105**, 51.

HART, F. D. (1966): Lessons Learnt in a Twenty-year Study of Ankylosing Spondylitis. Proceedings of the Royal Society of Medicine, **59**, 456.

Lancet Editorial (1962): Treatment of Ankylosing Spondylitis. Lancet, **2**, 703.

ROSE, G. K. (1961): Surgical Management of Ankylosing Spondylitis. Rheumatism, **17**, 63.

Osteochondritis

COMPERE, E. L., JOHNSON, W. E. & COVENTRY, M. B. (1954): Vertebra Plana (Calvé's Disease) due to Eosinophilic Granuloma. Journal of Bone and Joint Surgery, **36A**, 969.

Spondylolisthesis

HENDERSON, E. D. (1966): Results of the Surgical Treatment of Spondylolisthesis. Journal of Bone and Joint Surgery, **48A**, 619.

LAURENT, L. E. & EINOLA, S. (1961): Spondylolisthesis in Children and Adolescents. Acta Orthopaedica Scandinavica, **31**, 45.

NEWMAN, P. H. (1963): The Etiology of Spondylolisthesis. Journal of Bone and Joint Surgery, **45B**, 39.

ROMBOLD, C. (1966): Treatment of Spondylolisthesis by Posterolateral Fusion, Resection of the Pars Interarticularis, and Prompt Mobilisation of the Patient. Journal of Bone and Joint Surgery, **48A**, 1282.

Tumours

ROZA, A. C. DA (1964): Primary Intraspinal Tumours. Journal of Bone and Joint Surgery, **46B**, 8.

SISSONS, H. A. (1959): Tumours of the Vertebral Column. In *Modern Trends in Diseases of the Vertebral Column*. London: Butterworth.

CHAPTER FIVE
The Shoulder Region

General

MOSELEY, H. F. (1969): *Shoulder Lesions*. Edinburgh: Livingstone.

Arthritis

See bibliography for Chapter Two.

Dislocation

ADAMS, J. C. (1950) : Recurrent Dislocation of the Shoulder. In *Techniques in British Surgery* (ed. Maingot). Philadelphia : Saunders.

MOSELEY, H F. (1961) : *Recurrent Dislocation of the Shoulder.* Edinburgh: Livingstone.

REEVES, B. (1966) : Arthrography of the Shoulder. Journal of Bone and Joint Surgery, 48B, 424.

ROWE, C. R. (1962) : Acute and Recurrent Dislocations of the Shoulder. (Instructional Course Lecture, American Academy of Orthopaedic Surgeons.) Journal of Bone and Joint Surgery, 44A, 998.

Lesions of the Tendinous Cuff

BLOMSTEDT, B. (1961) : Treatment of Tendinitis Calcarea. Acta Chirurgica Scandinavica, 121, 151.

DEBEYRE, J., PATTE, D. & ELMELIK, E. (1965) : Repair of Ruptures of the Rotator Cuff of the Shoulder. Journal of Bone and Joint Surgery, 47B, 36.

HAMMOND, G. (1962) : Complete Acromionectomy in Treatment of Chronic Tendinitis of Shoulder. Journal of Bone and Joint Surgery, 44A, 494.

LINGE, B. VAN, & MULDER, J. D. (1963) : Function of the Supraspinatus Muscle and its Relation to the Supraspinatus Syndrome. Journal of Bone and Joint Surgery, 45B, 750.

MACNAB, I. & HASTINGS, D. (1968) : Rotator Cuff Tendinitis. Canadian Medical Association Journal, 99, 91.

STAMM, T. T. (1963) : A New Operation for Chronic Subacromial Bursitis. Guy's Hospital Reports, 112, 1.

Frozen Shoulder

CHARNLEY, J. (1959) : Periarthritis of the Shoulder. Postgraduate Medical Journal, 35, 384.

LUNDBERG, B. J. (1969) : The Frozen Shoulder. Acta Orthopaedica Scandinavica Supplementum No. 119.

NEVIASER, J. S. (1962) : Arthrography of the Shoulder Joint : Study of the Findings in Adhesive Capsulitis of the Shoulder. Journal of Bone and Joint Surgery, 44A, 1321.

Sterno-clavicular and Acromio-clavicular Joints

American Academy of Orthopaedic Surgeons (1962) : Treatment of Complete Acromio-clavicular Dislocation. (Instructional Course Lecture.) Journal of Bone and Joint Surgery, 44A, 1008.

BURROWS, H. J. (1951) : Tenodesis of Subclavius in the Treatment of Recurrent Dislocation of the Sterno-clavicular Joint. Journal of Bone and Joint Surgery, 33B, 240.

CHAPTER SIX

The Upper Arm and Elbow

Infections of Bone

See bibliography for Chapter Two.

Tumours of Bone

See bibliography for Chapter Two.

Arthritis

See bibliography for Chapter Two.

Osteochondritis Dissecans

ROBERTS, N. W. (1957): Osteochondritis Dissecans. Journal of Bone and Joint Surgery, **39B**, 219.
ROBERTS, N. & HUGHES, R. (1950): Osteochondritis Dissecans of the Elbow Joint. Journal of Bone and Joint Surgery, **32B**, 348.
SMILLIE, I. S. (1960): *Osteochondritis Dissecans.* Edinburgh: Livingstone.

Tennis Elbow

CYRIAX, J. (1969): *Text-book of Orthopaedic Medicine, Vol. I* (5th ed.). London: Cassell.
SPENCER, G. E. & HERNDON, C. H. (1953): Surgical Treatment of Epicondylitis. Journal of Bone and Joint Surgery, **35A**, 421.
TEGNER, W. S. (1959): Tennis Elbow. Postgraduate Medical Journal, **35**, 390.

Ulnar Neuritis

McGOWAN, A. J. (1950): The Results of Transposition of the Ulnar Nerve for Traumatic Ulnar Neuritis. Journal of Bone and Joint Surgery, **32B**, 293.
OSBORNE, G. (1959): Ulnar Neuritis. Postgraduate Medical Journal, **35**, 392.
VANDERPOOL, D. W., CHALMERS, J., LAMB, D. W. & WHISTON, T. B. (1968): Peripheral Compression Lesions of the Ulnar Nerve. Journal of Bone and Joint Surgery, **50B**, 792.

CHAPTER SEVEN

The Forearm, Wrist and Hand

General

BOYES, J. H. (1971): *Bunnell's Surgery of the Hand.* Oxford: Blackwell Scientific Publications.
CAPENER, N. (1956): The Hand in Surgery. Journal of Bone and Joint Surgery, **38B**, 128.
PARRY, C. B. WYNN (1966): *Rehabilitation of the Hand*, 2nd ed. London: Butterworth.
PULVERTAFT, R. G. (ed.) (1966): *The Hand* (Vol. 7 of *Clinical Surgery.*) London: Butterworth.
PULVERTAFT, R. G. & REID, D. A. C. (1963): Surgery of the Hand in Great Britain. British Journal of Surgery **50**, 673.
RANK, B. K., WAKEFIELD, A. R. & HUESTON, J. T. (1968): *Surgery of Repair as Applied to Hand Injuries*, 3rd ed. Edinburgh: Livingstone.
ROBINS, R. H. C. (1961): *Injuries and Infections of the Hand.* London: Arnold.

Infections of Bone

See bibliography for Chapter Two.

Tumours of Bone

See bibliography for Chapter Two.

Volkmann's Ischaemic Contracture

SEDDON, H. J. (1956): Volkmann's Contracture: Treatment by Excision of the Infarct. Journal of Bone and Joint Surgery, **38B**, 152.

Deformities

BARSKY, A. J. (1951) : Congenital Anomalies of the Hand. Journal of Bone and Joint Surgery, 33A, 35.
ENTIN, M. A. (1958) : Reconstruction of Congenital Abnormalities of the Upper Extremities. Journal of Bone and Joint Surgery, 41A, 681.
HENRY, A. & THORBURN, M. J. (1967) : Madelung's Deformity. Journal of Bone and Joint Surgery, 49B, 66.

Arthritis

CALNAN, J. S. & REIS, N. D. (1968) : Artificial Finger Joints in Rheumatoid Arthritis. Annals of Rheumatic Disease, 27, 207.
FLATT, A. E. (1968) : The Care of the Rheumatoid Hand (2nd ed.) St Louis : The C. V. Mosby Co.
GOLDNER, J. L. & CLIPPINGER, F. W. (1959) : Excision of the Greater Mult-angular Bone as an Adjunct to Mobilisation of the Thumb. Journal of Bone and Joint Surgery, 41A, 609.
KESSLER. I. (1966) : Posterior Synovectomy for Rheumatoid Involvement of the Hand and Wrist. Journal of Bone and Joint Surgery, 48A, 1085.
MARMOR, L. (1965) : Surgical Treatment of the Rheumatoid Hand. Proceedings of the Royal Society of Medicine, 58, 567.
MATTSSON, H. S. (1969) : Arthrodesis of the First Carpo-metacarpal Joint for Osteoarthritis. Acta Orthopaedica Scandinavica, 40, 602.
MURLEY, A. H. G. (1960) : Excision of the Trapezium in Osteoarthritis of the First Carpo-metacarpal Joint. Journal of Bone and Joint Surgery, 42B, 502.
NALEBUFF, E. A. (1969) : Metacarpo-phalangeal Surgery in Rheumatoid Arthritis. Surgical Clinics of North America, 49, 823.
NALEBUFF, E. A. (1969) : Surgical Treatment of Tendon Rupture in the Rheumatoid Hand. Surgical Clinics of North America, 49, 811.
VAINIO, K. (1967) : Surgery of the Rheumatoid Hand. In Modern Trends in Orthopaedics (5) (ed. Graham). London : Butterworth.

Kienböck's Disease

GILLESPIE, H. S. (1961) : Excision of the Lunate Bone in Kienböck's Disease. Journal of Bone and Joint Surgery, 43B, 245.
LEE, M. L. H. (1963) : The Intra-osseous Arterial Pattern of the Carpal Lunate Bone and its Relation to Avascular Necrosis. Acta Orthopaedica Scandinavica, 33, 43.
AGERHOLM, J. C. & GOODFELLOW, J. W. (1963) : Avascular Necrosis of the Lunate Bone Treated by Excision and Prosthetic Replacement. Journal of Bone and Joint Surgery, 45B, 110.

Infections of the Hand

BAILEY, D. (1963) : The Infected Hand. London : Lewis.
LOWDEN, T. G. (1964) : Prevention and Treatment of Hand Infections. Postgraduate Medical Journal, 40, 247.
PIMM, L. H. & WAUGH, W. (1957) : Tuberculous Tenosynovitis. Journal of Bone and Joint Surgery, 39B, 91.
SNEDDON, J. (1971) : The Care of Hand Infections. London : Edward Arnold.
STONE, N. H., HURSCH, H., HUMPHREY, C. R. & BOSWICK, J. A. (1969) : Empiric Selection of Antibiotics for Hand Infections. Journal of Bone and Joint Surgery, 51A, 899.

Tumours

BUTLER, E. D., HAMILL, J. P., SEIPEL, R. S. & LORIMIER, A. A. DE (1960) : Tumors of the Hand. American Journal of Surgery, 100, 293.

Carpal Tunnel Syndrome

BOULTER, P. S. (1959) : The Carpal Tunnel Syndrome. Postgraduate Medical Journal, **35,** 406.

NISSEN, K. I. (1959) : Pain in the Arm and the Carpal Tunnel Syndrome. Postgraduate Medical Journal, **35,** 379.

PHALEN, G. S. (1966) : The Carpal Tunnel Syndrome. Journal of Bone and Joint Surgery, **48A,** 211.

Ganglion

McEVEDY, B. V. (1962) : Simple Ganglia. British Journal of Surgery, **49,** 585.

Dupuytren's Contracture

HONNER, R., LAMB, D. W. & JAMES, J. I. P. (1971) : Dupuytren's Contracture. Journal of Bone and Joint Surgery, **53B,** 240.

HUESTON, J. T. (1965) : Dupuytren's Contracture. Annals of the Royal College of Surgeons of England, **36,** 134.

LETTIN, A. W. (1964) : Dupuytren's Diathesis. Journal of Bone and Joint Surgery, **46B,** 220.

McFARLANE, R. M. & JAMIESON, W. G. (1966) : Dupuytren's Contracture. Journal of Bone and Joint Surgery, **48A,** 1095.

Tendon Injuries

BROOKS, D. M. (1970) : Problems of Restoration of Tendon Movements after Repair and Grafts. Proceedings of the Royal Society of Medicine, **63,** 67.

HALLBERG, D. & LINDHOLM, A. (1960) : Subcutaneous Rupture of Extensor Tendon of Distal Phalanx of Finger (Mallet Finger). Acta Chirurgica Scandinavica, **119,** 260.

JAMES, J. I. P. (1970) : Suture or Tendon Graft ? Journal of Bone and Joint Surgery, **52B,** 203.

McKENZIE, A. R. (1967) : Function after Reconstruction of Severed Long Flexor Tendons of the Hand. Journal of Bone and Joint Surgery, **49B,** 424.

MADSEN, E. (1970) : Delayed Primary Suture of Flexor Tendons Cut in the Digital Sheath. Journal of Bone and Joint Surgery, **52B,** 264.

MAYER, L. (1971) : Suture or Tendon Graft ? (editorial). Journal of Bone and Joint Surgery, **53B,** 1.

PULVERTAFT, R. G. (1961) : Tendon Grafts. Journal of Bone and Joint Surgery, **43B,** 421.

STARK, H. H. & WILSON, J. N. (1962) : Mallet Finger. Journal of Bone and Joint Surgery, **44A,** 1061.

CHAPTER EIGHT
The Hip Region

Congenital Dislocation

BARLOW, T. G. (1968) : Congenital Dislocation of the Hip. Hospital Medicine, **2,** 571.

CARTER, C. & WILKINSON, J. (1964) : Persistent Joint Laxity and Congenital Dislocation of the Hip. Journal of Bone and Joint Surgery, **46B,** 40.

CARTER, C. O. & WILKINSON, J. A. (1964) : Genetic and Environmental Factors in the Etiology of Congenital Dislocation of the Hip. Clinical Orthopaedics, **33,** 119.

CHIARI, K. (1970) : Pelvic Osteotomy for Hip Subluxation. Journal of Bone and Joint Surgery, **52B,** 174.

CHRISTENSEN, I. (1969): Anteversion Deformity and Derotation Osteotomy in Congenital Dislocation of the Hip. Acta Orthopaedica Scandinavica, **40,** 62.

HENDERSON, R. S. (1970): Osteotomy for Unreduced Congenital Dislocation of the Hip in Adults. Journal of Bone and Joint Surgery, **52B,** 468.

MCKIBBIN, B. (1970): Anatomical Factors in the Stability of the Hip Joint in the Newborn. Journal of Bone and Joint Surgery, **52B,** 148.

PEMBERTON, P. A. (1958): Osteotomy of the Ilium with Rotation of the Acetabular Roof for Congenital Dislocation of the Hip. Journal of Bone and Joint Surgery, **40A,** 724.

RITTER, M. A. & WILSON, P. D. (1968): Colonna Capsular Arthroplasty: Long-term Follow-up. Journal of Bone and Joint Surgery, **50A,** 1305.

SALTER, R. B. (1967): Congenital Dislocation of the Hip. In *Modern Trends in Orthopaedics* (5) (ed. Graham). London: Butterworth.

SALTER, R. B. (1969): An Operative Treatment for Congenital Dislocation and Subluxation of the Hip in the Older Child. In *Recent Advances in Orthopaedics* (ed. Apley). London: Churchill.

SMITH, W. S., PONSETI, I. V., RYDER, C. T. & SALTER, R. B. (1966): Congenital Dislocation of the Hip in the Older Child (Symposium) (Instructional Course Lectures, American Academy of Orthopaedic Surgeons). Journal of Bone and Joint Surgery, **48A,** 1390.

SOMERVILLE, E. W. (1967): The Results of Treatment of 100 Congenitally Dislocated Hips. Journal of Bone and Joint Surgery, **49B,** 258.

TREVOR, D. (1968): The Place of the Hey Groves-Colonna Operation in the Treatment of Congenital Dislocation of the Hip. Annals of the Royal College of Surgeons of England, **43,** 241.

WYNNE-DAVIES, R. (1970): Acetabular Dysplasia and Familial Joint Laxity: Two Etiological Factors in Congenital Dislocation of the Hip. Journal of Bone and Joint Surgery, **52B,** 704.

Arthritis (Inflammatory)

ADAMS, J. A. (1963): Transient Synovitis of the Hip Joint in Children. Journal of Bone and Joint Surgery, **45B,** 471.

EYRE-BROOK, A. (1960): Septic Arthritis of the Hip and Osteomyelitis of the Upper End of the Femur in Infants. Journal of Bone and Joint Surgery, **42B,** 11.

HARDINGE, K. (1970): The Etiology of Transient Synovitis of the Hip in Childhood. Journal of Bone and Joint Surgery, **52B,** 100.

LLOYD-ROBERTS, G. C. (1960): Suppurative Arthritis in Infancy. Journal of Bone and Joint Surgery, **42B,** 706.

OBLETZ, B. E. (1960): Acute Suppurative Arthritis of the Hip in the Neonatal Period. Journal of Bone and Joint Surgery, **42A,** 23.

Arthritis (Degenerative)

ALVIK, I. (1963): Arthrodesis and Arthroplasty of the Hip Joint. Acta Orthopaedica Scandinavica, **33,** 253.

AUFRANC, O. E. (1967): Mould Arthroplasty of the Hip. In *Modern Trends in Orthopaedics* (5) (ed. Graham). London: Butterworth.

CHARNLEY, J. (1961): Arthroplasty of the Hip: A New Operation. Lancet, **I,** 1129.

COVENTRY, M. B. (1969): Osteotomy of the Hip for Degenerative Arthritis. Mayo Clinic Proceedings, **44,** 505.

GUDMUNDSSON, G. (1970): Intertrochanteric Displacement Osteotomy for Painful Osteoarthritis of the Hip. Acta Orthopaedica Scandinavica, **41,** 91.

HIRSCH, C. & GOLDIE, I. (1968): Osteotomy in Osteoarthritis of the Hip Joint. Acta Orthopaedica Scandinavica, **39,** 182.

KOLLBERG, G. & LUNDHOLM, G. (1965): The Voss Operation in Osteo-arthritis of the Hip. Acta Orthopaedica Scandinavica, **36**, 82.

McKEE, G. K. & WATSON-FARRAR, J. (1966): Replacement of Arthritic Hips by the McKee-Farrar Prosthesis. Journal of Bone and Joint Surgery, **48B**, 245.

MERLE D'AUBIGNÉ, R. (1969): Arthroplasty in the Treatment of Degenerative Osteoarthritis of the Hip. In *Recent Advances in Orthopaedics* (ed. Apley). London : Churchill.

NISSEN, K. I. (1963): The Arrest of Early Primary Osteoarthritis of the Hip by Osteotomy. Proceedings of the Royal Society of Medicine, **56**, 1051.

RING, P. A. (1968): Complete Replacement Arthroplasty of the Hip by the Ring Prosthesis. Journal of Bone and Joint Surgery, **50B**, 720.

ROBSON, P. N. & MIERT, P. J. Van (1962) Treatment of Osteoarthritis of the Hip by Interstitial Cobalt 60 Irradiation. British Journal of Surgery, **49**, 624.

SANDER, S. & HALL, K. V. (1962): Denervation of the Hip Joint. Acta Chirurgica Scandinavica, **124**, 106.

SCOTT, J. C. (1963): Pseudarthrosis of the Hip. Clinical Orthopaedics, **31**, 31.

Perthes' Disease

AXER, A. (1965): Subtrochanteric Osteotomy in the Treatment of Perthes' Disease. Journal of Bone and Joint Surgery, **47B**, 489.

CATTERALL, A. (1971): The Natural History of Perthes' Disease. Journal of Bone and Joint Surgery, **53B**, 37.

EVANS, D. L. & LLOYD-ROBERTS, G. C. (1958): Treatment in Legg-Calvé-Perthes' Disease. Journal of Bone and Joint Surgery, **40B**, 182.

RATLIFF, A. H. C. (1967): Perthes' Disease : A Study of Thirty-four Hips Observed for Thirty Years. Journal of Bone and Joint Surgery, **49B**, 102.

Slipped Upper Femoral Epiphysis and Coxa Vara

BLOCKEY, N. J. (1969): Observations on Infantile Coxa Vara. Journal of Bone and Joint Surgery, **51B**, 106.

BORDEN, J., SPENCER, G. E. & HERNDON, C. H. (1966): Treatment of Coxa Vara in Children by Means of a Modified Osteotomy. Journal of Bone and Joint Surgery, **48A**, 1106.

DUNN, D. (1964): The Treatment of Adolescent Slipping of the Upper Femoral Epiphysis. Journal of Bone and Joint Surgery, **46B**, 621.

FAHEY, J. J. & O'BRIEN, E. T. (1965): Acute Slipped Capital Femoral Epiphysis. Journal of Bone and Joint Surgery, **47A**, 1105.

FAIRBANK, T. J. (1969): Manipulative Reduction in Slipped Upper Femoral Epiphysis. Journal of Bone and Joint Surgery, **51B**, 252.

NEWMAN, P. H. (1960): The Surgical Treatment of Slipping of the Upper Femoral Epiphysis. Journal of Bone and Joint Surgery, **42B**, 280.

RIDDELL, D. M. & PEARSON, J. R. (1966): The Treatment of Slipped Upper Femoral Epiphysis by Subtrochanteric Osteotomy. British Journal of Surgery, **53**, 753.

SALENIUS, P. & KIVILAAKSO, R. (1968): Results of Treatment of Slipped Upper Femoral Epiphysis. Acta Orthopaedica Scandinavica Suppementum No. 114.

CHAPTER NINE

The Thigh and Knee

Infections of Bone
See bibliography for Chapter Two.

Bone Tumours

LEE, E. S. & MACKENZIE, D. H. (1964): Osteosarcoma. British Journal of Surgery, **51**, 252.
Also see bibliography for Chapter Two.

Arthritis

BENTLEY, G. & GOODFELLOW, J. W. (1969): Disorganisation of the Knees Following Intra-articular Hydrocortisone Injections. Journal of Bone and Joint Surgery, **51B**, 498.

HARRIS, W. R. & KOSTUIK, J. P. (1970): High Tibial Osteotomy for Osteo-arthritis of the Knee. Journal of Bone and Joint Surgery, **52A**, 330.

JACKSON, J. P., WAUGH, W. & GREEN, J. P. (1969): High Tibial Osteotomy for Osteoarthritis of the Knee. Journal of Bone and Joint Surgery, **51B**, 88.

JONES, G. B. (1968): Arthroplasty of the Knee by the Walldius Prosthesis. Journal of Bone and Joint Surgery, **50B**, 505.

PLATT, G. & PEPLER, C. (1969): Mould Arthroplasty of the Knee. Journal of Bone and Joint Surgery, **51B**, 76.

POTTER, T. A. (1969): Arthroplasty of the Knee with Tibial Metallic Implants of the McKeever and MacIntosh Design. Surgical Clinics of North America, **49**, 903.

SHIERS, L. G. P. (1961): Hinge Arthroplasty for Arthritis. Rheumatism, **17**, 54.

STEVENSON, F. H., CHOLMELEY, J. A. & JORY, H. I. (1958): Tuberculosis of the Knee: Results with Chemotherapy. Tubercle, **39**, 1.

WILKINSON, M. C. (1962): Partial Synovectomy in the Treatment of Tuberculosis of the Knee. Journal of Bone and Joint Surgery, **44B**, 34.
Also see bibliography for Chapter Two.

Chondromalacia of Patella

CROOKS, L. M. (1967): Chondromalacia Patellae. Journal of Bone and Joint Surgery, **49B**, 495.

OUTERBRIDGE, R. E. (1964): Further Studies on the Etiology of Chondromalacia Patellae. Journal of Bone and Joint Surgery, **46B**, 179.

WILES, P., ANDREWS, P. S. & BREMNER, R. A. (1960): Chondromalacia of the Patella. Journal of Bone and Joint Surgery, **42B**, 65.

Injuries of the Menisci

BONNIN, J. G. (1956): Internal Derangements of the Knee Joint and Allied Conditions. In *Modern Trends in Orthopaedics* (2). London: Butterworth.

RIX, R. R. (1962): **Accuracy of Diagnosis of Torn Meniscus** in the Knee. Journal of the American Medical Association, **180**, 60.

SMILLIE, I. S. (1970): *Injuries of the Knee Joint*, 4th ed. Edinburgh: Livingstone.

Osteochondritis Dissecans ; Loose Bodies

GREEN, J. P. (1966): Osteochondritis Dissecans of the Knee. Journal of Bone and Joint Surgery, **48B**, 82.

MURPHY, F. P., DAHLIN, D. C. & SULLIVAN, C. R. (1962): Articular Synovial Chondromatosis. Journal of Bone and Joint Surgery, **44A**, 77.

SMILLIE, I. S. (1957): Treatment of Osteochondritis Dissecans. Journal of Bone and Joint Surgery, **39B**, 248.

SMILLIE, I. S. (1960): *Osteochondritis Dissecans.* Edinburgh: Livingstone.

STOUGAARD, J. (1964): Familial Occurrence of Osteochondritis Dissecans. Journal of Bone and Joint Surgery, **46B**, 542.

Recurrent Dislocation of Patella

BOWKER, J. H. & THOMPSON, E. B. (1964) : Surgical Treatment of Recurrent Dislocation of the Patella. Journal of Bone and Joint Surgery, **46A,** 1451.

CARTER, C. & SWEETNAM, R. (1960) : Recurrent Dislocation of the Patella and of the Shoulder. Journal of Bone and Joint Surgery, **42B,** 721.

HEYWOOD, A. W. B. (1961) : Recurrent Dislocation of the Patella. Journal of Bone and Joint Surgery, **43B,** 508.

CHAPTER TEN
The Leg, Ankle and Foot

General

GIANNESTRAS, N. J. (ed.) (1970): Static Problems of the Foot (Symposium). Clinical Orthopaedics, **70,** 2.

JONES, F. WOOD (1949) : *Structure and Function as Seen in the Foot.* London : Baillière, Tindall and Cox.

LEWIN, P. (1959) : *The Foot and Ankle.* London : Henry Kimpton.

WESTIN, G. W. (1965) : Tendon Transfers about the Foot, Ankle and Hip in the Paralyzed Lower Extremity. (Instructional Course Lecture, American Academy of Orthopaedic Surgeons.) Journal of Bone and Joint Surgery, **47A,** 1430.

Rupture of Calcaneal Tendon

HOOKER, C. H. (1963) : Rupture of the Tendo Calcaneus. Journal of Bone and Joint Surgery, **45B,** 360.

Osteomyelitis

See bibliography for Chapter Two.

Tumours

See bibliography for Chapter Two.

Vascular Lesions

MOZES, M., RAMON, Y. & JAHR, J. (1962) : The Anterior Tibial Syndrome. Journal of Bone and Joint Surgery, **44A,** 730.

SEDDON, H. J. (1966) : Volkmann's Ischaemia in the Lower Limb. Journal of Bone and Joint Surgery, **48B,** 627.

Arthritis

JOPLIN, R. J. (1969) : Surgery of the Forefoot in the Rheumatoid Arthritic Patient. Surgical Clinics of North America, **49,** 847.

MARMOR, L. (1964) : Surgery of the Rheumatoid Foot. Surgery, Gynecology and Obstetrics, **119,** 1009.

Also see bibliography for Chapter Two.

Congenital Club Foot

BEATSON, T. R. & PEARSON, J. R. (1966) : A Method of Assessing Correction in Club Feet. Journal of Bone and Joint Surgery, **48B,** 40.

CLARK, J. M. P. (1968) : Surgical Treatment of Club Foot. Proceedings of the Royal Society of Medicine, **61,** 779.

DWYER, F. C. (1964) : The Relationship of Variations in the Size and Inclination of the Calcaneum to the Shape and Function of the Whole Foot. Annals of the Royal College of Surgeons of England, **34,** 120.

EVANS, D. (1961) : Relapsed Club Foot. Journal of Bone and Joint Surgery, **43B,** 722.

FRIPP, A. T. & SHAW, N. E. (1967): *Club Foot.* Edinburgh : Livingstone.

McCAULEY, J. C. (1966) Clubfoot. Clinical Orthopaedics, **44,** 51.

SINGER, M. (1961): Tibialis Posterior Transfer in Congenital Club Foot. Journal of Bone and Joint Surgery, **43B,** 717.

SWANN, M., LLOYD-ROBERTS, G. C. & CATTERALL, A. (1969): The Anatomy of Uncorrected Club Feet. Journal of Bone and Joint Surgery, **51B,** 263.

WYNNE-DAVIES, R. (1964): Family Studies and the Cause of Congenital Club Foot. Journal of Bone and Joint Surgery, **46B,** 445.

WYNNE-DAVIES, R. (1964): Talipes Equinovarus. Journal of Bone and Joint Surgery, **46B,** 464.

Accessory Bones

O' RAHILLY, R. (1953): A Survey of Carpal and Tarsal Anomalies. Journal of Bone and Joint Surgery, **35A,** 626.

Pes Planus

GRICE, D. S. (1952): An Extra-articular Arthrodesis of the Subastragalar Joint for Correction of Paralytic Flat Feet in Children. Journal of Bone and Joint Surgery, **34A,** 927.

ZACHARIAE, L. (1963): The Grice Operation for Paralytic Flat Feet in Children. Acta Orthopaedica Scandinavica, **33,** 80.

Painful Heel

LAPIDUS, P. W. & GUIDOTTI, F. P. (1965): Management of Painful Heel. Clinical Orthopaedics, **39,** 178.

Forefoot and Toes

CHOLMELEY, J. A. (1958): Hallux Valgus in Adolescents. Proceedings of the Royal Society of Medicine, **51,** 903.

COCKIN, J. (1968): Butler's Operation for Over-riding Fifth Toe. Journal of Bone and Joint Surgery, **50B,** 78.

DOVEY, H. (1969): The Treatment of Hallux Valgus by Distal Osteotomy of the First Metatarsal. Acta Orthopaedica Scandinavica, **40,** 402.

FOWLER, A. W. (1958): Excision of the Germinal Matrix: A Unified Treatment for Embedded Toe-nail and Onychogryposis. British Journal of Surgery, **45,** 382.

FOWLER, A. W. (1959): A Method of Forefoot Reconstruction [for claw toes]. Journal of Bone and Joint Surgery, **41B,** 507.

GIBSON, J. & PIGGOTT, H. (1962): Osteotomy of the Neck of the First Metatarsal in the Treatment of Hallux Valgus. Journal of Bone and Joint Surgery, **44B,** 349.

KESSEL, L. & BONNEY, G. (1958): Hallux Rigidus in the Adolescent. Journal of Bone and Joint Surgery, **40B,** 668.

LLOYD-DAVIES, R. W. & BRILL, G. C. (1963): The Aetiology and Out-patient Treatment of Ingrowing Toe-nails. British Journal of Surgery, **50,** 592.

NISSEN, K. I. (1948): Plantar Digital Neuritis. Journal of Bone and Joint Surgery, **30B,** 84.

SMILLIE, I. S. (1960): *Osteochondritis Dissecans.* Edinburgh : Livingstone.

TAYLOR, R. G. (1951): The Treatment of Claw Toes by Multiple Transfers of Flexor into Extensor Tendons. Journal of Bone and Joint Surgery, **33B.** 539.

Index

(Where bold type is used it indicates the main reference)

A

Abdominal disorders simulating hip disease, 353
  simulating spinal disease, 220
Abscess, Brodie's, **75**, 401
  paraspinal, 187, 189
  psoas, 187
  retropharyngeal, 154
Accessory bones in foot, 414
Acetabuloplasty, 326
Achondroplasia, 107
Aclasis, diaphysial, 84, **104**
Acromegaly, 126
Acromio-clavicular joint, dislocation of, 242
  examination of, 225
  osteoarthritis of, 241
  subluxation of, 242
Active exercises, 19
Acute lumbago, 184, 204, **207**
Adolescent coxa vara, 346
  kyphosis, 198
Albers-Schönberg disease, 36
Albright's syndrome, 110
Amputation, congenital, 37
Amyoplasia congenita, 36
Andry, Nicolas, 1
Aneurysmal bone cyst, 101
Angina pectoris simulating shoulder disease, 244
Ankle, arthritis of, gouty, 407
  haemophilic, 407
  neuropathic, 407
  pyogenic, 405
  rheumatoid, 405
  tuberculous, 405
  Charcot's disease of, 407
  disorders of, 405
  (classification), 398
  examination of, 393
  osteoarthritis of, 406
  recurrent subluxation of, 407
Ankylosing spondylitis, 63, **195**, 218
  cervical spine involvement in, 157
  sacro-iliac joints affected in, 218
Antero-lateral decompression of spinal cord, 190

Apophysitis of calcaneus, 98, **425**
  of tibial tubercle, 98, **388**
Arm, upper, disorders of, 248
  (classification), 248
Arterial insufficiency in lower limb, 403
  in upper limb, 165, **271**
  occlusion, 165, 271, 403
  simulating disease of hip, 353
  of spine, 221
Arteriography, 12, **394**
Arterio-venous fistula, congenital, 36
Arthritis, **42**
  degenerative, 55
  gonococcal, 43
  gouty, **58**
    of ankle, 407
    of toe joints, 440
  haemophilic, **60**
    of ankle, 407
    of elbow, 256
    of knee, 372
  hypertrophic, 55
  infective, 43
  neuropathic, **62**
    of ankle, 407
    of elbow, 257
    of knee, 373
  of rheumatic fever, 63
  osteo-, **55** (*see* osteoarthritis)
  post-traumatic, 55
  pyogenic, **43**
    of ankle, 405
    of elbow, 253
    of hip, 329
    of joints of hand, 277
    of knee, 365
    of shoulder, 227
    of wrist, 276
  rheumatoid, **46**
    of ankle, 405
    of elbow, 254
    of hand joints, 278
    of hip, 332
    of knee, 365
    of shoulder, 228
    of spine, 192
    of wrist, 278
  septic, 43

Arthritis, suppurative, 43
  transient, of hip, 328
  tuberculous, **51**
    of ankle, 405
    of elbow, 254
    of hip, 334
    of knee, 368
    of sacro-iliac joint, 218
    of shoulder, 228
    of sterno-clavicular joint, 242
  types of, 42
Arthrodesis, **26**
  indications for, 26
  methods of, 26
  position for, 27
Arthrography, 12
Arthrogryposis multiplex congenita, 36
Arthroplasty, **28**
  indications for, 28
  of elbow, 254, 255
  of finger joints, 280
  of hip, 327, 333, **340**
  of knee, 367
  of metatarso-phalangeal joint, 434
  methods of, 28
Athetosis, 141
Axonotmesis, 144

B

Back, disorders of, 178
    (classification), 178
  examination of, 173
  pain, postural, 215
Baker's cyst (of knee), 391
Biceps tendinitis, 240
  tendon, long, rupture of, 239
    tenosynovitis of, 240
Biliary disorders simulating shoulder
    disease, 244
  simulating spinal disease, 220
Bone abscess, chronic, **75**, 401
  accessory (in foot), 414
  cyst, 100
  fibrous dysplasia of, monostotic, 101
    polyostotic, 109
  grafts, 30
  infection of, pyogenic, 69
    syphilitic, 79
    tuberculous, 76
  rarefaction of (causes), 127
  tumours of, **81**
    in lower limb, 362, 402
    in upper limb, 250, 270, 295
Bow leg, 386
Brachial pain, causes of, 160
  plexus injuries, 146

Brodie's abscess, **75**, 401
Bryant's triangle, 313
Bursa, trochanteric, tuberculosis of, 35
Bursitis, **128**
  olecranon, 261
  post-calcaneal, 424
  prepatellar, 389
  semimembranosus, 390
  subacromial, 236, 238
  trochanteric, 351

C

Calcaneal apophysitis, 98, **425**
  paratendinitis, 423
  tendon, rupture of, 400
Calcaneus, apophysitis of, 425
  disease of, causing painful heel, 423
  ' osteochondritis ' of, 98, **425**
Calcified deposit in medial ligament of
    knee, 392
  in supraspinatus tendon, 236, 238
Callosities, 432
Calvé's disease of spine, 97, **201**
Capsular arthroplasty of hip, 327
Caries sicca, 228
Carpal tunnel, compression of median
    nerve in, 296
Carpo-metacarpal joint of thumb, osteo-
    arthritis of, 283
Cartilage, semilunar, cyst of, 377
  discoid, 378
  tear of, 374
Causalgia, 145
Cerebral palsy, 137
Cervical rib, 165
  spine, ankylosing spondylitis of, 157
    disorders of, 152
      (classification), 151
    examination of, 148
    osteoarthritis of, 157
    pyogenic infection of, 156
    subluxation of, 168
    tuberculosis of, 153
    tumours involving, 170
  spondylolisthesis, 65, **168**
  spondylosis, 157
Charcot's osteoarthropathy, **62**
  of ankle, 407
  of elbow, 257
  of knee, 373
Cholecystitis simulating shoulder dis-
    ease, 244
  spinal disease, 220
Chondroma, 82
  multiple, 106
  of hand bones, 295

Chondromalacia of patella, 374
Chondromatosis, multiple, 82, **106**
  synovial, 66
    of elbow, 260
    of knee, 382
Chondrosarcoma of bone, 82, **91**, 105, 107
  in hand, 295
Cineradiography, 13
Claudication, intermittent, 403
Clinical examination, methods of, 5
Club foot, congenital, 409
  hand, 37
Clutton's joints, 374
Coccydynia, 216
Coccygeal pain, 216
Codman's triangle, 89
Coeliac disease, 119
  rickets in, 119
Colonna operation (for congenital dis-
  location of hip), 327
Compound palmar ganglion, 293
Conduction tests, 14
Congenital club foot, 409
  deformities, 35
    causes of, 35
  dislocation, 64
    of hip, 321
  high scapula, 153
  short neck, 153
Constriction rings, 37
Contracture, Dupuytren's, 298
  Volkmann's ischaemic, 271
Contrast radiography, 12
Cooper, Sir Astley, 1
Coxa plana, 342
  vara, 350
    adolescent, 346
    congenital, 351
    epiphysial, 346
Cranio-cleido dysostosis, 36
Cretinism, 127
Crutch palsy, 307
Cubitus valgus, 252
  varus, 253
Cup arthroplasty, **28**, 340
Cushing's syndrome, 126
Cyst, Baker's, 391
  bone, 100
  of lateral meniscus, 377
  popliteal, 390

D

Dactylitis, syphilitic, 80
  tuberculous, 76
Decompression of spinal cord, 190
Deep x-ray therapy, 24

Deformity, acquired, 38
  congenital, 35
    causes of, 35
  fixed, estimation of, 8, 316
  Madelung's, 276
  of elbow, 252
  of foot, 409
  of hip, 321
  of knee, 385
  of neck, 152
  of spine, 181, 185
  of toes, 433
  of wrist, 276
  treatment of, 42
De Quervain's tenovaginitis, 304
Diagnosis of orthopaedic disorders, 5
Diaphysial aclasis, 84, **104**
Diathermy, short-wave, 20
Disc, prolapsed (cervical), 161
  (lumbar), 202
Discoid lateral meniscus, 378
Discrepancy of limb length, 33
Dislocation, 64
  congenital, 64
    of hip, 321
  habitual, of patella, 385
  of acromio-clavicular joint, 242
  of sterno-clavicular joint, 242
  pathological, 65
    of hip, 330, 331, 332
  recurrent, 65
    of patella, 383
    of shoulder, 230
    of sterno-clavicular joint, 242
  spontaneous, 65
  traumatic, 64
Drugs, use of, 21
Dupuytren's contracture, 298
Dyschondroplasia, 82, **106**, 295, 402
Dysplasia of bone, fibrous, monostotic,
    101
    polyostotic, 109
Dysraphism, spinal, **141**, 180

E

Ecchondroma, 82
Ectrodactyly, 37
Elbow, arthritis of, haemophilic, 256
    neuropathic, 257
    pyogenic, 253
    rheumatoid, 254
    tuberculous, 254
  Charcot's disease of, 257
  deformities of, 252
  disorders of, 252
    (classification), 248

Elbow, examination of, 245
  loose bodies in, 259
  osteoarthritis of, 255
  osteochondritis dissecans of, 258
  osteochondromatosis of, 260
  tennis, 261
Electrical stimulation of muscles, 19
  tests, 14
Electrodiagnosis, 14
Electromyography, 16
Enchondroma, 82
Environmental factors in congenital
  deformity, 35
Eosinophilic granuloma, 123
  simulating vertebral osteochon-
    dritis, 201
Epicondylitis, 261
Epiphysiodesis, 33, 387
Epiphysis, slipped upper femoral, 346
Equalisation of leg length, 33
Erb's palsy, 146
Ewing's tumour, **92**
  of femur, 363
  of tibia, 403
Excision arthroplasty, 28
Exercises, active, 19
Exostosis, multiple, 84, **104**
  subungual, 444

F

Fanconi's syndrome, 118
Fascial space infections (of hand), 286
Fasciitis, plantar, 426
Fatigue fracture of metatarsal, 428
Femur, osteomyelitis of, 361
  osteotomy of, displacement, 339
    McMurray, 339
    rotation, 326
  short, congenital, 37
  syphilitic infection of, 362
  tumours of, 362
Fibroma, 130
Fibrosarcoma of bone, 92
  of soft tissue, 131
Fibrositis, 129
  cervical, 171
  lumbar, 217
  thoracic, 217
Fibrous dysplasia, monostotic, 101
  polyostotic, 109
Fibula, osteomyelitis of, 401
  tumours of, 402
Finger, 'trigger,' 305
Flat foot, 417
  anterior, 427
Foot, accessory bones of, 414

Foot, deformities of, 409
  disorders of, 409
    (classification), 398
  examination of, 393
  flat, 417
    anterior, 427
  strain, 419
  valgus, 417
Forearm, disorders of, 269
  (classification), 268
  examination of, 264
Forefoot, pain in, 427
Fracture, stress, of metatarsal, 428
Fragilitas ossium, 104
Freiberg's disease of metatarsal, 98, **441**
Fröhlich type of hypopituitarism, 126
'Frozen' shoulder, 240
Functional disorders, 16

G

Ganglion (of foot), 433
  (of hand), 297
  compound palmar, 293
Gargoylism, 36
Gaucher's disease, 124
General affections of the skeleton, 103
  (classification), 103
Genetic factors in skeletal disorders, 35,
    38
Genu valgum, 385
  varum, 385
Giant-cell tumour (osteoclastoma), **84**
  of femur, 363
  of humerus, 250
  of radius, 271
  of tibia, 402
  of ulna, 271
  (of tendon sheath), 131, **296**
Gigantism, 125
Girdlestone pseudarthrosis, 340
Gleno-humeral joint, disorders of, 227
Gout, **58**, 440
Gouty arthritis, **58**
  of ankle, 407
  of great toe joint, 440
Grafts, bone, 30
  tendon, **32**, 303
Granulomatosis, lipoid, 122
  eosinophilic, 123
Gynaecological disorders simulating
  spinal disease, 221

H

Haemangioma, 130
Haemophilic arthritis, **60**

Haemophilic arthritis of ankle, 407
  of elbow, 256
  of knee, 372
Hallux rigidus, 438
  valgus, 433
Hammer toe, 437
Hand, bone tumours in, 295
  disorders of, 276
    (classification), 269
  examination of, 264
  fascial spaces of, anatomy of, 286
    infection of, 286
  joints of, arthritis of, 277, 278, 283
  rheumatoid disease of, 278
  soft-tissue tumours in, 295
  tendon injuries in, 300
Hand-Schüller-Christian disease, 123
Harrington's rods in scoliosis, 183
Heat treatment, 20
Heel, painful, 423
  pad, tender, 426
Hemivertebra, 180, 184
Hereditary factors in disease, 38
Hip, arthritis of, pyogenic, 329
    rheumatoid, 332
    simulating spinal disease, 221
    transient, 328
    tuberculous, 334
  disease, extrinsic disorders simulating, 352
  dislocation of, congenital, 321
    pathological, 330, 331, 332
  disorders of, 321
    (classification), 320
    simulating disease of knee, 392
  examination of, 308
  osteoarthritis of, 336
  osteochondritis involving, 342
  Perthes' disease of, 342
  snapping, 352
  synovitis of, traumatic, 328
History, importance of, in diagnosis, 5
Hodgkin's disease, 96
Humerus, osteomyelitis of, 248
  tumours of, 250
Hurler's syndrome, 36
Hydrarthrosis, syphilitic, 374
Hyperparathyroidism, 124
Hypopituitarism, 126
Hysterical disorders, 17

I

Idiopathic scoliosis, 181
  steatorrhoea, 122
    osteomalacia in, 122
Infantile paralysis, 133

Infection of bone, 69
  pyogenic, 69
  syphilitic, 79
  tuberculous, 76
  of hand, 286
Ingrowing toe nail, 442
Injections, treatment by, 20
Injuries, 35
Innominate osteotomy, 327
Intermittent claudication, 403
Internal derangements of joints, 65
  of knee, 374
Interpretation of clinical findings, 16
Intervertebral disc, prolapse of (cervical), 161
  (lumbar), 202

J

Joint(s), acromio-clavicular, disorders of, 241
  dislocation of, 64
  gleno-humeral, disorders of, 227
  internal derangements of, 65
  interposition of soft tissue in, 65
  loose bodies in, 66
  metatarso-phalangeal, arthritis of, 438
  movement, examination of, 8
  of toes, arthritis of, 438
  sacro-iliac, disorders of, 218
  sterno-clavicular, disorders of, 242
  subluxation of, 64
  subtalar, arthritis of, 421, **423**
  swelling, determining the cause of, 8
  tarsal, arthritis of, 421
  trapezio-metacarpal, arthritis of, 283
Jones, Sir Robert, 4

K

Kienböck's disease of lunate bone, 97, **284**
Klippel-Feil syndrome, 153
Knee, arthritis of, haemophilic, 372
    neuropathic, 373
    pyogenic, 365
    rheumatoid, 365
    tuberculous, 368
  Baker's cyst of, 391
  Charcot's disease of, 373
  deformities of, 385
  disease of, extrinsic disorders simulating, 392
  disorders of, 365
    (classification), 360
  examination of, 354

Knee, internal derangements of, 374
  loose bodies in, 381
  medial ligament of, ossification in, 391
    calcified deposit in, 392
  osteoarthritis of, 369
  osteochondritis dissecans of, 379
Knock knee, 385
Köhler's osteochondritis of navicular
  bone, 97, **421**
Kyphosis, **185**
  adolescent, 198
  in ankylosing spondylitis, 198
  senile, 113

L

Landmarks of surgery in nineteenth
  century, 2
Leg, disorders of, 400
  (classification), 398
  lengthening, 33
  shortening, 33
Legg-Perthes' disease, 97, **342**
Letterer-Siwe disease, 123
Leukaemia, 96
Ligamentous strain, lumbar, 215
  sacro-iliac, 219
Limbs, measurement of, 309
Lipoid granulomatosis, 122
Lipoma, 130
Liposarcoma, 133
Lister, Joseph, 3
Little's disease, 137
Local affections of bone, 97
  heat, 20
Localised nodular tenosynovitis, 295
Long, Crawford, 3
Loose bodies, intra-articular, **66**
  in elbow, 259
  in knee, 381
Lorain type of hypopituitarism, 126
Lordosis, 185
Lower limbs, measurement of, 309
Lumbago, acute, 184, 204, **207**
Lumbar and sacral anomalies, 180
  ligamentous strain, 215
Lunate bone, Kienböck's disease of, 97
  284
Lupus erythematosus, arthritis in, 49
Lymphadenoma, 96

M

McMurray's femoral osteotomy, 339
  test for torn meniscus, 359

Madelung's deformity, 276
Malignant tumours of bone, 86
  of soft tissue, 131
Mallet finger, 301
Manipulation, 22
  dangers of, 24
  empirical, 23
  for chronic pain, 23
  for correction of deformity, 22
  for joint stiffness, 22
March fracture, 428
Massage, 20
Measurements in clinical examination, 8
Median nerve, compression of, 296
Medical Research Council grading of
  muscle power, 9
Meningocele, **141**, 181
Meniscus (of knee), cyst of, 377
  discoid 378
  tears of, 374
Metastatic tumours in bone, 95
  in hand, 295
Metatarsal, osteochondritis of, 98, **441**
  stress fracture of, 428
Metatarsalgia, 427
Metatarsalgia, Morton's, 427, **429**
Metatarso-phalangeal joint, gouty
  arthritis of, 440
  osteoarthritis of, 438
Metatarsus primus varus, 433
Mid-palmar space, anatomy of, 289
  infection of, 292
Morton, W. T. G., 3
Morton's metatarsalgia, 427, **429**
Movements of joints, examination of, 8
  passive, 19
Multiple chondromatosis, 106
  exostoses, 104
  myeloma, 93
  of femur, 364
  of humerus, 251
Muscle, electrical stimulation of, 19
  power, estimation of, 9
Myelocele, 141, 181
Myelo-meningocele, 141, 181
Myelography, 12
Myeloma, multiple, 93
  of femur, 364
  of humerus, 251
Myelomatosis, 93
Myositis ossificans, 108

N

Navicular bone, osteochondritis of, 97,
  421

Neck, disorders of, 152
  (classification), 151
  simulating disease in hand, 306
  examination of, 148
  short, congenital, 153
Nelaton's line, 314
Nerve conduction tests, 14
  injuries, peripheral, 144
  median, compression of, in carpal
    tunnel, 296
  ulnar, neuritis of, 263
Neurapraxia, 144
Neuritis, brachial, 158, 160
  plantar digital, 429
  ulnar, 263
Neurofibroma, 130
  multiple, 108
Neurofibromatosis, 108
  scoliosis in, 184
Neuroma, plantar interdigital, 429
Neuropathic arthritis, 62
  of ankle, 407
  of elbow, 257
  of knee, 373
Neurotmesis, 144
Non-operative treatment, methods of, 18
Nutritional osteomalacia, 120
  rickets, 116

O

Olecranon bursitis, 261
Ollier's disease, 82, 106, 295, 402
Onychogryposis, 444
Os tibiale externum, 414
  trigonum, 414
Osgood-Schlatter's disease, 98, 388
Osteitis, 68
  pyogenic, 69
  syphilitic, 79
Osteitis deformans (Paget's disease), 110
  sarcoma complicating, 88
Osteitis fibrosa cystica, generalised, 124
  localised (bone cyst), 100
Osteoarthritis, 55
  of acromio-clavicular joint, 241
  of ankle, 406
  of cervical spine, 157
  of elbow, 255
  of hip, 336
  of knee, 369
  of metatarso-phalangeal joint, 438
  of shoulder, 229
  of spine, 193
  of tarsal joints, 421
  of trapezio-metacarpal joint, 283

Osteochondritis of wrist, 281
Osteoarthropathy, Charcot's, 62
  of ankle, 407
  of elbow, 257
  of knee, 373
Osteoarthrosis, 55
Osteochondritis dissecans, 67
  affecting ankle, 67
  affecting elbow, 258
  affecting hip, 67
  affecting knee, 379
  affecting metatarsal head, 441
Osteochondritis juvenilis, 97
  Calvé's, of spine, 201
  common sites of, 97
  of femoral head, 342
  of lunate bone, 284
  of metatarsal head, 441
  of navicular bone, 421
  of spine, 198
  Scheuermann's, of spine, 198
Osteochondroma, 82
  multiple, 104
Osteochondromatosis, synovial, 66
  of elbow, 260
  of knee, 382
Osteochondrosis, 97
  (see osteochondritis)
Osteoclasis, 25
Osteoclastoma, 84
  of femur, 363
  of fibula, 402
  of humerus, 250
  of radius, 271
  of tibia, 402
  of ulna, 271
Osteodystrophy, parathyroid, 124
  renal, 118
Osteogenesis imperfecta, 104
Osteogenic sarcoma, 88
  of femur, 363
  of humerus, 251
  of tibia, 403
Osteoid osteoma, 102
Osteoma, simple, 82
  osteoid, 102
Osteomalacia, 10, 120
  in idiopathic steatorrhoea, 122
  nutritional, 120
    biochemical changes in, 121
Osteomyelitis, acute, 69
  chronic, 74
  complicating open fracture, 70
  haematogenous, 69
  joint infection complicating, 69
  of femur, 361
  of forearm bones, 269
  of humerus, 248

Osteomyelitis of spine (cervical), 156
  (thoracic or lumbar), 191
  of tibia, 401
Osteo-periostitis, syphilitic, 80
Osteopetrosis, 36
Osteoporosis, causes of, 127
  senile, 113
Osteosarcoma, **88**, 251, 363, 403
Osteotomy, **25**
  corrective, 252, 249, 350, 387
  displacement, 339, 436
  indications for, 25
  innominate, 327
  McMurray, 339
  rotation, 326
  Schanz, 328
  technique of, 26
  varus, 345

P

Paget's disease, 110
  sarcoma complicating, 112
Painful arc syndrome, 235
  heel, 423
Palmar aponeurosis, contracture of, 298
Pancoast's tumour, 167
  as cause of pain in upper limb, 307
Paralysis, infantile, 133
  in peripheral nerve lesions, 144
  in poliomyelitis, 133
  in spina bifida, 141
  spastic, 137
Paraplegia in vertebral tuberculosis, 76
  (cervical), 155
  (thoracic or lumbar), 187, 189
Paratendinitis (in forearm), 275
  calcaneal, 423
Parathyroid osteodystrophy, 124
Paresis, spastic, 137
Passive joint movements, 19
Pasteur, Louis, 3
Patella, avulsion fracture of, 388
  chondromalacia of, 374
  habitual dislocation of, 385
  recurrent dislocation of, 383
Patellar tendon, rupture of, 388
Pathological dislocation, 65
  of hip, 331, 332
Pellegrini-Stieda's disease, 391
Pelvic disorders simulating hip disease, 353
  simulating spinal disease, 220
  girdle, tumours of, 215
  osteotomy, 327
Periostitis, syphilitic, 80
Peripheral nerve injuries, 144

Peritendinitis (in forearm), 275
Perthes' disease of hip, 97, **342**
Pes cavus, 415
  planus, 417
Phocomelia, 37
Physiotherapy, methods of, 18
Pituitary diseases, 125
Plantar digital neuritis, 429
  fasciitis, 426
  warts, 430
Plasma cell tumour, 93
Pleurisy simulating shoulder disease, 244
Poliomyelitis, 133
Polyarthritis, rheumatoid, 46
Polydactyly, 37
Polyostotic fibrous dysplasia, 109
Popliteal cysts, 390
Postural back pain, 215
Pott's disease of spine, 76, **186**
  paraplegia, 187, 188
Prepatellar bursitis, 389
Prolapsed intervertebral disc (cervical), 161
  (lumbar), 202
  simulating disease in hand, 268, 307
  simulating hip disease, 352
Prosthetic replacement of finger joints, 280
  of hip, 340
Pseudarthrosis of hip, 340
Pseudocoxalgia, 342
Psoas abscess, 187
Psoriasis, arthritis in, 49
Psychogenic disorders, 16
Pulp space, anatomy of, 286
  infection of, 291
Pyogenic arthritis, **43**
  of ankle, 405
  of elbow, 253
  of hip, 329
  of joints of hand, 277
  of knee, 365
  of shoulder, 227
  of wrist, 276
  infection of spine (cervical), 156
  (thoracic or lumbar), 191

Q

Quadriceps, rupture of, 387

R

Radiation, infra-red, 20
  therapy, deep, 24
Radiographic examination, 10
Radiotherapy, 24

Radius, osteomyelitis of, 269
  tumours of, 270
Rarefaction of bone, causes of, 127
Recklinghausen's disease (hyperpara-
    thyroidism), 124
    (neurofibromatosis), 108
Recurrent dislocation or subluxation, 65
  of ankle, 407
  of patella, 383
  of shoulder, 230
  of sterno-clavicular joint, 242
Referred symptoms, investigations of, 9
Reiter's syndrome, 49
Renal calculus simulating spinal disease,
    220
  infection simulating spinal disease, 220
  rickets, 118
Replacement arthroplasty of finger
    joints, 280
  of hip, 340
Rest, place of, in treatment, 18
Reticulosis, skeletal, 122
Rhabdomyosarcoma, 133
Rheumatic fever, arthritis of, 63
Rheumatoid arthritis, 46
  of ankle, 405
  of elbow, 254
  of hand joints, 278
  of hip, 332
  of knee, 365
  of shoulder, 228
  of spine, 192
  of wrist, 278
  tendon lesions in, 279
  polyarthritis, 46
Rib, cervical, 165
  tumours of, 215
Rickets, biochemical changes in, 121
  coeliac, 119
  infantile, 116
  nutritional, 116
  renal, 118
    tubular, 118
  vitamin-resistant, 117
Roentgen, 4
Rotation osteotomy of femur, 326
Rotator cuff of shoulder, tear of, 232
Rupture of calcaneal tendon, 400
  of extensor pollicis longus, 302
  of long tendon of biceps, 239
  of quadriceps apparatus, 387
  of supraspinatus tendon, 232

S

Sacro-iliac joints, ankylosing spondylitis
    affecting, 218
  arthritis of, pyogenic, 219

Sacro-iliac joints, arthritis of, rheuma-
    toid, 219
  simulating hip disease, 353
  tuberculous, 218
  disorders of, 218
  examination of, 173
  osteoarthritis of, 219
  strain of, 219
Salter's pelvic osteotomy, 327
Sarcoma of bone, endothelial, 92
  Ewing's, 92
    of femur, 363
    of tibia, 403
  osteogenic, 88
    complicating Paget's disease, 88
    of femur, 363
    of humerus, 251
    of tibia, 403
  synovial, 132
Scapula, congenital high, 153
  tumours of, 215
Schanz osteotomy, 328
Scheuermann's osteochondritis of spine,
    97, 198
Schlatter's disease of tibia, 388
Schoemaker's line, 314
Sciatica, 173, 174
  as symptom of prolapsed interverte-
    bral disc, 202
  causes of, 205, 206
Sciatic scoliosis, 184, 204
Scoliosis, 181
  compensatory, 185
  idiopathic structural, 181
  in neurofibromatosis, 109, 184
  sciatic, 184, 204
  secondary, 183
  structural, 181
Scope of orthopaedic surgery, 4
Scurvy, infantile, 115
Semilunar cartilage, cyst of, 377
  discoid, 378
  tears of, 374
Semimembranosus bursitis, 390
Senile osteoporosis, 113
Sever's disease of calcaneus, 98, 425
Shelf operation for congenital disloca-
    tion of hip, 326
Short-wave diathermy, 20
Shoulder, adhesive capsulitis of, 240
  arthritis of, pyogenic, 227
    rheumatoid, 228
    tuberculous, 228
  disease, extrinsic disorders simulating,
    243
  dislocation of, recurrent, 230
  disorders of, 227
    (classification), 227

Shoulder, examination of, 222
  'frozen,' 240
  movements of, 224
  osteoarthritis of, 229
  periarthritis of, 240
Silastic prosthesis, 280
Sinography, 13
Slipped upper femoral epiphysis, 346
Snapping finger, 305
  hip, 352
Soft tissue, inflammatory lesions of, 128
  tumours of, 130
Spastic paralysis, 137
  paresis, 137
Spina bifida, **141**, 180
Spinal cord, compression of (cervical),
  169
  (thoracic or lumbar), 213
  decompression of, 190
  tumour of (cervical), 170
  (thoracic or lumbar), 212
  dysraphism, **141**, 180
  fusion, 195
Spine (cervical), ankylosing spondylitis
  affecting, 157
  disorders of, 152
  (classification), 151
  examination of, 148
  osteoarthritis of, 157
  osteomyelitis of, 156
  pyogenic infection of, 156
  rheumatoid arthritis of, 192
  subluxation of, 168
  tuberculosis of, 153
  tumours involving, 170
Spine (thoracic or lumbar), Calvé's
  disease of, 201
  congenital anomalies of, 180
  disease of, extrinsic disorders simu-
    lating, 220
  disorders of, 180
  (classification), 178
  examination of, 173
  fusion of, 195
  movements of, 175
  osteoarthritis of, 193
  osteochondritis of, 198, 201
  osteomyelitis of, 191
  pyogenic infection of, 191
  rheumatoid arthritis of, 192
  Scheuermann's disease of, 198
  tuberculosis of, 186
  tumours of, 212
Spondylarthrosis, 193
Spondylitis, ankylosing, 63, **195**, 218
  pyogenic, cervical, 156
  thoracic or lumbar, 191
  tuberculous, cervical, 153
  thoracic or lumbar, 186

Spondylolisthesis, cervical, 168
  lumbar, 209
Spondylosis, cervical, 156
  thoracic or lumbar, 193
Spondylolysis, 208
Sprengel's shoulder, 153
Steatorrhoea, idiopathic, 122
Stereoscopic radiography, 12
Sterno-clavicular joint, arthritis of, 242
  dislocation of, 242
  disorders of, 242
  examination of, 225
Sternum, tumour of, 215
Still's disease, 49
Straight leg raising test, 176
Strain, foot, 419
  ligamentous, lumbar, 215
  sacro-iliac, 219
Strength-duration curves, 14
Stress disorders, 16
  fracture of metatarsal, 428
Subacromial bursitis, 236, 238
Subluxation, congenital, 64
  recurrent, 64
  of ankle, 407
  of sterno-clavicular joint, 242
Subphrenic abscess simulating shoulder
  disease, 244
Subungual space, anatomy of, 286
  infection of, 291
  exostosis, 444
Supraspinatus, minor tear of, 236
  syndrome, 235
  tendinitis, 236
  tendon, calcified deposit in, 236
  torn, 232
Syndactyly, 37
Synostosis, radio-ulnar, 37
Synovectomy (hand), 280
  (knee), 366
Synovial chondromatosis, 66
  of elbow, 260
  of knee, 382
Synovioma, 132
Syphilis of bone, 79
Syphilitic hydrarthrosis, 374
  metaphysitis, infantile, 79
  osteo-periostitis, 80

T

Talipes calcaneo-valgus, 413
  equino-varus, 409
Tarsal joints, arthritis of, 421
Tender heel pad, 426
Tendinitis, biceps, 240
  supraspinatus, 236

Tendinous cuff of shoulder, rupture of, 232
  strain of, 236
Tendo calcaneus (achillis), rupture of, 400
Tendon, biceps, rupture of, 239
  calcaneal, rupture of, 400
  grafts, 33
  injuries (in hand), 300
  lesions in rheumatoid arthritis, 48, 279
  quadriceps, rupture of, 387
  sheath (of hand), anatomy of, 289
    infection of, 292, 293
    tumour of, 296
  supraspinatus, rupture of, 232
    inflammation of, 236
    strain of, 236
  transfer, 31
Tennis elbow, 261
Tenosynovitis, 128
  biceps, 240
  calcaneal, 423
  frictional (in forearm), 275
  infective (in hand), 292, 293
  localised nodular, 295
  rheumatoid, 278
Tenovaginitis, 129
  De Quervain's (at wrist), 304
  stenosans, digital, 305
Test of function, 9
  electrical, 14
  McMurray's, 359
  straight leg raising, 176
  Thomas's, 317
  Trendelenburg's, 318
Thenar space, anatomy of, 289
  infection of, 292
Thigh, disorders of, 361
  (classification), 360
Thomas, Hugh Owen, 4
Thomas's test for fixed flexion at hip, 317
Thumb, absence of, 37
  'trigger,' 305
Tibia, Brodie's abscess of, 401
  osteomyelitis of, 401
  syphilitic infection of, 401
  tumours of, 402
Tibial tubercle, apophysitis of, 388
  avulsion of, 388
Toe(s), deformities of, 433
  disorders of, 433
  hammer, 437
  nail, deformed, 444
    ingrowing, 443
    under-riding, 438
Tomography, 12
Torticollis, 152

Total replacement of hip, 340
Trapezio-metacarpal joint, osteoarthritis of, 283
Trendelenburg's test, 318
Trigger finger, 305
  thumb, 305
Tubercle, tibial, apophysitis of, 388
  avulsion of, 388
Tuberculosis of bone, 76
  of spine, 76, 186
    (cervical), 153
Tuberculous arthritis, 51
  of ankle, 405
  of elbow, 254
  of hip, 334
  of knee, 368
  of sacro-iliac joint, 218
  of shoulder, 228
  bursitis, 129
    trochanteric, 351
  spondylitis, 186
    (cervical), 153
  tenosynovitis, 293
Tumour, bone, 81
  in lower limb, 362, 402
  in upper limb, 250, 270, 295
  metastatic, 95
  'dumb-bell', 170, 212
  giant-cell, of bone, 84
    of tendon sheath, 296
  Pancoast's, 167, 307
  soft-tissue, 130
  spinal, 170, 212
  thoracic inlet, 167, 307

U

Ulna, osteomyelitis of, 269
  tumours of, 270
Ulnar neuritis, 263
Ultrasonic therapy, 20

V

Valgus foot, 417
Vascular disease in lower limb, 403
  in upper limb, 165, 271
  simulating disease of hip, 353
  of spine, 221
Venography, 13
Verruca plantaris, 430
Vertebra plana, 201
Vertebral anomalies, congenital, 180
  infections, 156, 191
  osteochondritis, 198, 201
  tuberculosis, 186
    (cervical), 153

Visceroptosis simulating spinal disease, 220

Vitamin-resistant rickets, 117

Volkmann's ischaemic contracture, 271

Von Recklinghausen's disease (hyperparathyroidism), 124

(neurofibromatosis), 108

Wrist, arthritis of, rheumatoid, 278

deformity of, Madelung's, 276

disorders of, 276

(classification), 269

examination of, 264

Kienböck's disease of, 97, **284**

osteoarthritis of, 281

W

Wart, plantar, 430

Wrist, arthritis of, pyogenic, 276

X

X-ray examination, 10

therapy, 24

Printed by T. & A. Constable Ltd., Edinburgh